MAKING HEALTH PUBLIC

Making Health Public examines the relationship between media and medicine, considering the fundamental role of news coverage in constructing wider cultural understandings of health and disease. The authors advance the notion of 'bio-mediatization' and demonstrate how health knowledge is co-produced through connections between dispersed sites and forms of expertise. The chapters offer an innovative combination of media content analysis and ethnographic data on the production and circulation of health news, drawing on work with journalists, clinicians, health officials, medical researchers, marketers, and audiences. The volume provides students and scholars with unique insight into the significance and complexity of what health news does and how it is created.

Charles L. Briggs is a professor in the Department of Anthropology at the University of California, Berkeley, USA. His work combines linguistic and medical anthropology with socio-cultural anthropology and folkloristics.

Daniel C. Hallin is a professor in the Department of Communication at the University of California, San Diego, USA. His work concerns journalism, political communication, and the comparative analysis of media systems.

Praise for this book:

"This fresh, vivid, and surprising book will change how you think about the massive circulation of news about health and disease. Drawing on extensive knowledge and research, Briggs and Hallin show how the tight suturing of biomedicine and the media powerfully affects our culture, our politics, and our identities."

Steven Epstein, *Northwestern University, USA*

"No work within media theory until now has seriously explored how media and health domains might be transforming each other. Briggs and Hallin call for serious attention to how 'the media' is enacted deep in professional domains, and their intervention promises to take debates about mediatization to a new, more sophisticated level. Their book offers a remarkable combination of quantitative and qualitative methodologies applied to an impressive media sample and a wide-ranging set of interviews. This may well prove to be one of the most significant empirical studies of media and society in the past two decades."

Nick Couldry, *London School of Economics and Political Science, UK*

MAKING HEALTH PUBLIC

How news coverage is remaking media, medicine, and contemporary life

Charles L. Briggs and Daniel C. Hallin

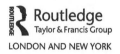
Routledge
Taylor & Francis Group

LONDON AND NEW YORK

First published 2016
by Routledge
2 Park Square, Milton Park, Abingdon, Oxon OX14 4RN

and by Routledge
711 Third Avenue, New York, NY 10017

Routledge is an imprint of the Taylor & Francis Group, an informa business

British Library Cataloguing-in-Publication Data
A catalogue record for this book is available from the British Library

Library of Congress Cataloging-in-Publication Data
Names: Briggs, Charles L., 1953– author. | Hallin, Daniel C., author.
Title: Making health public : how news coverage is remaking media,
medicine, and contemporary life / Charles L. Briggs and Daniel C. Hallin.
Description: Milton Park, Abingdon, Oxon ; New York, NY : Routledge,
2016. | Includes bibliographical references and index.
Identifiers: LCCN 2015045012| ISBN 9781138999879 (hardback : alk.
paper) | ISBN 9781138999862 (pbk. : alk. paper) | ISBN 9781315658049
(e-book)
Subjects: LCSH: Mass media in health education. | Health promotion. |
Medicine—Vocational guidance.
Classification: LCC RA440.5 .B75 2016 | DDC 362.1—dc23
LC record available at http://lccn.loc.gov/2015045012

ISBN: 978-1-138-99987-9 (hbk)
ISBN: 978-1-138-99986-2 (pbk)
ISBN: 978-1-315-65804-9 (ebk)

Typeset in Bembo
by Book Now Ltd, London
Printed and bound in Great Britain by
Ashford Colour Press Ltd, Gosport, Hampshire

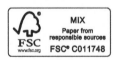

CONTENTS

FIGURES

TABLES

PREFACE

This book focuses on the United States, but the project that produced it began in the middle of a nightmare that unfolded in a rainforest in Venezuela. Having worked with people classified as "the indigenous Warao ethnic group" in the Delta Amacuro rainforest of Venezuela since 1986, Charles stumbled into a major epidemic of cholera during a chance visit in November 1992. A preventable and treatable bacterial infection, cholera cases predictably were concentrated in areas that lacked potable water and sewage facilities and had only minimal access to health care. Some five hundred people died there from cholera in less than two years.

The Regional Health Service responded primarily in two ways. First, they rushed medical personnel and supplies to the area. Second, they attempted to control the political fallout sparked by widespread news coverage that emerged as thousands of refugees, many quite ill from an unsightly diarrheal disease, who were camped on the outskirts of small cities adjacent to the rainforest, became visible to the local and national press. Officials and journalists collaborated in crafting a story that blamed the epidemic largely on "indigenous culture" rather than on structural factors sustained by unsustainable policies, ones that also produced unconscionably high rates of child mortality. The experience left him deeply curious about how news coverage of health emerges and what its impact on politicians, health officials and practitioners, patients, and publics might be. Epidemics that emerged in subsequent years, most recently Ebola, only contributed to this interest.

Charles contacted Dan, who had focused on news media for decades and also had conducted research in Latin America. At first Dan was lukewarm, given that his interest was in political—not medical—news. Dan then attended a session of an informal seminar that Charles had organized with graduate and undergraduate students at the Center for Iberian and Latin American Studies (CILAS) at the University of California, San Diego. Analyzing a group of health new stories from the United States and Venezuela, his eyes opened wide and he remarked—"this is the most political news there is!" That was October of 2003, and we've been at it ever since.

During a trip to Mexico, Charles discussed the project with a distinguished medical anthropologist, Argentine-Mexican scholar Eduardo Menéndez, who had published work discussing health and media. Together we launched a pilot project; Menéndez collaborated with Renée Di Pardo on the Mexican side and Charles and Dan in the United States. Menéndez recruited a leading scholar of critical epidemiology, Hugo Spinelli, who collaborated with Anahi Sy in developing an Argentine component at the Instituto de Salud Colectiva of the Universidad Nacional de Lanús in Buenos Aires. Clara Mantini-Briggs, a Venezuelan public health official who played a key role in cholera control efforts during the epidemic in Delta Amacuro, joined Charles in studying Venezuelan health news. Charles also studied Cuban health news. Although this broader comparative project informs the argument we present here, we decided that the issues were too complex to tackle such a broad range of cases, so *Making Health Public* focuses on the United States, although we place US coverage in global context in the Conclusion.

The more we looked at the US news media—newspapers, radio, television, and the emerging Internet and social media venues—the more health news seemed to be everywhere. And when a health crisis emerged, such as an epidemic or a large case of food contamination, the stream became a raging flood. Journalists covered a very large range of topics, from new scientific discoveries, diseases, vaccines, drugs, and devices, testing, prevention, treatment protocols, scandals, policy issues, pregnancy and birth, nutrition, and a steady stream of articles about health "risks" and ways to improve wellbeing. And health stories touched on business, sports, travel, politics, immigration, economics, education, and many other areas. They ranged from highly technical pieces explaining complex scientific and medical issues to light, upbeat, news-you-can-use pieces to advice and question-answer columns. They were crafted by journalists who worked on many different beats, some generalists, some consumer, business or political reporters, some specialized health journalists, and some occupying the unique role of physician-reporters.

We soon found the task nearly overwhelming. The problem was not just the quantity and variety of the coverage. The issue was more that we couldn't get an analytic hold on the problem. Our own training and experience as scholars in different fields—anthropology, particularly of language and medicine for Charles and media studies and political science for Dan—was helpful. We specialized respectively in ethnography and critical discourse analysis and historical and institutional approaches and quantitative content analysis. The problem lay more in how to break the magical hold of the scientific and medical content, the way that we—even after reading, viewing, and listening to thousands of health stories—continue to be seduced by the powerful sense of looking over the shoulders of a reporter who is looking over the shoulders of leading researchers, clinicians, epidemiologists, and policymakers, thereby gaining privileged access to people with big, specialized vocabularies and special ways of seeing.

Slowly, we came to see that each story models knowledge as much as health, teaching lessons about what counts as medical facts, who makes them, who can interpret them, how they should travel beyond the walls of clinics and hospitals, what laypersons need to know and what they should do with this material. One reason that questions of the production, circulation, and reception of knowledge are so important is that producing knowledge also creates nonknowledge: what counts as ignorance or superstition instead of facts; where biomedicine ends and alternative forms begin; and the dangers associated with illegitimate actors pretending to produce health knowledge, resulting in resistance, noncompliance, self-medication, and misinformation.

Given the importance of these questions, we began to ask ourselves who decides them: when researchers, clinicians, corporate officials, federal regulators, and patients all seem to speak, all ventriloquized by a journalist, where does one voice end and another begin, and how do they come together? Who gets to shape the basic story line about a particular phenomenon? We found a lot of PR/media professionals, either in health institutions or contracted by them; what were they doing there and how were they helping to shape research and clinical practice? To be sure, there are a lot of standard journalistic practices that shape how these stories are researched and written, but the power of biomedicine reshapes them in complex and somewhat unique ways in health news.

It was clear that we would never be able to answer such questions by just reading, watching, and listening to stories: we had to be there when they were being made, and we had to listen to all of the parties talking about their roles. We accordingly interviewed a vast range of health and media professionals, asking them to walk us through their daily labor of connecting—and, in part, making—the different social worlds that stories bridge. And we soon learned that making health news is part of a much larger process, one that occurs in biotechs, pharmaceutical corporations, clinics, hospitals, research labs, social movement and environmental organizations, and other sites as much as newsrooms, far beyond the points at which specific stories are being researched and written. We came to see that drugs, epidemics, discoveries, treatments, and such do not come into being and then subsequently get "represented" by journalists; rather medical subjects and objects are co-produced by media and medical professionals all along the way. Nonprofessionals—including patients as well as readers and viewers—are deeply involved as well, so we did interviews, focus groups, and ethnography, enabling us to think about lay involvement in making and receiving health news.

There were small literatures in a range of fields that focused specifically on news coverage of health. At the same time that we learned a great deal from previous work in this area, we found that it did not provide us with the analytical traction that we sought. Much was based on content analysis alone, thereby failing to capture features, sites, and actors who seldom if ever make it into the content of stories. Much research privileged the power of biomedicine, focusing primarily on a particular disease and assessing how well journalists or audiences reproduced biomedical knowledge of it. We were more interested in how making health news makes medicine than in whether journalists correctly "translated" or shamelessly "sensationalized" what doctors and researchers said. As a result, we kept dismantling assumptions and fashioning new tools until we established a new approach and a set of concepts that, we felt, finally were sufficient to do the work of analyzing rather than reproducing the commonsense ways we are taught to receive health news, which are even reflected in skeptics' claims that health reporting is just PR for big pharma and massive health maintenance organizations (HMOs).

Reading this book will thus take as much *unthinking* as thinking, as much letting go of deeply ingrained ideas about relationships between science, medicine, and media as learning new techniques for reading or viewing each new story that comes along. We wrote this book for all the people who help make health news stories, meaning clinicians, public health professionals, epidemiologists, journalists, activists, and laypersons, as well as the anthropologists, sociologists, and scholars in science, technology, and society (STS), media, and journalism studies. Part I lays the foundations, providing the analytic apparatus we developed and introducing readers to the medical and media professionals who make the stories and to the broad types of stories that have been reported from the 1960s to the present and how they are reported. Part II takes a very different course, telling deeper and more focused stories in three different areas: the H1N1 or "swine flu" epidemic of 2009, news coverage of biotech and pharmaceutical corporations, and how racial and ethnic difference are projected in health news and ways that they are hidden from view.

We do not have a story to pitch; as it were, we come, to paraphrase Shakespeare, neither to praise nor to bury health journalists or the people whose work they report. Our goal is different. We believe that news coverage of health is much more important than most professionals and scholars think—we have come to see the ways that it plays a crucial role in how we inhabit our bodies and interact with one another in clinics and hospitals, in shaping our most basic features, desires, and habits. We do not try to convince readers that health news stories operate as tools for enhancing public scientific and medical literacy or Trojan horses that beguile people into buying more pills and more expensive procedures. We think it more important to help equip health and media professionals, policymakers, scholars, and laypersons to be more critical of the ways that we are all recruited to take our assigned roles in producing, circulating, and receiving health knowledge. We start from the radical assumption that all of us make valuable knowledge about health and that no population should be stigmatized as lacking the capacity even to understand medical facts—and receive inferior healthcare as a result. We thus hope that by teaching people to read health stories in new and critical ways, *Making Health Public* will help scholars ask new sorts of questions and open up for all of us new, collaborative possibilities.

ACKNOWLEDGMENTS

When you've been at a project for a long time, there are a lot of people to thank. Our deepest debt, certainly, is to the hundreds of journalists, clinicians, public health practitioners, researchers, PR/marketing specialists, and laypersons who shared with us their experiences and views of what we term biomediatization. Busy people took time to grant interviews, share texts, participate in focus groups, and just let us watch them work, talk, and interact with media. In keeping with informed consent protocols and institutional rules that structure communication in many media and health institutions, most are given pseudonyms here; we regret that we cannot thank them by name. We just have to leave it at: many thanks for helping us enter your worlds and for sharing with us their complexities and contradictions.

Many institutions have helped us. The project was born in conversations with Latin American colleagues, springing from a common puzzlement over why health news proliferates in so many countries and over how we might combine anthropology, media studies, Latin American Social Medicine and critical epidemiology, and other fields in thinking more critically about it. Conversations with Eduardo Menéndez were particularly crucial; they formed the basis for a pilot project, funded by UCMEXUS-CONACYT. Menéndez and Renée Di Pardo led research on the Mexican side and Charles and Dan in California. Meetings with Hugo Spinelli in Buenos Aires, Quito, and Berkeley sharpened the comparative dimension, including the interface between social medicine and media studies; Anahi Sy developed the Argentine collaboration. In addition to participating actively in the Venezuelan component of the larger research project, Clara Mantini-Briggs helped organize and lead US focus groups and work with students on US and Venezuelan materials. Thanks to the support of the remarkable health communication scholar Mohan Dutta, Charles' research in Singapore in 2014 was supported by the National University of Singapore and the National University of Singapore Society. The Vanderbilt Television News Archive provided an indispensible source for locating national network and cable news stories.

The initial site for the California team was the Center for Iberian and Latin American Studies of UC San Diego, where students and faculty began to puzzle collectively over health news stories. Ramón Gutiérrez, Director of the Center for Race and Gender, provided crucial financial support, enabling us to recruit Cecilia Rivas and Rob Donnelly as research assistants. Elizabeth Kelley participated as a Graduate Student Researcher on the Berkeley side, providing important contributions to the biotech/pharma chapter. Undergraduate Elidia Esqueda grasped the importance of *Los Angeles Times* articles on Latina teen pregnancies, which she analyzed in her Honor's Thesis. Other UCSD faculty lent support. The indefatigable Ana Celia Zentella kindly introduced Charles and Clara to a Latino/a congregation at a small church north of La Jolla. The long process of transitioning between mountains of results and an emerging manuscript was crucially facilitated by the Center for Advanced Study in the Behavioral Sciences, Stanford University, which provided Dan a fellowship in 2011–12.

At UC Berkeley, the Undergraduate Research Apprenticeship Program provided a context in which some 6–12 Berkeley undergraduates participated actively most semesters, locating materials, participating in coding and analysis, transcribing interviews, keeping track of their own consumption of health media, and sharing their insights. They included: Margeaux Akazawa, Stefania Arteaga, Kanelle Barreiro, Zion Barrios, Courtney Borba, Cody Bouscaren, Dixie Brea, Rosana Carranza, Eric Chàvez, Joan Chen, Rachael Erlich, Natalie Friess, Jazmine García Delgadillo, Lauren Gruber, Karen Hernández, Andrew Ignacio, Wyatt Lienhard, Maria Lolas Ojeda, Stephanie Lechuga, Monica Moncada, Shannon Najmabadi, Jessica Neasbitt, Jessica Parra-Fitch, Lina Pervez, José Polio, Chantiri Ramírez, Colleen Raspberry, Farha Rizvi, Jessica Robles, Elizabeth Rocha, Kaley Rodríguez, Laura Carolina Rodríguez-Adjunta, Jesús Rondón, Trilce Santana, Ashley Sorgi, Danae Sterental, Elizabeth Vargas, and Juan Carlos Villaseñor. Deidre Clyde, Johnson Co, and Erica Magill made particularly outstanding contributions. At UC San Diego, undergraduates Yvonne Hsiung, Tanja Pantoja, Annalise Romoser, and Elizabeth Loft provided important help, and graduate student researchers Marisa Brandt, Brie Iaterola, and Yi Hong Sim played key roles in parts of the content analysis.

The Human Subjects programs at UC Berkeley and UC San Diego separately reviewed and approved our project.

We would like to thank audiences at the following institutions for insightful comments on presentations of this work: The University of British Columbia, University of Chicago, Cornell University, University of Cuenca, Emory University, Finmark University, University of Göttingen, University of La Habana, University of Helsinki, Hong Kong University, Indiana University, Keio University, King's College London, University of Leeds, Merteens Institute (Royal Netherlands Academy of Arts and Sciences), National University of Singapore, University of Pennsylvania, Sofia University, Stanford University,

Tartu University, UC Berkeley, UC Riverside, UC San Diego, UC San Francisco, USC Annenberg School of Communication, Yale University, and York University. We have presented papers at annual meetings of the American Anthropological Association, International Communication Association, International Pragmatics Association, Society for Medical Anthropology, Western States Folklore Society, and conferences sponsored by the Centre for Research on Socio-Cultural Change, the Observatorio Latinoamericano de Salud, and the Wenner-Gren Foundation for Anthropological Research, Inc. Charles presented preliminary versions of two chapters at a meeting held by the Cultural Logic of Facts and Figures: Objectification, Measurement and Standardization as Social Processes (CUFF) of the Department of Social Anthropology at the Norwegian University of Science and Technology, which also provided funding for editorial assistance kindly provided by Jill Hannum and help from UC Berkeley student Nicholas Alexander Behney in checking references.

We wish to thank colleagues who have kindly read parts of the manuscript and offered insightful comments, especially Leo Chávez, Nick Couldry, Mohan Dutta, George Lipsitz, Mark Nichter, and Jane Rhodes.

Finally, our families continued to live with us while we continued to work so long on this project. Clara, Feliciana, Gabi, and Gabriel supported Charles, each in their different ways. Ruth, Amelia, and Nicholas similarly supported Dan, with Ruth and Nicholas providing expertise in the preparation of the visual images. The project was born about the same time Amelia was, and covered the first twelve years of her life.

INTRODUCTION

News coverage of health constitutes one of the most visible features of the contemporary world. The avalanche of recent news stories about Ebola provides just a small indication of the proliferation of health coverage. H1N1 ("swine flu"), avian flu, SARS, and other epidemics similarly became the biggest stories of their day. Beyond epidemics, the US daily news is filled with reports of new drugs, tests, treatments, or devices, health insurance policies (particularly "Obamacare"), and changes in the identification of risk factors or treatment and dietary guidelines (see Figure 0.1). Health stories range across many genres, from consumer to business to political reporting, and they vary in tone from highly positive stories about miracles of biomedical technology to exposés of regulatory failure or physicians whose drug recommendations have been swayed by perks and gifts. "Hype," including marketers' and journalists' roles in creating it, even figures in news stories themselves. A day seldom goes by on which *The New York Times* fails to publish a health story; three to five stories are common, with one often appearing on the front page. Despite declines in the size and power of traditional media, health news thrives across platforms.[1] The editor of one metropolitan newspaper told us that his paper's management had a list of five topics, one of which had to appear on the front page every day; health was on that list. In on-line news platforms, meanwhile, health is considered one of the key "verticals" or special-interest subject areas around which audiences and advertiser bases can be built.

According to audience surveys, health is a rare category that "is of strong interest to readers and viewers across the hard news/soft news spectrum" (Hamilton 2004:79). Forty-seven percent of viewers of the *MacNeil-Lehrer News Hour* and similar percentages of *Oprah* viewers and *People* magazine readers say they follow health news closely. On television, health-related stories compete with economics and politics for top billing in terms of frequency, placement, and audience appeal. The Tyndall Report (n.d. a) listed NBC's science correspondent, Robert Bazell, trained in immunology, as the second most-used network correspondent

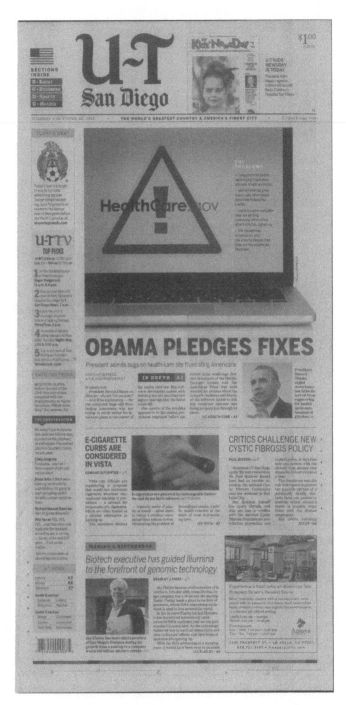

FIGURE 0.1 Health news takes up the entire front page of the *San Diego Union-Tribune*, 22 Oct. 2013 in, it suggests, "the world's greatest country and America's finest city."

during the first decade of the twenty-first century. Health news averages about 1,000 minutes a year on network news, about comparable to economic or war coverage, more than crime stories and much more than such areas as the environment, race, and immigration (Tyndall Report n.d. b).[2] In addition to CNN's Dr. Sanjay Gupta, all the national network television news organizations have MDs as medical editors; ABC's Dr. Richard Besser, pediatrician and epidemiologist, was the acting director of the Centers for Disease Control and Prevention (CDC) when the H1N1 or "swine flu" pandemic began.

Incorporating other types of professionals is a highly unusual practice within journalism, suggesting that biomedicine continues to enjoy special cultural authority. Medical drama serials, like *Grey's Anatomy* and *House,* garner large audiences; the *Dr. Oz Show* ranks among the top shows in daytime television, with 2.9 million viewers in 2011 (Block 2012). Dr. Oz had 3.46 million Twitter followers in 2014 and leads the list of celebrities whose presence on a magazine cover will move copies (Haughney 2012). Gupta had 1.83 million Twitter followers. Health is prominent in Yahoo and Google News; and health-focused blogs, websites, and other venues proliferate (Tan 2007). Health institutions hire ex-journalists to shape news coverage of their activities and the issues that concern them. Health journalism's relationship with advertising—so apparent on television, web versions of newspapers, and the social media—is as visible as it is complex. Although types of health media and the size of audiences vary between countries, the pervasiveness of health in the media is a global phenomenon.

Despite its cultural prominence, health news has been largely ignored as an object of scholarly analysis. Bruno Latour begins his influential *We Have Never Been Modern,* one of the classic works of Science and Technology Studies (STS), by referring to his own enactment of "modern man's form of prayer": reading "my daily newspaper" (1993[1991]:1–2). Referencing news articles on the ozone layer, AIDS, computers, frozen embryos, forest fires, whales, contraceptives, and high-definition television enables him to launch his argument regarding the purification process that separates nature from society, science from politics, and the hybridization that implicitly connects what he calls nature/culture. Nevertheless, Latour never tells readers which newspaper he was reading, let alone analyzes how journalists and news audiences might form part of the actor-networks he traces. His ethnographic presence in laboratories (Latour and Woolgar 1979) does not lead him to see that PR/media professionals may be working there alongside scientists in the production of scientific knowledge and culture.

This averted gaze is all the more striking in view of how STS scholars have fruitfully suggested that notions of information and mediated modes of representation are deeply ingrained in recent transformations of science and medicine. Clarke *et al.* (2003) trace a shift roughly in the mid-1980s from *medicalization,* the increasing extension of medical practices and forms of authority into wider spheres of life (Zola 1972), to what they term *biomedicalization.* This term describes the greater interpenetration of biomedicine into other social structures, such as industry, the state, and the mass media, the increasingly central role of science and technology, the proliferation and diversification of flows of biomedical knowledge through public channels, and this process' influence on identities and modes of self-construction (see also Rose 2007). Their wide-ranging discussion of the "Transformations of Information and the Production and Distribution of Knowledges" points to the centrality of communicative and related practices and technologies in *constituting*—not just representing—biomedicalized objects and subjects.

While attending to how "Information on health and illness is proliferating through all kinds of media, especially in newspapers, on the Internet, in magazines, and through direct-to-consumer prescription and over-the-counter drug advertising" (2003:177), Clarke *et al.* do not challenge the foundational conceptual separation between technoscience versus information and media. Media theorist Jesús Martín Barbero (1987) suggests that adopting "communication" and "media" as analytic points of departure obscures how their definitions are shaped by and shape entrenched, unexamined meanings hardwired into other commonsense terms, like society, the State, and citizenship. He argues that we should bracket preconceptions regarding the meaning and scope of "media" and "communication" and see how they get defined in particular settings for specific motives.

Martín Barbero's move could not be more important for our project. The concept of "health communication," for example, generally assumes the separability of medicine and public health versus communication and media. Health professionals often complain that journalists "sensationalize" or "oversimplify" biomedical knowledge, suggesting that these "distortions" are motivated by the desire to boost newspapers sales or advertising revenues. They frequently claim that journalists should, like themselves, be centrally motivated by the goal of educating "the public," of bringing evidence-based medicine to wider audiences. The journalists that we have interviewed sometimes identify with such pedagogical efforts and in turn accuse health professionals of being too jargon-filled or uninspiring to be effective communicators. Other journalists espouse variations of the professional ideology of journalistic objectivity (Schudson 2003), suggesting that their primary duty is to decide what's newsworthy (Gans 1979), play a watchdog function of uncovering malfeasance, look out for "the public's" interests—or simply entertain and enlighten in a non-instrumental way. Note how these views of health journalism revolve around what Thomas Gieryn (1983) termed "boundary-work," the construction of boundaries that separate science from non-science and partitioning scientific knowledge into particular disciplinary domains. Communication is assumed to start with preexisting medical objects (such as disease categories) and subjects (such as clinicians, researchers, and patients) and create words and images to portray them. These words and images are deemed immaterial, only *representing* such things as viruses and prevention strategies; their effects are limited to orienting people who lack scientific knowledge through training as health professionals or scientists. This way of defining health communication ties it slavishly to medicine and public health and casts it in a subordinate, marginal role.

This situation bears a remarkable similarity to Derrida's critique of Saussure's portrayal of speaking and writing. For Saussure, oral communication embodies presence; writing simply represents signs without partaking in the foundational "thought-sound" (1959 :112) association. Speech is thus productive and primary, writing derivative and secondary. For writing to serve its function, an ideally iconic relationship must be fulfilled—speaking and writing must match one-for-one. Similarly, the relationship between biomedicine and journalism most commonly projected in both scholarship and public and professional discourse about health news masks metaphysical assumptions as simple empirical facts. It is likewise constituted through hierarchically ordered binary oppositions between preexisting medical objects and the representation of those objects by journalists. The former, created by authoritative actors in privileged, dedicated spaces—labs, epidemiologists' offices, and the like—is primary, constitutive, and autonomous. News emerges only afterwards and in lower-status media production sites.

What would happen if we imagined "the media" as taking up residence in clinics, hospitals, pharmaceutical corporations, and public health offices, seeing health professionals as embedded in media spheres? This situation would afford possibilities for studying what we call *biomediatization*, the co-production of medical objects and subjects through complex entanglements between epistemologies, technologies, biologies, and political economies. *We argue here that this process is not a thought-experiment but an important feature of the contemporary world.*

Public spotlights and scholarly peripheries

We focus on an object that is pervasive and yet, curiously, has been largely overlooked as an analytic focus by scholars in medical anthropology, STS, and media and journalism studies alike: health news. It is a boundary-object, one held in common by actors occupying distinct social spheres but inflected in different vocabularies by each (Star and Griesemer 1989). Latour is hardly alone among STS scholars in viewing medical and science news as undeserving of serious study. Anthropologists and STS scholars have examined new objects, subjects, and forms of knowledge, such as medical and scientific technologies, pharmaceuticals, clinical trials, practices of organ transplant, and the migration of logics associated with emergency preparedness into public health.[3] Media objects, mainly newspaper articles, are frequently invoked to attest to the currency and importance of these phenomena, but scholars seldom reflect on how their making might form part of the *production* of medical and scientific objects and subjects. STS's own boundary-work thus places the analysis of science and health news beyond its borders. For example, as we show in Chapter 4, the H1N1 virus emerged as a public object through the mobilization of a network of media and health professionals who had been exchanging logics and practices through years of collaboration, even while journalists and health professionals generally project their work as embodying distinct—if not opposing—perspectives, interests, and types of professional training.

These same beliefs about the distinctness of health and media are reflected in anthropology in the separation between medical anthropologists and media anthropologists, which helps prompt inattention to health news in the discipline.[4]

There is now an emerging focus on the anthropology of the news.[5] Health news, however, seldom draws the attention of media anthropologists; since health issues get medicalized, they seem best left to medical anthropologists. We suggest that bringing together perspectives from medical, linguistic, and media anthropology holds the potential not only for significantly enriching these research areas but for making broader contributions.

Similarly, in media and journalism studies, health news has never been a central part of research agendas. The literature includes important work, including by Lupton (1997, 2012) and Blakeley (2006), and early works on health journalism like Nelkin (1995), Signorielli (1993), and Karpf (1988), together with significant work on entertainment media, including Friedman (2004) and Turow (2010). Other significant works have been few and far between (e.g., Lawrence 2004). For the most part, media studies scholars have left the study of media and health to researchers in the subfield of health communication; their work is generally shaped by the field of public health and largely isolated from media and journalism studies more broadly. Medical sociologist Clive Seale, in one of the few monographs on media and health, noted that:

> the few attempts to summarize the media health field as a whole have been striking in their omission of the broad range of theoretical perspectives and analytical approaches developed in the media studies field. There appear to have been no sustained attempts to conceptualize media health as a case study within larger media processes, or to compare media health coverage with that in other areas.
>
> *(2002: 25)*

Our book addresses this gap head on, also using perspectives from anthropology and other fields, at the same time that it explores why this hiatus has emerged and persisted.

There is a scholarly cadre, scattered across many disciplines, that has produced interesting work on health news, particularly HIV/AIDS, Ebola, genetics, cancer, and influenza. Researchers have identified processes in which coverage of epidemics, which often follow a formulaic "outbreak narrative" (Wald 2008), moves from an initial sense of alarm to strategies for "containing" threats and distancing readers/viewers from them (see Ungar 1998; Joffe and Haarhoff 2002). Scholars point to how modes of framing stories often introduce notions of the Other, such as by locating Ebola in African bodies and impoverished landscapes. Some work, such as Martin Bauer's (1998), goes on to see how the proliferation of health news has medicalized society itself, reshaping conceptions of bodies and social relations through understandings of the power of biomedicine.

Nevertheless, many scholarly works in this area, as Seale (2002: 25) observes, focus on single diagnostic categories, thereby presupposing the objectifying work that such categorization presumes (see Bowker and Star 1999; Conrad 1992). Articles often begin with a summary of the biomedical "facts," thereby reproducing biomedical and public health agendas. A common concern is with "inter-reality distortion"—how journalists "distort" clinical, genetic, and epidemiological knowledge. This formulation extends the boundary-work that reproduces constructions of "the media" as a bounded realm containing media institutions, professionals, and readers/viewers and yet somehow exists apart from "biomedicine," a totalizing category critically engaged by medical anthropologists. As Seale (2002) and Mohan Dutta (2008) suggest, constructing health communication as hypodermic injections of knowledge into the minds of ignorant laypersons erases its political performativity, meaning its capacity to produce hierarchically ordered classes of actors and forms of knowledge rather than simply to represent what is already known. Inattention to the performative power of health news also emerges from how scholars working in this area generally rely on textual analysis and/or surveys in lieu of ethnography, such excellent exceptions as Klinenberg (2002) notwithstanding.

Scholars such as Deborah Lupton (1995, 2012) and Paula Treichler (1999) have forged critical perspectives that look analytically at how textual and visual representations shape understandings of diseases, patients, and populations. Mohan Dutta (2008; Dutta and Basu 2011) forged a "culture-centered critical health communication" approach that draws on subaltern, postcolonial, and decolonial studies in criticizing the Eurocentric bias of dominant approaches and the exclusion of health knowledge produced by populations targeted by top-down health communication approaches. Despite interesting examples, health news has not formed a principal focus for researchers working in this tradition. In general, the dominant literature on health media has largely revolved around content analyses shaped by preexisting notions of "health" and "communication." These underpinnings, we suggest, interact to curtail analysis of the production of biomedical objects and subjects and how logics and practices are dispersed between institutional and other sites, thereby engendering complex, hybridized phenomena. In this book, we combine the analysis of media texts with ethnographic research across a wide range of different kinds of actors and sites involved in the production of health news—in media, but also clinics, businesses, government agencies and more—in critically examining how health stories are produced and how they work, including how they separate, in Pierre Bourdieu's terms (1993), such "social fields" as journalism, medicine, and public health and organize the types of knowledge they produce hierarchically.

The performative role of biocommunicable models

The production and circulation of biomedical knowledge, in which all of us participate, is, as Clarke *et al.* (2003) and others stress, complex, non-linear, and widely dispersed. Nevertheless, it is projected as following a number of cultural models for the production, circulation, and reception of health knowledge. They are not unconscious or hidden, discernible only by scholars. Indeed, we show that health journalism often incorporates these models quite visibly into news reporting, providing simultaneously two distinct if interrelated perspectives on health.

Even as a health news story conveys biomedical content, providing "information" about a "new" disease, treatment, risk factor, or the like, it also projects how knowledge about the phenomenon emerges and circulates and who should attend to it and how. We refer to these projections as "biocommunicable models."

Consider the measles outbreak that began at Disneyland in California in 2015. A typical story, on NBC News,[6] reported that a spike in measles cases could be

> blamed partly on parents who refused to vaccinate their children because of what doctors call misguided concerns over the shot's safety. But medical experts say the vaccine, the only way to protect against measles, has virtually no side effects, and a CDC campaign aims to drive this point home.

Several weeks later, the CNN website had a story titled "5 myths surrounding vaccines—and the reality,"[7] accompanied by a "First Person" article by a mother who recounts her daughter's experience with measles and urges other parents to comply with pediatricians' vaccination recommendations.[8] A story like this reports various forms of "biomedical information," such as summaries of existing research on the safety of vaccines. But the story it tells is as much about communication as about biomedical science: it interprets the outbreak of disease as a failure of what we call biocommunicability, projecting a strongly normative model of how health knowledge ought to circulate, and of the roles that different kinds of actors should play in that process.

Reporting of the 2015 measles outbreak represented a particularly strong example of what we call the *biomedical authority* model of biocommunicability: physicians and biomedical researchers are presented as authoritative sources of information; laypersons are urged to attend to and follow their advice and are warned of the consequences of failing to play that role. Journalists, meanwhile, cast themselves either as passive listeners or as assistants in the dissemination of information. This model is often taken as common sense, and may in part account for the lack of scholarly interest in health news as an object of study: if health news is doing "nothing more" than passively transmitting information from scientists to lay audiences, then it doesn't seem a particularly important object of study. Even in a story like this, however, where the biomedical authority model seems to apply quite strongly, if we foreground the performative role of health journalism, rather than understanding it narrowly in terms of the transmission of information, powerful and important dimensions of the work of communication comes into focus, work that deserves to be examined and perhaps in some ways contested. As we shall see, moreover, the medical authority model is by no means the only model of biocommunicability present in health news. It competes and combines with other models. The complexity of ideological projections of biocommunicability in health news is closely related to the historical transformations analyzed by Clarke *et al.* (2003)—the increasing imbrication of biomedicine with other social fields, and its increased internal complexity. A key part of our methodology in this book is to foreground this performative role of health communication, and we will do this both in the analysis of media texts and in our ethnographic research on the understandings and practices of the actors involved in the production of health news.

Mediatization and biomedicalization

The conceptual framework of this book centers on two neologisms: biocommunicability and biomediatization. Each of these words is a mouthful, but we hope readers will be convinced that they help us to see a familiar but surprisingly complex phenomenon in a new way. What we call "biomediatization" involves the simultaneous operation of two processes which might, on the surface, appear mutually exclusive, and whose relationship has certainly been little explored: mediatization and biomedicalization.

Mediatization refers to transformations occurring as media become increasingly central to social life.[9] Research on mediatization emerged particularly in the field of political communication, though it has expanded rapidly into other areas. Political communication scholars have described a transformation in which older logics of political action centering on institutions like parties and trade unions were displaced and transformed by new, mediatized forms of politics. As political candidates were increasingly "marketed" to publics, conceived of as aggregations of individual consumers, politics became personalized and individualized, and professionals trained in media-related skills were increasingly central to the practice of politics (Mazzoleni 1995; Mazzoleni and Schulz 1999; Schulz 2004). Jesper Strömbäck (2008) argues that mediatization involves four phases, from early phases in which political actors increasingly rely on and interact with media while remaining culturally and institutionally separate to a final phase he calls "pre-mediatization," in which media logics are incorporated into the culture and practice of political actors.

In some accounts, this process is understood as a kind of zero sum transformation in which media institutions become increasingly autonomous and powerful and eventually dominate other institutions. Pierre Bourdieu's (1996) polemical little book *On Television* makes this kind of argument, and Strömbäck (2008: 240) writes that in the fourth phase of mediatization, "the media and their logic can be said to *colonize* politics." Media institutions have become more autonomous and more powerful in important ways, and they do challenge the autonomy and authority of other social fields, including medicine. Dominique Marchetti, one of the few to look systematically at media/medicine interactions, writes of a transformation in France from a closed world in the 1950s—one in which medical specialists controlled the public flow of information about medicine, working with a small group of specialist reporters, who for the most part deferred to them—to a new reality in the 1980s when health news was increasingly "subjected to the ordinary laws of the production of public information" (2010:15; translation ours). These "laws" or practices opened the discussion of medical issues to a wider range of voices and gave journalists a more active, mediating role. Nevertheless, the most recent scholarship on mediatization has increasingly questioned the notion of a simple shift of power toward "the media" and called for a more sophisticated understanding (Deacon and Stanyer 2014; Couldry 2012). Health news provides rich territory for advancing more complex understandings of mediatization.

Sociologists and anthropologists of medicine have advanced arguments about *biomedicalization* that are parallel in many ways to media studies work on mediatization, centering on an expansion of the social and cultural influence of biomedicine. Medical logics have penetrated other spheres; we have come to think of eating, leisure, sex, and education in biomedical terms. On the surface, mediatization and biomedicalization seem to contradict one another, and an interesting question arises about how they intersect: are media colonized by an increasingly powerful biomedical field, or is biomedicine penetrated and colonized by the media? We will try to show in this book that grasping the nature and power of this process requires going beyond such simple binaries to take apart the forms of boundary-work that continually shore up what seem to be autonomous domains even as medical-media hybrids become increasingly embedded in daily life. The better question is not which sphere has more power but rather how the complex inter-penetration of media and medicine has reshaped each domain.

Historically, as Clarke *et al.* (2003) and others have articulated it, biomedicalization is a complex process, entailing internal changes in biomedical fields as, for example, research science and pharmaceutical industries become more powerful relative to individual clinicians. It also involves increased interpenetration between medicine and other social fields as medicine has become entangled with the market and the state, and more central to forms of governance, producing what these authors describe as a growing "heterogeneity of production, distribution, and access to biomedical knowledges" (Clarke *et al.* 2003:177). This transformation is related both to mediatization—to an increasing entanglement of biomedicine with various forms of media—and at the same time with other entanglements—commercialization, politicization, we could say—which hybridize medicine and blur its boundaries.

Mediatization is complex in parallel ways. Media institutions and practices too have become increasingly multiple and complex, intertwined with other social fields and subject to boundary disputes even as—to some extent precisely because—of the increased penetration of media into many other social fields. In the case of politics, for example, when politicians began using television to reach voters directly and hiring advertising and public relations professionals to run their campaigns, this process threatened the central mediating role of *journalists*, who responded in a variety of ways to reassert some measure of control over the flow of communication, deepening the process of mediatization (Hallin 1992). The mediatization of politics, to an important degree, involved an appropriation *by political actors* of media personnel and practices that enhanced, rather than under-mined their power over public communication, even as it transformed politics and made media logics more central.

Similarities between journalism and biomedicine, two complex, interconnected social fields, are an important theme of this book. Both are forms of knowledge production. Both are seen as professions, expected to be governed, as Kenneth Arrow (1963:859) put it in a famous article on medicine and the market, by a "collectivity orientation,"[10] standing above the self-interested behavior expected of ordinary economic actors to serve the interests of patients or readers, and society as a whole. Both have lost autonomy in important ways, however, particularly in relation to the market,[11] even as their centrality to social and cultural life has increased. Both have seen their professional authority questioned and have been embroiled in boundary disputes and ethical debates.

We explore here the complex exchange and partial hybridization of logics and professional practices between media and biomedicine that results from the simultaneous processes of biomedicalization and mediatization; this is one of the key reasons we consider health news to be a fruitful object from the point of view of social theory, highly interesting for scholars both of the media and of health and medicine. The contemporary biomedical field is unquestionably highly mediatized, and it is important to understand what this means in its full complexity. Health information circulates increasingly, and health issues are discussed in mediated public forums that involve wide ranges of actors and discursive logics; clinicians, research scientists, and public health officials interact intensively with public relations professionals, journalists, politicians, "patient advocates," and lay activists (Clarke *et al.* 2003; Heath, Rapp, and Taussig 2004; Marchetti 2010).

In terms of Strömbäck's (2008) formulation, biomedicine can be seen as characterized by the deepest form of mediatization, in which media personnel and logics are fundamentally integrated into institutions and practices of another social field. Clinical and public health institutions—from small community clinics to governmental agencies at all levels and international organizations—all have journalists on their staffs. "Media training" teaches health professionals, particularly those occupying the most visible posts in their organizations, the practices and logics associated with journalism and public relations. Public health officials sometimes devote almost half of their time to responding to press inquiries and attempting to insert their "messages" into media venues. The shift from a risk conception of health to an emphasis on "preparedness," beginning before 2001 but enhanced by the post-9/11 emphasis on bioterrorism and biosecurity, has increased this interpenetration. The CDC also funds "scenarios" or "exercises" that simulate epidemics, bioterrorist attacks, or other health "emergencies" in which journalists employed by the US Department of Homeland Security and public health and security agencies of state and local governments work side-by-side with those employed by media organizations in producing simulated press releases, press conferences, and news reports.

In the pharmaceutical and medical device industries, increasingly central to the production and circulation of medical knowledge, economic growth is founded simultaneously on scientific research, business models, and communication strategies; advertising and public relations professionals participate centrally in efforts to "create patient populations" as much as to create drugs (Dumit 2012: 163) and "facilitate adoption and awareness among regulators, payers, medical influencers and patients alike by conditioning the market for acceptance of new concepts" (Dumit 2012: 64). The penetration of media logics and personnel into the co-production of biomedical knowledge is strong enough that Dumit, who advances an important argument about the role of pharmaceutical marketing in creating a new model of "mass health," makes the case that "it is marketers, not scientists or clinicians, who decide what information, knowledge and facts are worthy as opposed to worthless" (2012: 88–89).

The centrality of market considerations does not, however, impose a single, unifying logic that displaces or fully assimilates those associated with scientific discovery and humanistic conceptions of medicine. Our ethnographic interviews with marketers, journalists, scientists, clinicians, health officials, and patients lead us to conclude that marketers and journalists collaborate with these other social actors in attempting to produce the sense that distinct and often colliding perspectives and interests can be reconciled. Such conflicts and scandals are a regular feature of health news, and, as we see in our discussion of pharma and biotech coverage (Chapter 5), health news often focuses on apparent violations of the boundaries that separate domains and knowledge forms. Benson and Neveu (2005: 6), who apply Bourdieuian field theory to the analysis of journalism, observe that journalism is "a crucial mediator among all fields."[12] Far from playing the passive role of transmitting information from science to the lay public, journalists play active, constitutive roles in defining, policing, and bridging the boundaries between these fields.

If biomedicine is deeply mediatized, however, clearly it is also true that media are deeply biomedicalized. The widespread incorporation of media personnel and logics into biomedicine may blur the boundaries of biomedical professions, but they also account to a significant degree for the enormous social and cultural influence of biomedicine. This is manifested across many dimensions, from direct to consumer advertising to the involvement of pharmaceutical company public relations professionals in "disease awareness" campaigns and patient advocacy organizations and the production of on-line health information. Certainly the news media are no exception; the vast quantity of health news documented at the beginning of this chapter, and the example of reporting of the 2015 measles epidemic, cited earlier in this chapter, both illustrate this. So do the CDC preparedness exercises described above, in which journalists participate alongside public health and security officials. Journalists rely heavily on public relations professionals employed by research, clinical, and public health institutions. This familiar reliance on "information subsidies" (Gandy 1980) goes deeper than in many other areas of coverage, with, for example, the Kaiser Family Foundation sponsoring significant amounts of health journalism. Both non-profit and commercial health institutions produce increasing quantities of sponsored content for media outlets. Network television news is heavily dependent on direct-to-consumer advertising and makes prominent use of physician-correspondents, whose unusual hybrid professional role we explore in detail.

Early research on health and science journalism often used the phrase "two cultures" regarding journalism and biomedicine.[13] Journalists and scientists were understood to see the world quite differently, and this was interpreted as a source of misunderstandings. This "cultural" difference purportedly explained what was perceived to be "distortion" in the proper transmission of scientific information. Journalism and biomedicine do have different institutional structures; the two-cultures framework, in the best of the research that uses it, at least has the virtue of taking journalism seriously as a distinct form of cultural production, which much writing on journalism from public health perspectives fails to do. But the simultaneous and interrelated realities of mediatization and biomedicalization mean that such simple dichotomies cannot capture the nature of the interaction between the news media and biomedicine. Both are complexes of heterogeneous cultural forms that have been deeply influenced by one another and whose basic modes of practice presuppose one another.

We thus propose dropping the "two cultures" trope; rather we draw on a concept associated with STS and analyze the *co-production*[14] of both health coverage and the medical subjects and objects it reports. This phenomenon points to a further analytic reason that we think health news forms a particularly important site for critical inquiry: the relationship between nature/science/medicine and language/communication is less a chasm than a border along which new biomedical objects and subjects—and the ways we come to know and talk about them—are produced. This is what we mean when we use the term *biomediatization*. In putting forward this concept we advance a radical claim here: the new epidemics that so frequently infect us today—including "swine flu" (H1N1), Ebola, avian influenza (H5N1), and "epidemics" of diabetes and obesity—along with the promise of new wonder drugs and treatments—*are co-produced by health and media professionals*. Our argument is not "social constructionist," if this term would suggest that we believe that viruses, bacteria, cancers, and their effects are merely imagined. We are rather interested in how biologies are connected from the get-go with their media manifestations as they are dispersed via articles in biomedical journals, newspapers, television broadcasts, websites, tweets, and complex entanglements of professional logics and practices. The shock that people so frequently express when this foundational hybridization becomes evident rests on boundary-work, on the continual construction of medicine and media as autonomous domains, which requires overlooking or misrecognizing the processes we document here. Biomediatization is not just about the production of articles, broadcasts, websites, and tweets, that is, things that are contained with the sphere of "the media": basic notions of health, disease, citizenship, immigration, ethno-racial categories, and of "the state" are also getting constructed in the process.

The genesis of an unusual collaboration

Our collaboration is unique, in that it brings together a medical and linguistic anthropologist, Briggs, and a media and journalism scholar, Hallin. We knew different bodies of literature, and in this book we put these literatures into dialogue. Integrating contrastive research strategies has been just as important as combining different analytic frameworks. Scholarly readers' receptivity is shaped both by the methodologies they deem appropriate and by the criteria they use in evaluating them. Many media scholars, for example, demand rigorous sampling and coding techniques. Qualitative sociologists and anthropologists are more likely to engage with work based on in-depth interviewing and ethnography. Thus Hallin offered forms of framing analysis commonly employed in media studies and political communication, including quantitative content analysis. Briggs used ethnography, discourse analysis, and interviewing. Quantitative content analysis can be extremely useful for uncovering patterns across large and diverse bodies of media content. It is inevitably narrow and thin in its capacity to reveal the structure of meaning in news texts, however, and for this other forms of interpretive analysis have greater power. Rather than simply juxtapose perspectives, we have worked together for over a decade to the extent that Briggs has participated in quantitative analyses and Hallin has conducted ethnographic interviews. Our book is thus unusual with respect not only to its range of research strategies but also to the degree to which we have integrated them.

The research that underlies this book has three main components. First, we compiled a vast body of news content, including several systematic samples (described in detail in subsequent chapters). The earliest phase of our research focused on a metropolitan newspaper, the *San Diego Union-Tribune* (*SDU-T*). This was our local newspaper when the collaboration began, which facilitated carrying out a multi-method study, not only analyzing news content but also interviewing reporters and their "sources"—other actors involved in the co-production of news—and doing some audience reception analysis. We collected the entire corpus of health-related stories for 2002 and the first half of 2003, then coded stories from the first six months of 2002, totaling 1,206, for analysis. Other systematic samples included 357 network television news stories from April 2009 through June 2012; a sample of 400 articles from the *NYT* and *Chicago Tribune* (*CT*) covering the 1960s through the 2000s; and a sample of coverage of the 2009 H1N1 epidemic in the *NYT, New York Post, USA Today, SDU-T,* and *Atlanta Journal-Constitution.* We also collected a much larger corpus of news media content that we used for the qualitative discourse analysis, including newspapers, various forms of broadcast (network, cable, local and daytime television, and National Public Radio (NPR)), Internet-based media, ethnic media (especially Univisión, *El Latino*, a Spanish daily newspaper in San Diego, and a radio station, Radio Hispana), as well as monitoring comments on major stories in blogs and on-line forums. We generally monitored on a daily basis the *NYT, SDU-T, San Francisco Chronicle,* NPR, and network and local news; we also searched news databases and Internet sources for content on particular stories or themes.

Our focus is principally, though not exclusively, on what are usually called "mainstream media." The contemporary media system is increasingly fragmented and decentered, and media study today is inevitably limited in its ability to capture the full complexity of the information and discourses that circulate across its different components. Nevertheless, as Andrew Chadwick (2013: 59) put it in an influential recent book on the interaction of "old" and "new" media, "television, radio and newspapers are still, given the size of their audiences and their centrality to public life, rightly referred to as 'mainstream.'" These media, as Chadwick observes in *The Hybrid Media System,* have important presences of their own on-line, their content is widely recirculated by other Internet-based media, and to a very significant extent they provide the reference point for the diverse representations that circulate in "legacy" and "new" media alike. The content and practices of mainstream news media are, however, incomprehensible today without reference to the wider field of public communication, ranging from direct-to-consumer advertising to discussion of news content in on-line health-related forums. We will examine many examples of the importance of these interactions.

The media we focus on retain great power to set the terms of public debate. They are directed both toward mass publics and policymakers. Many health and public relations professionals we interviewed stressed that their interactions with reporters were often intended to influence policymakers and funders as much as the mass public. They are what might be termed full-spectrum media, in the sense that they include a wide range of genres of news, directed to different kinds of audiences and connected to different social purposes, including personal health coverage, business reporting, political reporting on health policy, and investigative journalism. If we were primarily interested in health-related choices at the individual level, we might have chosen to focus on other kinds of media. Though newspapers and television play important roles in individual health decisions (Kelly *et al.* 2010), we might have focused more on Internet sites like Web MD or on-line forums on which people affected by particular diseases or belonging to particular health-related sub-communities share information. Our principal focus, however, is not the effect of media on individual behavior but their role in the constitution and circulation of *public* understandings of health and medicine; and for this purpose newspapers and television—including their digital versions, on-line comments sections, and integration with social media—remain at the center of the analysis.

We conducted a broad ethnographic inquiry between 2003 and the present, the second major component of our research. Because of our interest in the relation of mediatization and biomedicalization, and our understanding of health news as co-produced by actors from different domains, our ethnography covered many different kinds of sites and actors. We interviewed reporters, producers, and editors.[15] Our most systematic interviewing of print journalists in the United States was at *The New York Times* and the *San Diego Union-Tribune,* where we spoke with journalists who report health news for various "desks" (science, metropolitan, lifestyle, business, national, and international) and their editors. We also spoke with radio journalists and television reporters and producers from local news organizations to national network news and CNN. Most of our interviewees work for English-language media, but we interviewed five Spanish-language newspaper, radio, and television journalists in Spanish as well.

We also interviewed a host of health professionals. Five were clinicians who had never spoken with a journalist or taken media training but had ideas about the material that their patients bring from the media, Internet, and social media to their examining rooms. Twelve were sources, including administrators at non-governmental organizations (some clinically focused, others not), who had been mentioned in specific stories; they detailed for us how they ended up "in the media" and what they thought about the process. We also interviewed seven health officials, whose jobs involve extensive public communication, including responding to reporters' inquiries and attempting to "feed information" to the media. We also spoke with scientists, clinical researchers, administrators of clinics, hospitals, and health maintenance organizations (HMOs), and public health officials from local, county, and state health offices to high officials in the CDC and other organizations, as well as employees of the Pan American Health Organization and the World Health Organization.

Without the interviews we conducted, we would never have seen how deep the amalgamation of health and media institutions runs, and how much the exchange of practices and logics shapes what people do and how they do it. This process also helped us document boundary-work, the way health and media professionals project the sense that they follow different epistemologies, practices, and interests even as the overlaps and correspondences run ever deeper. In interviews, we focused on biocommunicable models, on basic conceptions regarding how knowledge about health is produced, circulates, and received, as well as on practices, revealing complex entanglements that complicated the cultural models.

When time and permission were both forthcoming, we extended contacts emerging from interviews into ethnography, enabling us to appreciate participants and practices we might have otherwise overlooked. Spending time in local and state public health offices helped us gauge how much time public officials devote to "the media" and how this work helps shape agendas. Sessions on health media held at meetings of clinical and public health professional associations and annual meetings and conferences for journalists also provided rich ethnographic venues. We interviewed six employees of consulting firms who provide media/PR services. Some of the most fruitful sites were those associated with media training and emergency preparedness "exercises" or "scenarios," both of which bring media and health professionals into extended dialogs that foster crucial overlaps and complementarities in their practices. Participating in courses and simulated "events" associated with bioterrorist attacks or the emergence of a new virus enabled Briggs to see first-hand how principles of "crisis and emergency risk communication" and practices rehearsed in biosecurity "exercises" trained media and health professionals to co-produce health discourse in very particular sorts of ways. Indeed, our concept of biomediatization emerged from the results of ethnographic observation and interviews.

Finally, documenting reception was challenging. The ethnography helped us overcome the subtle ways that our own assimilation of the linear, hierarchically ordered model had blinded us to the extent to which some of the principal receivers of health news are located *within* health organizations. We could see how journalists and administrators in health organizations keep close track of what appears in print, in broadcasts, and on blogs, websites, and social media and how minutely "reception" is linked to production. In gauging reception, we were greatly aided by the websites designed for audience commentary on print, radio, and television news stories, which also provide a means of tracking who is e-mailing, tweeting, or otherwise transmitting them. Polls and surveys commissioned by public health and other organizations have been useful. We conducted a number of focus groups over the years in which we presented print and/or television news stories and asked participants to comment; most were organized in the San Diego and San Francisco Bay areas.[16] The interviews and focus groups with Latinos/as in the former region were particularly useful, as people spoke both about how they responded to health news in relation to their own knowledge production and about reception practices. Given that this population is often stereotyped as a bastion of failed biocommunicability, their response illuminated how people position themselves vis-à-vis the subject positions by which they are interpellated. Nevertheless, we readily acknowledge that documenting reception on all of these fronts is challenging, and more can always be done.

Interviews and ethnography in health and media organizations raise complex issues of confidentiality, from the privacy of patient records to concern with the vulnerability of public officials to political and corporate pressure to issues of immigration status and economic exploitation. We spoke with a remarkable number and range of people and visited a great variety of sites. In each, we offered the option of anonymity to all participants, which could include the names of their organizations. Nearly everyone is accordingly given a pseudonym in this book, and some institutions, from small non-governmental organizations (NGOs) to major national television broadcasting corporations, have also been assigned fictitious names. In a few cases, we have listed a corporation or media/public relations firm as being in "a California biotech sector" in order to render it more difficult to identify interviewees and organizations. We faced tough issues of how to protect the anonymity of journalist interviewees at the same time that we were discussing their stories. For this reason, we avoid providing precise references to their articles, broadcasts, or websites when such links might deprive them of anonymity.

A look at what's to come

Chapter 1 develops the concept of biocommunicability, exploring the contrasting cultural models of health knowledge and its circulation that are projected in health news and other forms of health discourse. We also apply this same methodology to an analysis of the scholarly literature on health news, developing an argument that unexamined assumptions about biocommunicability have limited the ability of this field to develop a sophisticated understanding of health news.

Chapter 2 moves from texts to practices, drawing on interviews and ethnography to introduce the people who co-produce health news. Our goal is to replace stick figures and stereotypes—the idea that there is a single, fixed understanding of health and media relations associated with any of these roles—with the fascinating complexities and contradictions that individuals face in the course of their daily work of biomediatization.

Chapter 3 offers an overview of the major genres and frames in health coverage. We explore how journalists negotiate among competing ways of framing health issues, looking particularly at the distinction among biomedical, life-style, and social, environmental or political economy frames. We also look at how they negotiate breaches and challenges to medical authority.

The remaining three chapters are case studies, bringing together ethnography and analysis of news texts. Chapters 4 and 5 look at particular sites where important forms of biomediatization can be seen, and each highlights the intersection of biomedicine with another social field—with government and the practices of "security" in Chapter 4, and with capitalism in Chapter 5. Chapter 4 focuses on "risk communication" in the 2009 H1N1 pandemic and public health officials' and reporters' roles in creating emerging diseases as social objects. The H1N1 virus emerged in a context of great uncertainty, but a remarkably complex and resilient story was produced in just 24 hours. Public health officials largely succeeded in "containing" the discursive contagion that ensued, sidelining politicians and potential critics. This collaboration between public health officials and journalists reflects the incorporation of media logics into public health and of biomedicine into journalism. After exploring the role of bioterrorism "exercises" in shaping this co-production process, we close by contrasting H1N1 with the more recent Ebola outbreak.

Chapter 5 moves us to where biomedicine merges with the market as we examine news coverage of research by biotech and pharmaceutical corporations, the development of new drugs and devices, and scandals resulting in the withdrawal of treatments. Interviews with media consultants for these corporations point to the central part they play. Journalists, we argue, play a much more complex role in mediating between social fields and forms of knowledge than the literature on pharmaceutical marketing has captured, engaging in forms of boundary-work that help both to produce pharma as a boundary-object and to police the troubling hybridities that often result as science, medicine, and capitalism merge.

Chapter 6 examines the complex ways that race and ethnicity are treated in health news. Health news is generally structured around a "post-racial" vision that limits attention to race and ethnicity. We show that race and ethnicity are, nevertheless, thematized under certain circumstances. Often, racialized subjects are presented as deficient in terms of biocommunicability, blocked by "cultural barriers" from fulfilling normative models of health citizenship. We also examine the central and complex role of African American and Latino/a health and media professionals, who are often projected in this coverage as bridging biocommunicable gaps that separate racialized subjects from normative circuits of health communication.

At the same time that we offer what we believe to be the most comprehensive exploration of health news coverage to date, our book is not about that topic—if it is understood as a narrowly bounded domain in which journalists "translate" biomedical research, practice, and policy into objects that circulate within "the media." Rather, by joining critical perspectives on medicine and media, we hope to contribute much more broadly to understanding why both domains are so consequential in contemporary society and the rapidly shifting ways that they intersect in our daily lives, thereby prompting some of our deepest fears and desires. The tremendous power of this juxtaposition emerges precisely from its marginal position vis-à-vis the powerful domains of medicine and journalism. By demonstrating the nature of biomediatization and its centrality to contemporary life, we hope to open up a debate that is of vital importance to scholars, clinicians, policymakers, journalists, and "laypersons"—that is, to all of us.

Notes

1 Print health journalism has been affected by cutbacks in both staffing and the size of the "news hole," the amount of print space or airtime devoted to news content. Nevertheless, there is some evidence that this is not as consistent as in other areas (Schwitzer 2009).

2 One broad study of news across platforms found that in 2007–8, health news made up about 3.6 percent of the total "news hole"; the following year the percentage was much higher, as healthcare reform and the H1N1 pandemic were among the top news stories across most media (Kaiser Family Foundation/Pew Research Center 2009).

3 For examples see Dumit (2003) and Rapp (1999) on medical technologies; Fullwiley (2011), Montoya (2011), Rabinow (1999), and Rapp, Heath, and Taussig (2002) on genetics; Biehl (2005), Petryna, Lakoff, and Kleinman (2006), Petryna (2009), Hayden (2010), and Dumit (2012) on pharmaceuticals and clinical trials; Cohen (2002[2001]), Lock (2002), and Scheper-Hughes (2000) on practices of organ transplant; and Collier, Lakoff, and Rabinow (2004), Collier and Lakoff (2015), Lakoff (2008), Lakoff and Collier (2008), and Briggs (2011b) on logics of preparedness, to name just a few authors and research foci.

4 Media anthropology is now is graced by edited collections (Askew and Wilk 2002; Ginsburg, Abu-Lughod, and Larkin 2002) and a number of ethnographies (such as Abu-Lughod 2005; Larkin 2008; Mankekar 1999).

5 E.g., Hannerz (2004), Pedelty (1995), Bird (2010), and Boyer (2005, 2013).

6 19 Jan. 2015, http://www.nbcnews.com/health/health-news/measles-outbreak-spreads-california-other-states-n289091.

7 Ben Brumfield and Nadia Kounang, 5 Feb. 2015, http://www.cnn.com/2015/02/04/us/5-vaccine-myths/index.html.

8 Shelley Jonson Carey, "Measles Was No Big Deal – Until My Daughter Caught It." 17 Feb. 2015. http://www.cnn.com/2015/02/17/living/feat-measles-vaccine-first-person/.

9 For discussions of mediatization, see Couldry and Hepp (2013), Couldry (2012), Hepp (2012, 2013), Hjavard (2013), Lundby (2009), Landerer (2013) and Altheide and Snow (1979).

10 Arrow took this phrase from Talcott Parsons' (1951:463; also 1964) work on professionalization.

11 On commercialization and deprofessionalization in journalism, see Hallin (2000).

12 Mediatization and mediation are distinct concepts. Mediatization refers to a historical process at the structural level. Mediation refers to kinds of work that are done by particular actors or institutions. It is sometimes used to refer to the transmission of information, but we use it here to refer to the work of adjudicating among and synthesizing competing perspectives and claims to public attention.

13 See Nelkin (1995). Seale (2002:52–54) summarizes this perspective.

14 See Jasanoff (2004) on co-production. Marchetti (2010:10) also uses the term in writing about medicine and media.

15 More specifically, we interviewed seven television journalists, three radio, and ten newspaper reporters and three editors. All of these journalists had experience with social media; we also interviewed three journalists who worked on entirely digital media. These totals

exclude interviews conducted outside the United States, including with international journalists and health officials. Note that some journalists had worked in quite a variety of news media.

16 We conducted six focus groups in the San Diego area, three in the San Francisco Bay Area, and one in Los Angeles. Of these, four were conducted in Spanish and six in English, and all were between one and two hours in duration. Only one was held in a clinical setting; otherwise, they were conducted in such contexts as informal gatherings after church services, meetings of teacher–parent organizations, and living rooms. They ranged from four to forty participants; the average was 11, excluding the facilitators. An initial set of questions focused on media consumption in general, practices for seeking out health-related information, perceptions of health news, and which sources of health knowledge were deemed more reliable. In each case, we then presented a mix of newspaper and television health stories and then asked people to comment on them. They were drawn from Spanish and English newspapers and from CNN, local news, and national network news in English and, for Spanish, a San Diego affiliate of Univisión.

PART I

Toward a framework for studying biomediatization

PART I

Toward a framework for studying biomedicalization

1

BIOCOMMUNICABILITY

Cultural models of knowledge about health[1]

Consider the following syndicated article that ran in the *San Diego Union-Tribune* headed "Actress fights, and beats, RA with new drug therapy":

> Rheumatoid arthritis has afflicted humans for centuries. . . . But until recently, "all of the useful treatments have been stolen from other specialties," says Dr. Israeli Jaffe, a rheumatologist at Columbia's College of Physicians and Surgeons. . . .
>
> Ten years ago Kathleen Turner didn't know what she had when her feet and elbow started hurting. . . . Finally diagnosed through a simple blood test for rheumatoid factor, she "didn't know the questions to ask," Turner says. Gathering the facts piecemeal, she says, "I figured if this happened to me, a lot of people are suffering."
>
> To fill the gap today, she is backing RA Access. . . . [2]

The story went on to give information about the organization's "patient-friendly" website and phone number, and mentioned that it was sponsored by Immunex and Wyeth-Ayerst, as well as giving contact information for the Arthritis Foundation.

Being scientifically and medically literate involves a constant search for new information about bodies, diseases, drugs, and technologies, adding them to our store of knowledge and responding in appropriate ways—such as going to the doctor, avoiding a particular food, doing yoga, or getting exercise. When confronted with an article like the one above—or a television broadcast or an Internet or Facebook posting—we focus on the biomedical content, in this case, rheumatoid arthritis and its diagnosis and treatment. Nevertheless, this article is centrally concerned with the production and circulation of knowledge and information. It maps an idealized "flow" of health knowledge: researchers should produce knowledge as much as "useful treatments," which should be rapidly disseminated among physicians, enabling them to readily diagnose cases like Turner's. Laypersons similarly should know about diseases and symptoms, enabling them to ask questions of their physicians.

Our central argument is that such stories are teaching us in two quite different ways simultaneously, but we are conditioned to focus only on one, the biomedical dimension. In addition to informing us about a disease, we learn about a powerful cultural model that projects who produces scientific and medical knowledge, how it circulates, and who should receive it. We also learn who seems to be failing to play her or his assigned role. The heroes here are a rheumatologist who produces new knowledge and places it in circulation and Turner, a patient who relentlessly sought out the appropriate sources of knowledge to obtain a solution to her problem. Implicitly, the doctors she visited initially did not fulfill their duty, as physicians, to have up-to-date knowledge and use it effectively in their consulting rooms.

Given that there is no medical breakthrough here, what made this story news? The drama results from disruptions of the flow of information: rheumatoid arthritis specialists were not generating disease-specific treatments; Turner, further "downstream," was misdiagnosed (beginning with a podiatrist who recommended "bigger shoes") and had to "gather the facts piecemeal," seemingly having to teach her doctors. It is, however, a story with a happy ending: just as Turner beat rheumatoid arthritis, researchers, physicians, and patients now have the means of overcoming the failure of biomedical communication. But if knowledge should properly be produced by medical researchers and circulated to physicians who then use it to diagnose and treat their patients, why would potential patients need to access this knowledge directly? And what role do two corporations and a disease-specific advocacy group play?

Since we are taught to focus on the biomedical content, this second educational project is largely relegated to the background, enabling it to shape our thinking about health without being subject to the same sort of critical reflection. How can we bring the second pedagogical project into focus, opening up ways of thinking about how it interacts with biomedical content and its impact on audiences? Transforming common sense into an object of critical scrutiny is not easy, and we have developed some conceptual tools for guidance. One is the notion of a *biocommunicable cartography,* the projection in a particular story of a specific process of knowledge production, circulation, and reception. Such cartographies identify networks of actors—here researchers, physicians, patients, pharmaceutical corporations, and an NGO—and project specific expectations for the roles they play in producing, circulating, and receiving knowledge. These cartographies are cultural models woven into the words and images of stories themselves. Biocommunicable cartographies are not evident only in newspapers or even "the media" as a whole but also emerge in clinical interactions, health education "campaigns," and beyond, including health communication research.

Each story projects a unique assemblage of sites, actors, objects, modes of circulation, and forms of biocommunicable success and/or failure; nevertheless, if these were not intertextual—if they did not implicitly invoke other cartographies—

they would not resonate with us in the same way, nor would they remain in the background, enabling us to focus on the biomedical content. After examining thousands of news stories appearing in newspapers, on television and radio, and in Internet and social media venues we have identified a number of recurrent types, which we refer to as *biocommunicable models*. In this chapter we present the three types we have to found to be most recurrent. In using the term "model," we do not pretend to locate pure, ideal, or stable types. Indeed, particular stories—such as Turner's—often combine these models in complex and sometimes contradictory ways.

This chapter presents three predominant types of biocommunicable projections: the *biomedical authority, active patient-consumer*, and *public sphere* models. Each is complex and can be differentiated into sub-types, and they intersect in complex ways in particular biocommunicable cartographies.

Doctor knows best: biomedical authority/passive patient reception

In June 2010 public health officials in California launched a campaign to promote vaccination against whooping cough, extensively covered in health news on and off for several months. On 10 June the *San Diego Union-Tribune* (*SDU-T*) carried a front-page story that began:

> A whooping cough epidemic sweeping California has killed five infants this year, and health officials are urging the public to make sure all family members and caregivers are up-to-date on their vaccinations.
>
> Epidemiologists said a key to breaking what has been a three-to-five-year cycle of epidemics for whooping cough may be a booster shot that became available in 2005 for middle school children and adults.
>
> "We're really trying to raise awareness that it's important for parents, family members and caregivers to get a booster shot to provide a cocoon of protection around infants," said Ken August, spokesman for the California Department of Health.
>
> People should also not ignore a nagging cold that involves a cough, said Dr. John Bradley, director of infectious diseases at Rady Children's Hospital.[3]

This is an example of what we call the biomedical authority model of biocommunicability. All the sources cited are biomedical authorities, and the lay audience is projected as a passive receiver of the information they disseminate, which is summarized by a box accompanying the story. The assumption that medical science produces objective and highly specialized technical knowledge sets the medical realm off from many other realms of discourse, where more populist, relativist, or democratic communication ideologies prevail. The biomedical authority model imagines a hierarchically ordered, natural, necessarily linear trajectory that moves through space, time, and states of knowledge and agency, starting from the production of knowledge about health by biomedical authorities, its codification into texts (reports, scientific articles, pronouncements by public health officials, etc.), the translation of scientific texts into popular discourse (through health education, statements to reporters by health professionals, and media coverage), its dissemination through a range of media, and its reception by "the public," in this case by "parents, family members and caregivers."

Another version of this model appears in health advice columns. Preventing and curing Type 2 diabetes, writes Jane Brody in the *New York Times (NYT)*,

> requires a kind of intervention that only the potential and actual victims can provide: making better food choices, getting more exercise and—most important of all—avoiding excess weight or taking it off if it's already there. . . . One-third of the people with this disease do not know they have it.[4]

The exposition is didactic, and most of the information is presented without attribution, simply as fact—rather unusual in journalism. The voice of biomedical authority addresses its audience directly; the journalist's mediating role remains in the background. The article quotes one endocrinologist to establish the authority of the information, and it cites a Department of Health and Human Services study. Patients seldom speak in these articles, and there is hardly ever a human interest angle—a focus, that is, on stories of particular individuals who serve as exemplars, although many articles do include a photograph of a patient and/or one of the quoted professionals. Laypersons are sometimes interpellated as eavesdroppers, listening in on conversations that do not yet include us, sometimes instructed in a didactic mode, and sometimes, like the photographed patients, pictured as waiting to see how local physicians will bring us this new knowledge.

A 22 June 2011 "Healthy Living Report" on the ABC Evening News provides a rich example of the biomedical authority model in a story oriented toward health education. Its "peg" is the release of what anchor Diane Sawyer calls "a *giant* new survey" of diet and weight gain in which "researchers followed 120,000 people for two decades." Here ABC News Chief Health and Medical Director Dr. Richard Besser makes "a house call," bringing information on diet and weight gain to Edie, a slightly overweight middle-class woman (Figure 1.1). The didactic information is made entertaining by the "house call" device, in which Edie greets him and they surveil her kitchen, locating potato chips in the cupboard and potatoes in the refrigerator. To further liven up the dry numbers, a "Wild West" theme is added. "It's the showdown at the OK weight corral," Besser begins over music from an old Western, and he follows up by identifying "public enemies" in Edie's kitchen and reassuring us that "the cavalry [healthy foods] is nearby." Besser's words are reinforced by a superimposed image of graph lines, pictures of the foods that he has just identified, and a statistical projection of how many pounds each food will potentially add to or subtract from Edie's weight over a decade.

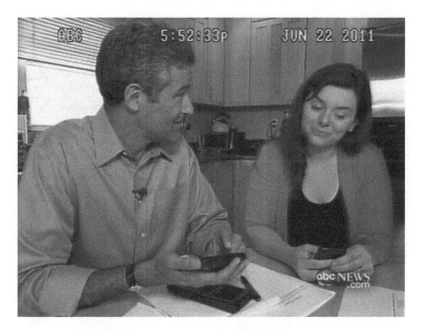

FIGURE 1.1 "Wow!" says Edie, as Richard Besser adds up the calories. ABC News, 22 June 2011.

On television, biocommunicable roles come alive in a new way, as the journalists step into the foreground as characters. A pediatrician and public health official as well as a journalist, Besser fuses media and medical roles, personalizing the latter. The role of passive patient-receiver, meanwhile, only implicit in our newspaper examples, comes alive as Edie opens her door to Besser. Her minimal lines (greeting Besser, giving her name, admitting that she likes potatoes, expressing sheepish surprise "Wow!"—when Besser projects her possible future weight gain), facial expressions, and bodily demeanor mark her subject-position. Practitioners of conversation analysis have suggested that utterances are characterized by "recipient design," meaning that such details as vocabulary, grammar, and inflection (or, more technically, prosody) are shaped in such a way as to project the cognitive and linguistic state of the receiver.[5] Here, Besser has shed his tie and jacket, uses a more colloquial vocabulary and Wild West idioms, suggesting an audience that needs entertainment and simplification to spark interest and enable them to understand his recommendations. Edie expresses ignorance of dietary recommendations and watches passively as Besser calculates the health implications. We all seem to be interpellated into her position as Besser frequently moves between conversing with her and voice-overs that direct the dietary warnings and recommendations to viewers.

Some stories project biomedical knowledge as flowing downward to fill a void, reaching lay audience members who lack knowledge. Others invoke competing circuits of information and involve exhortations to replace faux health beliefs with authoritative knowledge, often accompanied by admonitions to trust biomedical authority. "Health hoaxes . . . zip around cyberspace like flies around fresh meat," warns one article splashed across most of the front page of the Currents section of the *SDU-T* (Figure 1.2). The article details "the phony health scares exposed on a hoax-debunking Web site of the federal Centers for Disease Control and Prevention (CDC)" and advises readers to rely on web-based sources of health information properly inserted within established channels of dissemination of biomedical knowledge.[6] This framing of biomedical authority as displacing not just ignorance but superstition and information provided by illegitimate sources sometimes figures prominently in stories that focus on racial difference, as we discuss in Chapter 6.

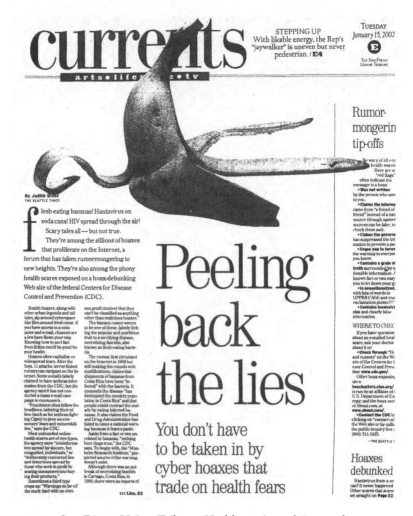

FIGURE 1.2   San Diego Union-Tribune Health section advises readers on proper channels for health information. *San Diego Union-Tribune*, 15 Jan. 2002.

Formerly, the biomedical authority model was clearly dominant. Nancy Lee shows that mid-twentieth-century health reporting typically admonished laypersons to rely exclusively on their family physician for health information. Lee (2007:117) quotes a 1930 article in *Hygeia*, a popular magazine published by the American Medical Association, which reflects the "doctor's orders" version of biocommunicability.

> The good patient, and he is the one who has by far the best chance of recovery, is he who obeys his medical adviser, seeks from him and not from his neighbors or from books in the library whose terms he does not understand the answer to his questions. . . . Confidence in one's physician is almost as important as confidence in one's confessor or in wife or husband.

In its pre-1960s form, this model projected a circuit of communication in which medical knowledge is produced by specialists and transmitted to patients by their primary-care physicians; it had no place for journalists as non-specialist mediators. That the AMA felt it necessary to publish a popular magazine in the 1930s, however, suggests that this effort to channel the flow of medical information and keep it out of the public arena ran counter to powerful social forces.

Historical transformations of US medicine, health education campaigns, the multiplication of actors and stakeholders (including media actors) involved in the circulation of medical knowledge, and the intensification of political, economic, and cultural conflicts over biomedicine have transformed this model of biocommunicability and eroded its dominance. Today it appears alongside, and sometimes in tension with, other biocommunicable models; at times it is present essentially as an absence, as a nostalgic contrast to the realities of biocommunicability in an era of neoliberal restructuring and politicization. It is, however, still profoundly important to an understanding of public communication about health and medicine. Its continuing importance is illustrated by the centrality of biomedical professionals—chiefly, researchers, public health officials, and physicians—as sources; they are the "primary definers"[7] whose voices dominate health and medical news. The linear, "hypodermic" model still informs health education and health promotion (and also much research in health communication), even as audiences have come to be seen as active, selective, and heterogeneous "consumers" of health information (Lupton 1995). Moreover, the biomedical authority model jumps back into prominence, as we see in Chapter 4, when authorities declare an epidemic or other health "emergency."

The biomedical authority model in research on health journalism

In the Introduction we observed that the study of health news is curiously isolated from wider trends in scholarship, mostly confined to the sub-field of health communication and little developed in other fields focused either on media or on medicine. We believe this is a result of an uncritical acceptance of the linear model of the flow of health news, which underpins the medical authority model.[8] One typical article, published in the *Journal of Health Communication*, introduces its research problem like this: "The reality of cancer does not always match public or individual perception of the disease. . . . One source with the potential to distort perception of cancer is news coverage" (Jensen *et al.* 2010:137). Summarizing the literature on cancer coverage, the authors write that "certain cancer sites were found to be covered disproportionate to their actual incidence and mortality rates, a phenomenon that came to be known as interreality distortion" (139).

Analyzing a research article of this sort in the same way as a news story, looking at the model of biocommunicability it projects, what we see is essentially a hierarchical model of linear transmission. Biomedical science is projected as producing knowledge that can be understood as a reflection of "reality." Knowledge is projected as flowing downward to a lay mass public; journalism, it would seem, is understood as significant as a research subject only because it plays a role in this process of transmission. The object of research on health journalism, then, is generally seen as assessing how accurately the media transmit biomedical information—or how much they "distort" it. This research generally has a negative tone toward journalism, presenting health news as an important vehicle of health education but generally a flawed one, whose main independent effect on the circulation of health information is understood as "distortion."

Examples of this focus on distortion in the transmission of scientific information are common in a wide range of the literature within and beyond the field of Health Communication. In "Distorting Genetic Research About Cancer: From Bench Science to Press Release to Published News," Brechman, Lee, and Cappella (2011:496) write, "Much of the research concerning how science is presented in the public press compares content between original science publications and mainstream news media." Statements culled from news reports and from press releases were presented to graduate students in genetics to be rated for their accuracy. Walsh-Childers, Edwards, and Grobmeyer (2011) used doctoral students in medicine to code magazine articles for their inclusion of and assessments of accuracy in stating thirty-three "key facts" about breast cancer. The hierarchical structuring of epistemologies and cultural fields is evident in the procedure of using medical students to judge journalism, rather than journalism students to evaluate medical research articles. (If the hierarchy seems self-evident, we should remember that public relations agencies are often involved in writing the articles to begin with; health journalists we interviewed often told stories about finding errors in journal articles sent to them prior to publication.)[9]

Starting with Lippmann and Merz (1920), media analysts have used comparisons between news representations and alternative accounts of reality to foreground the constructed nature of news, to establish that news cannot be understood simply as a mirror of reality, and thus to open the question of the social processes that account for its emphases and silences. The media rely heavily on the authority of highly developed bodies of knowledge produced by biomedical institutions to legitimize their representations and communicative authority, and it is reasonable to ask whether they are getting it right. It is clearly useful to document patterns in news coverage, like a focus on treatment over prevention found by Jensen *et al.* (2010), in an effort to make those involved in the process by which health news is produced aware of the patterns of emphasis and to generate reflection about the news decisions that produce them.

Comparisons between news coverage and epidemiological data also lead to hypotheses about processes that shape patterns of emphasis, which are potentially interesting for understanding the wider social process by which health knowledge is produced—but only, as we argue in subsequent chapters, if we move away from the model of linear transformation of information from biomedical science, through media to "the public," all imagined as distinct and separate spheres. Slater *et al.* (2008) and Jensen *et al.* (2010) argue that the differential representation of cancer types can be explained by the strength of organized media advocacy; we will see this process at work in many different contexts in the following pages. Menéndez and di Pardo (2009), coming from Latin American perspectives on medical anthropology and critical epidemiology, compare the content of Mexican newspapers with epidemiological data and find that, in 2002, HIV/AIDS constituted almost 15 percent of the press coverage in Mexico City, though it represented less than 1 percent of deaths in Mexico that year. HIV/AIDS coverage also focused heavily on women, though they represented a small number of cases. Cirrhosis and related liver diseases ranked fourth as a cause of death but was virtually unreported in the media. These findings open the way for discussion of a number of factors that may influence health journalism, ranging from organized advocacy, as in the case of breast cancer, to policy priorities, to liquor advertising.

If we stop here, however, we end up with a rather thin understanding of health news. The field of journalism studies long ago moved beyond the idea that media analysis is about exposing "bias" in media representations (Schudson 2003), just as the field of communication in general moved beyond understanding communication exclusively in terms of the transmission of information (Carey 1989). STS and the anthropology and sociology of medicine, meanwhile, developed a large body of research that demonstrates the inadequacy of what we call a *linear-reflectionist perspective* that envisions health news as transforming biomedical facts into popular discourse. STS scholars argue both that scientific knowledge cannot be understood as a simple "reflection of reality" unaffected by culture and society and that lay understandings of science and health cannot be reduced to misunderstandings or partial assimilations of scientific knowledge (Jasanoff *et al.* 1995). For the most part, we set aside in this book questions about whether health news reflects the "reality" of disease or whether journalists are "getting the science right" in order to develop a new framework for understanding the roles of the news media in the circulation of biomedical information and the constitution of cultural understandings of health, disease, and biomedicine.

The literatures we have discussed here understand health journalism from within public health perspectives, that is, they consider news coverage of health and medicine to be important because it affects individual health behavior and thus health outcomes. These health communication researchers understand the news media as a "health education service" (Brechman, Lee, and Cappella 2011:496) or as a "vehicle for dissemination of cancer control messages" (Stryker, Emmons, and Viswanath 2007:24). The dominance of a "health education" perspective in research on health news could be seen as one manifestation of biomedicalization, of the spread of biomedical ways of thinking into other social fields. It is obviously related to the fact that the field of health communication gets much of its US research funding from agencies like the National Institutes of Health. Certainly health education is one role that health journalism plays, of which health journalists are very conscious. However, as we document throughout this book, it is only one of many roles played by health journalism.

If we broaden our focus a bit and look at research on health news in another field, public understanding of science (POUS), interesting differences emerge regarding why it matters that journalism represent science accurately and what it would mean to do this. The PUOS literature includes many perspectives on this question, from the role of information in individual behaviors related to risk (somewhat closer to the health education focus of the health communication literature) to the judgments citizens make about policy issues related to science and technology to support for science as an institution to appreciation of science as a knowledge-producing practice. A policy perspective published in the journal *Public Understanding of Science* in 2001 distinguished between public understanding of *science*, in the sense of understanding the results of established science, and public understanding of *research*, in the sense of understanding research "as it is happening, including the set-backs, detours and disagreements, as well as the positive aspects of new discoveries and exciting new directions for exploration" (Field and Powell 2001:423).

Often the standards for representing science conflict, for example, between what we could call an instrumental conception of the news media (their role is to shape individual health behavior) and a representational conception (their role is to show science "as it really is"). Niederdeppe *et al.* (2010:246), coming from a health communication/public health perspective, criticize local TV news coverage of cancer for focusing on "novel or controversial" research rather than emphasizing "well-documented causes and known prevention methods"—a clear contrast with Field's and Powell's stress on promoting public understanding of "the positive role of controversy" in science.[10] In terms of biocommunicability, the former represents something closer to the biomedical authority model—a focus on controversy is seen as misleading patients and possibly leading to "noncompliance," while the latter represents a version of a public sphere model, understanding science as a process of open exchange and debate.

We argue throughout this book that health journalists do not simply *transmit* knowledge but *mediate* among different registers of knowledge, or competing perspectives on truth and value that contend in the field of health and medicine. Cancer, for example, and how it should be addressed as a public health issue is hardly an uncontested terrain. Sharply different perspectives on research priorities and strategies for prevention, screening, and treatment contend. News coverage of cancer sometimes focuses on what individuals can do to lower their own risk, sometimes on research priorities or disputes about clinical practice, sometimes on the implications of new research for the bottom lines of pharmaceutical companies, sometimes on regulatory and policy issues. A wide range of interests intervene in these debates, and the stakes are not only scientific and health-related but also economic, political, and cultural. Journalism does not, indeed, confine itself to transmitting "well-documented causes and prevention methods," in the words of Niederdeppe *et al.* (2010), to a lay audience. Many media professionals, as we discuss in Chapter 2, told us this is not the journalist's job at all but one for doctors and public health officials. And probably this is for the best, if we value broad public discussion of public health issues in the formulation of heath policy.

The patient-consumer model

The article on Turner and rheumatoid arthritis provides clear evidence of the biomedical authority model in the first half, with its quotations from a rheumatologist summarizing what biomedical science has learned about the disease. It projects an image of scientific progress with technologies that have "revolutionized treatment," directing readers to websites for access to authoritative information. But the linear, hierarchically organized model is complicated as the celebrity patient appears—and speaks—as an active seeker of information, moving from "gathering the facts piecemeal" to managing her own treatment and eventually becoming an advocate for patients. Turner steps into this role because the linear transmission of knowledge from science through physician to patient had failed. The process of biomedicalization involves a shift away from the individual physician as a primary actor and toward research scientists, large-scale institutions of the biomedical-industrial complex (particularly pharmaceutical corporations), and a multiplicity of mediated sites, including websites, electronic newsletters, and social media as well as "the traditional media." This change can be seen in the projection of biocommunicability in this story, as the physician is portrayed as the weak link. As Dumit (2012:78) argues, depicting physicians as ignorant or incompetent and thus requiring corporate-sponsored educational efforts enters significantly into pharmaceutical marketing strategies. Biocommunicable health is restored by the active patient-consumer, represented by Turner, teaming up with biomedical scientists, industry, and patient-advocacy groups. There are also key actors in this process not represented in the news story itself, including, of course, the journalist who wrote it, and also public relations consultants, one of whom we meet in Chapter 2.

Patient-consumer communicability significantly shifts relationships between health professionals and publics. Rather than posit passive receivers of authoritative information, the patient-consumer model imagines laypersons as individuals who make choices apart from the direct supervision of their physicians. Articles often pedagogically map the rational information acquisition/decision-making process that patient-consumers undertake. Besser's house call contrasts with a story by his CBS counterpart, Dr. Jon LaPook. On 29 July 2010, LaPook reported findings that calcium supplements recommended to prevent osteoporosis increased the risk of heart attack. Like Besser, LaPook personalized the story, reporting from a physician's office. Patient Lisa Kwok notes, "I think why this study concerns me is because of all the different factors I represent. And at some point we're going to have to make a decision as I get older." A soundbite from cardiologist Suzanne Steinbaum follows: "I think it's important for us to look at this study and re-think our practice. We shouldn't just recommend supplementation for all of our patients." LaPook then converses in studio with anchor Katie Couric. "So is this a real conundrum, John, for doctors?" Couric asks. "I mean what are they going to tell their patients about this?" "It is a conundrum, and this may represent a real sea change," LaPook replies. "I know, I have tons of patients, especially women after the age of 50, who are taking calcium supplements. And now I'm going to say, let's see if we can get it from food—not just dairy, but other things. . . . "Couric chimes in, "Like sardines ?" "Like sardines," LaPook continues, "figs, almonds, broccoli, soy beans. We're going to have a more complete list up on our web site. But the bottom line here, is, one size doesn't fit all, and doctors have to rethink what they just automatically were doing." "Alright," Couric concludes, "my doctor told me to get it from food just this morning." "And your doctor was right," LaPook replies.

In Besser's story, Edie is a passive receiver of information; Kwok appears as an active patient-consumer, displaying knowledge of her risk factors and speaking of the medical decisions that "we"—she and her doctor together—will make. She speaks for twelve seconds. Steinbaum speaks five; visually, they appear to be speaking as equals, presenting a similar relation to the new information. This projection of biocommunicability is reinforced by Couric, who as anchor typically stands in for the lay audience; she joins LaPook in generating the list of calcium-rich foods. This story, like the Turner story, is pegged to a disruption of biocommunicability, as changing science undercuts the advice physicians were giving to patients; in both stories, the journalists restore the circuit of information as Couric models the active patient-consumer and LaPook the ideal physician. As evident in Couric's role in providing content and reporting that she learned about the issue that morning from her doctor, biomedical authority and patient-consumer models intersect intimately.

The model of the active patient-consumer appears in a particularly strong form in much health reporting that is conceived as "service journalism," closely tied to consumer reporting. A 2005 front page of the *SDU-T* weekly Health section is titled "BETTER BIRTHS: Expectant mothers are doing their research to find the best hospitals and physicians" (Figure 1.3). "[M]any expectant mothers," the article reads, "are abandoning the idea that you deliver at whatever hospital your doctor works. They are going on-line, talking to friends and doing research to figure out which facility suits them best and then finding a doctor who works there."[11] No physicians are quoted; the voice of biomedical institutions is embodied not in medical experts

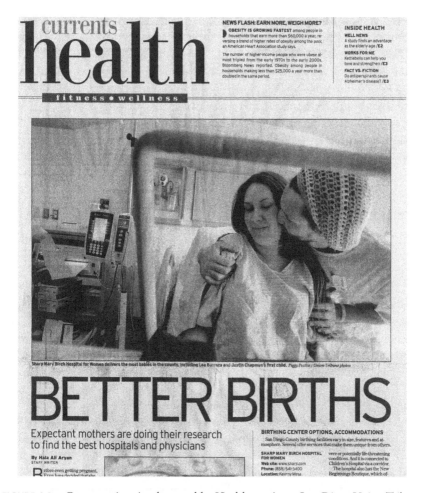

FIGURE 1.3 Consumerism in the weekly Health section. *San Diego Union-Tribune*, 3 May 2005.

but hospital administrators and public-relations officers. Patients "realize they have a choice and the right to get the care they expect," says one administrator. Sidebars list information resources, including websites, books, and magazines. Here the biomedical voice and the invisible presence of the reporter merge in biocommunicable projections of neoliberal health policies—medical care is oriented towards consumers making rational choices among available options. Patient-consumers frame what constitutes relevant and adequate knowledge, and journalists help consumers exploit the range of options apparently open to them. The goal is not simply avoiding illness but maximizing freedom, well-being, quality of life, and the future of one's children, becoming "the expert patient" (Dumit 2012:35).

Patient-consumer biocommunicability is prominent on the *Dr. Oz Show*. Dr. Mehmet Oz is a cardiothoracic surgeon who first appeared on *Oprah*, later creating one of the most successful shows on daytime television, with about 2,900,000 viewers daily in 2011 (Block 2012), 3,400,000 million unique viewers to his website in 2014 (second among daytime television shows), and 3,460,000 twitter followers (ahead of CNN's Dr. Sanjay Gupta with 1,830,000). Dr. Oz describes his show's purpose as empowering people to take control of their own health (Specter 2013):

> I want no more barriers between patient and medicine. I would take us all back a thousand years, when our ancestors lived in small villages and there was always a healer in that village—and his job wasn't to give you heart surgery or medication but to have a safe place for conversation. . . . Western medicine has a firm belief that studying human beings is like studying bacteria in petri dishes. Doctors do not want questions from their patients; it's easier to tell them what to do than listen to what they say. But people are on a serpentine path through life, and that's the way it's supposed to be. All I am trying to do is put a couple of road signs out there.

One important element of the *Dr. Oz Show,* that is found to some degree in highly commercialized consumer-oriented forms of health reporting, is a kind of leveling of knowledge hierarchies manifested in an emphasis on do-it-your-self health solutions and complementary and alternative medicine. Criticized for deviating from deference to scientific authority,[12] his show nevertheless incorporates elements of the biomedical authority model as Dr. Oz quizzes audience members on their health knowledge and chides them for their ignorance.

In the consumer and human interest genres, the patient-consumer model of bio-communicability appears in a highly positive form as a happy world where biomedical science—sometimes alongside complementary and alternative medicine—produces a cornucopia of choices that enables consumers to realize healthy life styles. Health news is one of the few categories in the US press where "good news" is at least as common as bad. This is in part why it is so popular with news organizations that have shifted toward market-driven models of practice, away from more hierarchical conceptions of news judgments in which journalists, as professionals, make judgments about what citizens need to know. Much health news fits into "life-style journalism" or "news you can use," attractive to news organizations because it is cheap to produce—much of it is syndicated material—and because it addresses readers as consumers, integrating advertising and editorial content (Underwood 1993). Patient-consumer reporting often naturalizes neoliberal models of biosociality and projections of the market as enhancing individual and public health.

A particularly explicit connection between patient-consumer biocommuni-cability and neoliberalism appeared in a syndicated column by George Will on obesity. Will writes,

> often the most effective dollars government spends pay for the dissemination of public health information. In an affluent society, which has banished

scarcity and presents a rich range of choice[s], many public health problems are optional—the consequences of choices known to be foolish.[13]

Will praises the Surgeon-General's Office as "sometimes . . . the government's most cost-effective institution" and presents the news-reading public as a composite of active governmental subjects, "middle class, broadly educated," each engaged in a search for news that s/he can use in making rational choices. Will models patient-consumer rationality by asking his readers to use a formula to calculate their Body Mass Index (BMI), in contrast to Besser's Edie, who watches while *he* calculates her projected weight gain. Patient-consumer biocommunicability defines citizenship for Will, which strongly implies individual responsibility for health problems. The government plays a limited role, consistent with neoliberal visions of efficiency—providing patient-consumers with "public health information [that] encourages moderation." Those who are not middle class, are outside of an information flow obviously not addressed to them, or do not experience neoliberal society as a "rich range of choice" are invisible—as they are also in the *SDU-T*'s report on "Better Births," and indeed almost always in its Tuesday Health section, as we will see in Chapter 6.

Patient-consumer biocommunicability positions journalists as advisors to patient-consumers, helping them manage the increased obligation to seek out health-related information associated with neoliberalism. But health news does not always present market relationships as free of contradiction. The rise of the biomedical-industrial complex and the deepening of medical/market entanglements juxtapose contrastive logics and value systems, sparking conflicts that appear in health news.[14] Neoliberal sensibilities coexist with nostalgia for the "residual value," in Williams' (1980) terms, associated with the doctor's orders model of all-knowing, "collectivity-oriented" biomedical professionals who once enjoyed our "generalized trust" (Arrow 1963:859). Health-related consumerism has complicated origins, springing in part from neoliberal restructuring of healthcare institutions, but in part also from new social movements in the 1970s, when languages of consumerism were invoked by lay activists challenging biomedical authority. *Our Bodies, Ourselves*, produced by the Boston Women's Health Collective (1971), was simultaneously a consumerist manifesto and a feminist challenge to physicians' control of women's health (Davis 2007). Journalists similarly fuse languages of consumerism and of political activism, as in an *SDU-T* editorial criticizing the California Medical Board's opposition to legislation requiring it to disclose convictions and completed investigations of physicians. "California patients ought to be entitled to the information they need to make informed decisions."[15] Here health professionals are demoted from privileged purveyors of scientific information to service providers to be evaluated like any other class of vendors.

In a column titled "What to Do If Treatment Isn't Clear," Jane Brody passes on a physician's advice to "ask pointed questions" and to be assertive, even if "some doctors may resent such an inquiry."[16] Here Brody implies a common projection of patient/physician relations as reflecting antagonism more than trust. Medical authorities may give conflicting advice or may be incompetent or inaccessible; they may resist their diminished biocommunicable power in the shift from vertically organized, linear to patient-consumer models. Researchers are also frequently blamed for conflicts in and disruptions of patient-consumer biocommunicability. An *NYT* article by Gina Kolata[17] adopts a familiar format of dividing health information into "myths" versus "facts," but here researchers themselves are portrayed as often succumbing to or promoting myths about diet and obesity. Kolata's story is pegged to a *New England Journal of Medicine* article that decries a lack of rigor in much nutritional research. (Kolata characterizes some of Besser's recommendations in the "Best & Worst Foods" story as either "myths" or "Ideas not yet proven TRUE OR FALSE.") References to conflicting studies are a staple of health coverage. "Here's some medical news you can trust," said a 2005 Associated Press story:[18] "A new study confirms that what doctors once said was good for you often turns out to be bad—or at least not as great as initially thought." Another front-page story asserted, "Patients often have the burden of deciding on treatment."[19] Such reporting reflects not only the decline of biomedical-authority biocommunicability but also the ambivalence of the neoliberal model, where the burden of choice and the absence of certainty can easily seem as terrifying as liberating. As Annemarie Mol (2008) suggests, the logic of choice and the language of rights can undermine the exchanges between patients and caregivers that emerge through a logic of care.

Many stories portray the information flowing to patient-consumers as unreliable due to conflicts of interest that arise from the mixture of market and medical logics. When physicians are characterized as *consumers* of information, the patient-consumer model fails to forestall the sense that fundamental principles of biomedicine and biocommunicability have been violated. The neoliberal model of active patient-consumers only appears as unproblematic when it embodies residual trust in science and professionalism, when consumer choices can be imagined as based on knowledge from objective, disinterested sources. Journalists waver among several stances, sometimes assuming the trustworthiness of biomedical knowledge, sometimes filling gaps resulting from its unreliability, scarcity, or excess—as in the case of stories on Internet health "rumors" or conflicting studies—and sometimes acknowledging frustration with the persistence of those gaps.

Such attention to gaps and obstacles also emerges in reporting that ridicules the celebration of consumer choice and self-realization, a stance that is often—as in critical commentary on Dr. Oz—portrayed as spilling beyond the proper bounds of medical science. One *NYT* article suggests that searching for weight-loss options might be less a process of expanding knowledge bases and choosing rationally among treatment options than, in the words of a physician interviewed, a search for "'one more fad for people who have spent their whole lives gaining weight effortlessly and now want to lose that weight effortlessly and quickly.'"[20] In "Destination: Wellness," reporter Jesse McKinley recounts his exploration of wellness tourism.[21] The impression that such services are largely frivolous gimmicks culminates in a statement by a workshop leader at "a venerable wellness resort," who responds to McKinley's disbelief: "We're just making this up.'" Rather than naturalizing or presupposing patient-consumer biocommunicability, McKinley exposes and ridicules it and yet, in the end, situates it culturally and economically as "a very lucrative" business (see Lau 2000).

Speaking as citizens: public sphere models of biocommunicability

> Kerri was 4 when she started having trouble walking. Justin was 5 when he got a nosebleed that would not stop. Danielle was 7 when her legs began to ache.
>
> During the 1980s, the children all lived, played and swam in the shadow of the Pelham Bay landfill. . . .

The *NYT* reported on 12 August 2013 that New York City settled a lawsuit brought by parents alleging that their children's leukemia was caused by the landfill in the Bronx, which the *Times* described as a "crime scene" where city workers took bribes and allowed illegal dumping.[22] The plaintiffs and the city both hired epidemiologists prepared to present opposite conclusions at the trial about whether there was a causal link between the pollution and the children's illnesses. It closes by quoting one mother, pictured in front of a chain-link fence surrounding the landfill as she relates asking health department officials how many of their children had leukemia:

> "And they said, 'None.' And I said, 'There are multiple children in the Catholic school and the public school that have leukemia, and you don't think there is anything wrong with that?'" she said of the area near the landfill.
>
> "And they didn't say anything."

This story follows journalistic practices common in certain types of political reporting, completely different from those discussed so far. No biomedical authorities are used as sources; the only ones referred to are the two epidemiologists on opposing sides in a legal battle. The norm of balance is nominally followed. But because the story clearly involves a scandal, and because of the human interest appeal of a mother who has lost a young child, she becomes the privileged speaker—and an unusual lay voice is heard in the news making a claim about biomedical knowledge.

In this example of what we call "public sphere" models of biocommunicability, readers are addressed not as patients or consumers, but as citizen-spectators (Muhlmann 2010) making judgments about collective decisions and social values.[23] The actors speak not as part of a linear transmission of information from science to the lay public, but in a battle between interested parties (the two epidemiologists) or as aggrieved citizens (the mother). The value of their words is judged not by scientific expertise but—in this particular example—by such criteria as sincerity, proximity to the experience of the audience, and "common sense." The increased interpenetration of the field of health with other social fields, and particularly with the market and state, is particularly evident in public sphere models because they often come into play when conflicts and scandals arise over these interactions. The other two principal models of biocommunicability involve multiple sub-genres, but public sphere models—arising at points of intersection and conflict between biomedicine and other social fields and between health reporting and other journalistic genres—are particularly diverse.

Standard political models

At one extreme, the norms of political communicability may completely push aside those associated with biomedicine. The report on the Bronx landfill provides an example. It is written by a New York City metro reporter who often reports on political scandal and who shared a Pulitzer Prize in 2009 for reports linking New York Governor Eliot Spitzer to a prostitution ring. Specialist healthcare reporters would likely object to the privileging of the mother's "anecdotal" epidemiological reasoning. Coverage of the Affordable Care Act debate in 2009–10 represented another, very different version, dominated by the voices of politicians. In a sample of *NYT* and *Chicago Tribune* health coverage from the 1960s to 2000s, we found that between 40 and 50 percent of stories addressed readers primarily in the role of citizen/policymaker (Hallin, Brandt, and Briggs 2013). Many of these were essentially routine public policy stories focusing on such subjects as Medicare funding or food safety regulation.

In other cases, the biomedical authority model refracts the norms of political reporting, producing hybrid forms. Pegged to the California governor's proposal to cut physician fees and other Medi-Cal payments, a front page *SDU-T* story titled "Medi-Cal 'death spiral' feared; Proposed fee cuts could further strain troubled program" (2 July 2003) addresses readers as citizens, not patients. The information circulated there is understood as important not because it affects choices by individual patients, but because it points to the danger of "intolerable strains on the health care system." It is a political story. It departs from common conventions of political reporting, however, beginning with a feature lead that focuses on one local physician, who appears in a photo, bending over a reclining patient; the doctor is portrayed in a positive and personalized way not normal for participants in political debate. It goes on to quote the president-elect of the California Medical Association (CMA), a physician who directs a chain of clinics, a local neurologist, and the San Diego Consumer Center for Health Education and Advocacy's director. The "diagnoses" given by these sources, all biomedical professionals, on the state of Medi-Cal are treated as authoritative statements, much as a conventional health story presents medical research. A measure of "balance" is introduced in the form of a quote from a Republican Assemblyman: "I don't disagree with what healthcare providers are saying. I'm a physician myself. But in this budget situation . . . a fiscally responsible budget requires spending reductions throughout." He argues that such decisions should be located in the sphere of public policy, not of medicine, inserting it into a flow of information governed by partisan balance rather than professional standing.

Elite public sphere models

As Nancy Fraser (1990) argues, public spheres are not unitary but layered, composed of separate communities that exchange views among themselves as well as interacting with one another through dominant institutions of the centralized public sphere. Biomedical professionals constitute an elite version of such a segmented public sphere. To its members, access depends on scientific, medical, or public health training and peer review. Health reporting, even when it focuses on public controversy, often accepts the legitimacy of this construction. It does not project an egalitarian public sphere, one in which any citizen can give an opinion on any issue, but represents debate taking place among credentialed experts, similar to other specialized, hierarchical areas of political reporting, such as national security reporting (Hallin, Manoff, and Weddle 1994). Thus the *NYT*, in a front page story, reports:

> With the government's blessing, a drug giant is about to expand the market for its block-buster cholesterol drug Crestor to a new category of customers: as a preventive measure for millions of people who do not have cholesterol problems. Some medical experts question whether this is a healthy move.[24]

The story quotes the deputy director of the Food and Drug Administration's (FDA) Center for Drug Evaluation and Research, a pharmaceutical company executive, three researchers, and a practicing cardiologist—representing different positions in the debate—and refers to a *Lancet* study. The journalist, following a standard convention, identifies financial ties that some of the researchers have to the manufacturer. This kind of reporting maps a flow of information confined to biomedical institutions, but assumes that debate within this specialized realm will be contentious, and possibly subject to "corruption" by political and economic interests. It also grants the public a right, if not of voice, at least to observe and judge.

As with other insiders to these debates, journalists may be active in inserting public sphere issues, as in a long front-page investigative *NYT* story, "Psychiatrists, Troubled Children and Drug Industry's Role."[25] It begins with a child who developed debilitating side effects from Risperdal; such leads are standard in investigative reporting, featuring a "worthy victim" to establish the newsworthiness of an ethical violation (Ettema and Glasser 1998). Her mother is paraphrased but not quoted; other sources are biomedical insiders: physicians, researchers, and pharmaceutical company representatives. The story revolves, however, around the *NYT*'s own analysis of Minnesota public records, showing relationships between the money psychiatrists received from drug makers and their prescription rates. Insider sources, like an American Psychiatric Association past president, who told the *NYT* that "psychiatrists have become too cozy with drug makers," help establish the exposé's legitimacy. Many sources, including doctors with high prescription rates and pharma spokespersons, probably would have preferred not to be dragged into the public sphere. Their statements appear not as authoritative expressions of scientific knowledge but as denials of economic motivation.

Many public sphere stories result primarily from actions of government agencies that generate biomedical controversy. They often modify this elite public sphere model, mixing conventions of political and science reporting and including limited voices from outside the sphere of biomedical specialists. When the Preventive Services Task Force recommended in 2011 that men should no longer receive prostate-specific antigen (PSA) blood tests for prostate cancer, the *NYT*'s Gardiner Harris, whose story ran as the right-hand lead (7 Oct. 2011),[26] noted that "advocates for those with prostate cancer promised to fight the recommendation," listing baseball player Joe Torre, financier Michael Milken, and former New York Mayor Rudolf Giuliani as "among tens of thousands of men who believe a PSA test saved their lives." His story went on to note that some pharmaceutical companies and doctors were likely to resist, due to the "lucrative" nature of the business of treating men with high PSA levels, and that some in Congress had called the plan "rationing," "although the task force does not consider costs in its recommendations."

This debate parallels a previous controversy over a 2009 Task Force recommendation to decrease breast cancer screenings. Journalists covered opposition from Republicans, who deemed the decision to be "rationing" healthcare, Tea Party activists, advocacy groups, and lay cancer survivors, as well as support from biomedical specialists. The issue was sufficiently politicized that it led White House officials to intervene in several subsequent FDA decisions deemed likely to promote political backlashes, leading to FDA/White House conflicts detailed as part of an *NYT* series on "the intersection of politics and science."[27] Like the breast cancer screening case, the PSA recommendation faced a high degree of public mobilization; journalists treated it as a public controversy. Nevertheless, specialist voices dominated the reporting. Harris' follow-up story reported that opponents "hoped to copy the success of women's groups that successfully persuaded much of the country two years ago" that the breast cancer recommendation was mistaken. Except one patient, all sources are physicians and researchers.

Social movement models

Another factor that draws health coverage into public spheres is the role of social movements. Theoretical writing about public spheres emphasizes the importance of social movements and civil society (Habermas 1996; Fraser 1990); research on the politics of health similarly emphasizes the role of social movements—the women's movement in the 1970s, for example, or the gay rights movement. Social movements have played important roles in shaping biocommunicability; mobilization around HIV/AIDS in the 1980s is particularly significant. Gay activists intervened into knowledge production about HIV/AIDS in the early days of the epidemic, challenging biomedical research and treatment, government policy, and media representations (Epstein 1996). This activist voice, with its privileging of forms of personal witnessing and distrust of biomedical authorities, came to be exported globally through the women's movement (Davis 2007) and HIV/AIDS-focused humanitarian interventions (Nguyen 2010). Social movement stories are only present to a limited extent in health news. Representatives from civil society and community groups constituted 4–7 percent of sources in various samples of content (Chapter 3). These stories are interesting, however, for ways they affect biocommunicable models and the tensions and ambivalences they embody.

Typical of this genre is an *NYT* article reprinted in the *SDU-T*,[28] which reports how the Alzheimer's Association and the American Bar Association (ABA) lobbied the federal government to change Medicare coverage to include Alzheimer's treatments. Given the public sphere orientation, denial of coverage emerges as not simply a biomedical but a political problem—"a form of discrimination against millions of people." The article recounts how an ABA lawyer used the Freedom of Information Act to obtain rules used by companies that review and reimburse Medicare claims to reject nearly all reimbursement requests for Alzheimer's patients and to reveal the existence of a "memorandum sent late last year from the government to the companies that review and pay Medicare claims." "The government," the article states, "gave no public notice of the new policy." A Medicare official, pressed to explain this communicable failure, responds: "'we saw it mainly as a technical matter.'" Governmental and biomedical institutions are criticized for creating a secret cartography of biomedical communication, designed to remain entirely within official and professional realms.

In public sphere stories that problematize biocommunicable failures, reporters collaborate (implicitly) with activists and researchers in providing alternative circuits for disseminating health information (Heath, Rapp, and Taussig 2004; Rapp and Ginsburg 2001). Since government officials have failed, journalists must intervene to re-situate issues in public spheres. Reporters thus implicitly construct themselves as bearing three crucial roles—deciding which knowledge should be public, finding information that has been withheld or improperly channeled and making it public, and constructing the boundaries of public discourse about health.

When public sphere coverage centers on social movements, the sources of health knowledge are frequently located outside of biomedical institutions. Efforts by "patients' advocates" to put a problem on public agendas and shape how knowledge is created about it are a common subject of health reporting, varying in the extent to which they are oppositional in their relation to governmental and professional authorities. The more oppositional version of this type of "patient advocate" intervention is evident in a series reporting the Autism Society of America's annual meeting, taking place in San Diego, "Mental Blocked: Patients and Researchers at Odds over Treatment."[29] It reported debates between researchers and activists critical of mainstream research; one charges, "You cannot simply believe what the medical establishment tells you." Here, activists stand outside of and in opposition to biomedical sectors, disrupting the biomedical authority model by shaping themselves as producers, co-producers, and/or collective, critical, knowledgeable receivers of health information (see Taussig, Rapp, and Heath 2003).

Social-movement-oriented stories sometimes involve portrayals of laypersons as producers of biomedical knowledge. In 2002, for example, the *SDU-T* reported efforts by Valley Center residents in North San Diego County to get the California Cancer Registry to investigate a suspected cancer cluster. Kerry Carr, "the mother of a teen-age son with leukemia," conducted an "informal survey" of local cancer cases.[30] Finding 17 children with cancer, Carr sparked meetings of community residents and "contacted health officials," leading to an investigation.[31] Public sphere biocommunicability often appears in reporting on environmental health threats. Biomedical authority and patient-consumer models generally characterize health problems as products of biology or individual behavior, following what Menéndez and Di Pardo (1996) refer to as the "hegemonic medical model." Environmental reporting, however, clearly involves social causality, thereby straining those models' boundaries. Much organizing has focused on environmental racism and justice—the differential location of sources of health-threatening pollution in communities of color (Bullard 1990; Szasz and Meuser 1997; Brown *et al.* 2011).

The Health and Environment Action Network (HEAN)[32] in San Diego, for example, is "very proactive in getting information to the media," one of its staff members, an employee with a background in political communication who previously worked for public relations and marketing firms, told us. HEAN is about 25 years old, focuses on social justice and environmental racism, and has some 5,000 members, including many residents of racialized and lower-income areas. A *SDU-T* article titled "County will take action against pollution suspect"[33] reported the decision of health officials to take legal action against a metal-plating shop, a target of HEAN's Toxic Free Neighborhoods campaign. Like other articles resulting from Network initiatives, it is visually interesting, including a large photo of a resident of the mainly Latino/a Barrio Logan, posing by an air quality monitoring device, the metal-plating shop behind (Figure 1.4). The photographer shoots the resident from a low angle, looking out at the camera—a pose of agency rarely found in images of non-professionals in health coverage.

Another story, "Kids Face Silent Danger: Health Experts Say Lead Pollution is Number 1 Environmental Threat,"[34] quoted "health officials and activists" and the mother of a boy diagnosed with lead poisoning. It pictured a HEAN activist testing for lead—a layperson producing biomedical information. HEAN's director clarified the organization's communicable positionality in an interview: "We don't pretend to be putting out hard scientific information. We're saying, 'let's take the information we've got, use a little common sense.' . . . It's that combination of science and demand for change. Or demand for action." As both stories suggest, organizations like HEAN establish their communicable positionality, in part, by working closely with biomedical professionals, including experts they recruit and public officials with whom they build alliances.

Public sphere reporting is often marked by ambivalence or qualification, particularly when involving laypersons stepping outside of the roles assigned them by biomedical authority and patient-consumer models and asserting rights to produce or to shape health knowledge. The *SDU-T*'s story on autism activists and researchers ended:

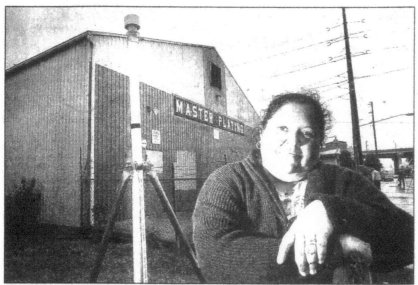

Elvia Martinez posed in the yard of her Barrio Logan home yesterday. In the background is a metal-plating shop that is suspected of being a source of the high toxic air pollution in the area. Next to her is a device that tests air quality. *Nelvin Cepeda / Union-Tribune*

► **AIR QUALITY**
CONTINUED FROM PAGE B1

laws."
   Elvia Martinez, who resides

ber, though they still exceeded
federal health limits.

is trying to close down Master
Plating Co. This comes after

FIGURE 1.4   The lay activist as producer of health knowledge. *San Diego Union-Tribune*, 8 Mar. 2002.

> Eric Courchesne . . . a leading autism researcher, rises. . . . A few parents shake Courchesne's hand. Many corner him later to ask more questions. Courchesne answers, but it's not an entirely satisfying experience for anyone.
>
> The science of autism is still mostly preoccupied by questions, blank spaces in search of answers. Until they are filled, there will be a sort of emptiness, one filled all too often by doubt and frustration.

Eventually, scientists—not activists—will fill these "blank spaces." An accompanying story, "With Rates Rising, Researchers Race to Find the Cause of Autism and Better Treatment," is mapped entirely through biomedical authority biocommunicability.[35]

In the cancer cluster stories, lay activists were granted authority partly because they did systematic research, and partly because a group of residents had been elected to a community advisory committee. At times they gained communicable standing by incorporating themselves into state- and expert-centered routines of knowledge production. They sometimes were presented according to conventions of political reporting, as protesting not against biomedical authority but bureaucracy. The production of knowledge by residents is framed in some cases as a response to "how long the government takes to do anything" and investigators' failure "to keep their promises."[36] Activists also gained standing from their personal, emotional stakes: another activist describes her involvement as "a natural outcome of watching my daughter get sick and die."[37] Some stories emphasized divisions among residents, however. Focusing on rifts within protest movements is a common trope in protest coverage (Gitlin 1980). Here divisions seemed to reflect some residents' ambivalences about what model of communicability to endorse, whether to defer to the governmental institutions and expert knowledge. Journalists also often contrasted lay perspectives with the views of experts who warned that the emergence of a cancer cluster is "a difficult and complex process to prove."[38] Lay involvement is presented as naïve, emotional, and "natural" in character, while real knowledge requires specialized procedures. Active participation in an economy of affect plays a key role in inducing reporters to transform lay intervention into the flow of health knowledge into news stories, but biocommunicable roles constructed in affective terms generally are context-specific, subordinate, and transient statuses. Biomedical professionals are expected to demonstrate empathy for these economies without entering into them.

Such articles open up alternative biocommunicable spaces in which laypersons can produce biomedical information and send it to researchers, clinicians, and governmental agencies; the latter are sometimes deemed to be defective receivers. Nevertheless, this space mainly emerges when biomedical authority and patient-consumer biocommunicabilities fail, thereby reinscribing the notion that they otherwise serve as the normal, desirable models. The ultimate truth-telling authority of experts is assumed—though not without some doubt. The "Inquiry Finds No Cluster of Cancers" article closes with the acknowledgment—by one of the few public health officials willing to be interviewed—"Health experts have conducted extensive environmental studies for clusters and usually no cause is determined." The egalitarian assumptions of the public sphere coexist in fundamental tension with the hierarchical assumptions of science and state authority, rendering this kind of health reporting deeply ambivalent.

Conclusion: the performative role of biocommunicable models

Biomediatization can be analytically separated into two fundamental features. It involves, on the one hand, *practices* that are heterogeneous and complex, spread across dispersed sites and processes of knowledge production, circulation, and reception. Some of these practices are seldom visible, others are largely discernible by insiders, and others become cultural icons. Here we have focused on cultural models that both shape and are shaped by these practices without ever fully merging with them; we have referred to these as *biocommunicable models*. The term biocommunicability contributes to efforts—evident in many humanities and social science disciplines—to grasp not only recent changes within the life sciences and medicine but how they have increasingly shaped identities, social relations, institutions, and fundamental ways of thinking and acting. It thus builds on the literatures on "biopolitics" (Foucault 1997), "biosociality" (Rabinow 1992), and "biomedicalization" (Clarke *et al.* 2003). As is the case with these other terms, the *bio* prefix in biocommunicality and biomediatization does not presuppose an autonomous, bounded, and ontologically distinct sphere of health or biomedicine. Indeed, we are precisely interested in seeing both how notions of health, disease, medicine, and the like are co-produced and in the boundary-work (Gieryn 1983) that seems to make them distinct.

Anthropologist Clifford Geertz (1972) provided a classic statement regarding ways that models interact with the phenomena they claim as their objects, which he described as their model of and model for qualities. Like all models, biocommunicable models are selective and simplifying. In their "models of" capacity, they pick out specific actors, objects, and processes and project them in particular roles as forming part of knowledge production, circulation, and reception. Laypersons may, for example, either be entirely absent from news stories, have a fleeting role, or be central—cast as passive receivers or active seekers and processors of information. Similarly, a classic type of biomedical authority story places the spotlight on articles in medical journals and Principal Investigators. Geert Jacobs (1999) argues that press releases are crucial to what gets covered in these stories and how it gets framed; their structure aims less at presenting "facts" than in "preformulating" news stories themselves. Health news is no exception here; biocommunicable authority models in particular help render the role of PR/media specialists in shaping health biomediatization invisible and powerful. The "model for" dimension projects how actors *should* be playing their proper roles in producing, circulating, and receiving knowledge. For example, rheumatoid arthritis researchers should be producing specialized knowledge that leads to the development of new treatments and then making these "facts" available to doctors; the latter should be sufficiently versed on new diagnostic tests and treatments that they can help patients effectively. Patients should not suffer ignorant physicians or have to educate them but should have ready access to "patient-friendly" materials to use in managing their emotions and making sure they receive proper treatment.

As "models of" and "models for," biocommunicable models are performative, in J. L. Austin's terms (1962), meaning that their use does not simply reproduce existing phenomena but helps to shape them. By providing biocommunicable cartographies, health news stories potentially structure how we think about diseases, drugs, or treatments by telling stories about how they came to be known, by whom, for whom the information is important and why, and what they should do with it. The "model for" capacity enables biocommunicable models to fashion futures, to project how a new discovery should reach doctors and patients or even how discoveries should be made and turned into cures. Biocommunicable cartographies are powerful, in part, because they interpellate us in particular ways, inviting some readers or viewers to enter the picture as doctors, researchers, or investors; most of us enter as laypersons who should pay attention and act and think in accordance with the knowledge they provide. People pictured as actors in stories may be placed on the outside by biocommunicable cartographies. The "Medi-Cal 'death spiral' feared" story, for example, interpellates readers as citizens who have the right to weigh in on decisions taken by their elected representatives; the low-income population directly affected by the proposed cuts is positioned as a *they* and not a *you*, talked about but not included as part of the implied audience, as excluded from the public sphere in which this debate is taking place. As Martín Barbero (1987) and many other media scholars have suggested, such media projections can simultaneous be hegemonic and yet not deterministic, modeling identities and social and political relations in ways that are constantly shaped by active processes of reception.

The performative power of biocommunicable models (and specific cartographies) rests on the way they generally constitute the background to biomedical figures. In biomedical authority stories, we are asked to become familiar with a new body of biomedical knowledge. If there are competing positions, we will expect the journalist to provide a "balanced" discussion that lays out how and why biomedical "experts" are divided. But we are not asked to decide whether doctors know best or whether physicians should study new recommendations. The biocommunicable background can, however, suddenly become the foreground. Stories that focus on "media hype" are particularly telling for two reasons. First, they suggest that biocommunicable trajectories are not just a vehicle for transporting medical knowledge but are themselves always part of the health news itself; what changes is how explicit or implicit they remain and how important they are in relation to the medical content. Second, "hype" is a negative term. Biocommunicability particularly comes into focus when something is wrong, when proper communication is blocked. If health news should not be hype, then it should be generated at biomedical sites by health professionals and be circulated and received faithfully and rationally. The label "hype" thus reveals the performativity of biocommunicability, but only at the cost of misrecognizing it.

The performative power of biocommunicable models is, to a great extent, what makes biomediatization work, what enables a diversity of actors—including journalists, patients, and PR/media consultants—to co-produce health knowledge. If biomediatization practices entangle us in complex ways in this process, it is the work of biocommunicable models to sort out the mess—to try to put each of us in our proper place. It is biocommunicability that seems to require media/medical boundary-work, separating knowledge-makers from circulators/translators from receivers or active, self-interested seekers. At the same time, however, we have explored in this chapter how the models seem to make messes of their own, generating fascinating multiplicities and contradictions. We are often interpellated by the same story as passive patients and as active patient-consumers, placed on the outside looking in, only then to be thrust into the center as consumers, producers of medical panic, or individuals who endanger their own or others' health through ignorance or willful resistance.

Biocommunicability is what makes health news so important, projecting it, in anthropologist Greg Urban's (2001) terms, as the metacultural force that keeps health knowledge flowing, including by revealing obstacles and drawing attention to efforts to get things moving properly again. Nevertheless, if our story ended with biocommunicability, we would simply reify the foundational separation of medicine and media it projects, if in multiple and complicated ways. Chapter 2 breaks new ground by going beyond the stories and behind the scenes to meet the people who engage actively in this co-production.

Notes

1 An earlier version of this discussion appeared in Briggs and Hallin (2007).
2 Susan Ferraro, 8 Mar. 2002:D3. The article was originally from the New York *Daily News*.
3 Lavelle, Janet. "Whooping Cough on the Rise: Adults, Children in State Urged to Get Booster Shot."
4 Jane E. Brody, "Personal Health: Diabetes Candidates Can Reduce the Risk," *New York Times* 15 Jan. 2002. Brody's Wednesday *NYT* health column is syndicated in the *SDU-T*, along with approximately 100 other newspapers.
5 See also Snow and Ferguson's (1977) classic work on what was once called "motherese" or "foreigner talk," which constructs the addressee as a child or foreigner.
6 Judith Blake, "Peeling Back the Lies," *SDU-T* 15 Jan. 2002:E1-E2.
7 The term comes from Stuart Hall *et al.* (1978).
8 A version of this section was first published in *Media, Culture & Society* (Hallin and Briggs 2015).
9 Seale (2002), who critiques this research perspective, summarizes many other examples.
10 Cole (1988) similarly criticizes the media not for overemphasizing conflict but for presenting the science of health risks as more certain than it is.
11 Hala Ari Aryan, 3 May 2005:E1.
12 For example in the *New Yorker* article cited above, and on *This Week Tonight with John Oliver*, 22 Jun. 2014.
13 "The Food We Eat Someday May Kill Us," *SDU-T,* 28 Feb. 2002:B12.
14 On consumerism and activism in general and specifically in the health fields, see West (2006), Cohen (2008), and Hoffman *et al.* (2011).
15 "Informed Patients: The Right to Know about Bad Doctors," 24 Jun. 2002:B1.
16 *SDU-T*, 15 Apr. 2002:D7.
17 "Many Weight-Loss Ideas Are Myth, Not Science, Study Finds," 31 Jan. 2013:A15.
18 Lindsey Tanner, "Don't Believe Everything Medical Studies Tell You," *SDU-T*, 13 Jul. 2005:A1.
19 Jan Hoffman, "Patients Often Have Burden of Deciding Treatment," *SDU-T*, 14 Aug. 2005:A1.
20 Tatiana Boncompagni, "Almost, Sort of Like a Workout," 12 Jul. 2012:E3.
21 30 Dec. 2012:TR1.
22 William K. Rashbaum, "Bittersweet Deal in 22-Year Fight Over Toxic Site in Bronx," A13.
23 We provide a more detailed treatment of public sphere models in Briggs and Hallin (2010).
24 Duff Wilson, "Plan to Widen Use of Statins Has Skeptics," 31 Mar. 2010:A1, 3.
25 Gardiner Harris, Benedict Carey and Janet Roberts, 10 May 2007:A1, 20.
26 "Panel's Advice on Prostate Test Sets Up Battle," A1.
27 Gardiner Harris, "White House and the F.D.A. Often at Odds," 3 Apr. 2012:A1, 14.
28 "In Shift, Medicare Has Begun Funding Alzheimer's Care," 31 Mar. 2002:A1.
29 *SDU-T*, 9 Jan. 2002:F1.
30 Christine Millay, "Cancer Inquiry Divides Valley Center Sides," 15 Mar. 2002:NC2, NI1.
31 Luis Monteagudo, Jr., "Incidence of Cancer Worrying Residents: Valley Center Cases Prompt Investigation," 12 Jan. 2002:NC1, NI1.
32 This is a pseudonym. Charles and Robert Donnelly interviewed HEAN's director and media coordinator in 2004.

33 8 Mar. 2002:B1.

34 *SDU-T,* 7 Jan. 2002:B1.

35 This story appeared shortly before the publication of Andrew Wakefield's paper in *The Lancet,* which became the principal scientific justification for claims that vaccines caused autism, until it was brought into question (by a British investigative journalist) and, in 2010, withdrawn. Over the years there was considerable debate among health journalists about whether to treat the vaccines/autism question as an issue open to debate or as an issue settled by science, with a shift toward the latter after 2010 (Brainard 2013; Clarke 2008). The 2014–15 measles outbreak produced a particularly strong rallying around medical authority by journalists, who strongly characterized fears about vaccine safety as "myths."

36 "Cancer Inquiry Divides Valley," op cit.

37 Mary Curran Downey, "Daughter's Death Gave Mom Role in Cancer Fight," 17 Feb. 2002:N2.

38 Christine Millay, "Inquiry Finds No Cluster of Cancers; Valley Center Probe Leaves Some Unsatisfied," 24 Apr. 2002:NI1.

2
THE DAILY WORK OF BIOMEDIATIZATION

In this chapter we turn from looking at the ideological "texts" of health news to the actors and their practices, foregrounding our ethnographic research to introduce people involved in the process of biomediatization. We sit with these actors as they try to make sense of the practices that position them in biomediatization processes and express their understandings of how it does and should work. Just as our research strategy shifts here from analysis of news texts to ethnography, so, too, does our writing style shift. This chapter has two voices, the first half written by Charles, the second by Dan, and the style is less analytic in an attempt to convey a more immediate sense of how biomediatization's actors spend their days and what keeps them up at night. Beyond providing a sense of some of the people who fill our newspapers, televisions, radios, computers, and phones with health news, we explore ethnographically the complexities of their work that do not fit smoothly into biocommunicable models. We begin with one of Charles's interviews.

It was one of those ethnographic moments that makes you feel absolutely stupid and yet turns out to be transformational. Media–cum–public relations firms are particularly well shielded, but I (Charles) had secured an interview with a public relations executive at Stratton-Domenici, a global media relations firm.[1] This offered a splendid opportunity to learn about the medical/media nexus from an individual whose full-time occupation consisted in pushing its boundaries in ways that continually reshape them.

Driving to a glitzy part of the biotech corridor, I passed an impeccable lawn and entered an underground garage beneath two tall, impressive buildings with glass facades that seemed to conflate nature and culture by turning architecture into reflections of the blue sky and surrounding scenery. When the elevator opened, I met a tanned man in his mid-30s with an athletic build who introduced himself as Jeff Harrison. Harrison, I later learned, completed his training in biology with a view to a career in medicine, but changed course: "it wasn't for me—I can't even watch my own blood be drawn!" Communications and public relations work for biotechs enabled him to continue learning "fantastic, phenomenal ideas. When I studied biology, the books I studied had been rewritten by a lot of these companies I'm working for." At the same time, his science background provided him with a competitive edge: "I brought the biology, the ability to understand what these scientists were talking about, to help translate it."

Once we were seated in two beautiful black leather chairs, I asked Harrison how he works with biotech corporations to initiate contact with journalists in transforming research results, corporate mergers, and FDA approval into news stories. His response quickly called my presuppositions regarding medical/media entanglements into question. The "general goals and objectives" that he helps his clients produce are often created years before a press release is written, he noted, almost dismissively. Harrison suggested that such planning unfolded differently in the case of a well-known disease, like prostate cancer, than a disease like myelodysplastic syndromes (MDS), where the number of patients is small and "most people don't know what MDS is."

MDS inhibits the growth of stem cells in bone marrow into fully developed red and white blood cells and platelets, leading to infection and anemia. It is called an "orphan disease," affecting a relatively small number of patients. Nevertheless, finding treatments that insurance companies and government agencies will reimburse, at extraordinary costs, lies at the forefront of pharmaceutical development. Here Harrison's work involves a "disease awareness campaign" that is "unbranded," that is, not tied to a company's name or a specific product. In such cases, corporate officials, physicians, patients, and sometimes a "celebrity spokesperson" collaboratively build visibility for the disease. (Actress Kathleen Turner's promotion of rheumatoid arthritis awareness, which we discussed in Chapter 1, provides an example.) Stratton-Domenici arranged speaking tours for the biotech's physicians and scientists and presentations at meetings of medical associations; meetings with journalists built knowledge of and trust in the client corporation and its "management team" long before any press coverage was desired. Investors formed a crucial audience, addressed through newspaper business pages and industry-oriented publications, websites, and other venues. Stratton-Domenici recruits medical writers and approaches the editors of leading medical journals.

What about that ephemeral but ubiquitous phenomenon often referred to as "the public," the ostensive target of most television, print, radio, and Internet media? "You don't really need that consumer audience until you're in Phase 3 trials, or you're seeking product approval." Then Harrison turns "disease awareness" into "a product launch announcement, some real hard news," pressing for the widespread coverage that he sidesteps until that point. Here biocommunicable models and discursive practices are woven together in a complex and shifting manner—for both interviewer and interviewee. Initially, it was the researcher—Charles—who invoked a linear, hierarchically ordered model. Harrison quickly dismissed this framework, outlining how Stratton-Domenici co-produces diseases, drugs, and devices with its clients. The "interview" turned into a basic course in biomediatization.

Does this mean that biocommunicable models are simply scholarly abstractions? To the contrary, Harrison's complex discussion over two hours revolved around biocommunicable models. The terms "educate" and "translate" emerged repeatedly, reiterating the linear model that would place the production of specialized biomedical knowledge in the hands of client scientists and require media specialists to circulate it. Stratton-Domenici's role is simply helping this natural process along:

> What we always say is, 'what are the facts, put them out there, let them have them', you know, because the last thing you want is rumors or some sort of assumptions or misperceptions running around. So it's good to be out there, [to] be as open and transparent as possible.

Even as he projects this linear flow, Harrison's strategy for prompting journalists to move from background education to producing stories—when the time is right—is to create the perception that this circuit has somehow gotten blocked,

> encouraging major news publications to cover a certain space that we don't think they're covering. You know, and that's the purpose of education, saying you know this is where the disconnect is, this is what people—your audience, *USA Today* or whatever publication it might be—they're not getting this. This is why we think you need education on it.

Biocommunicable failure becomes the "peg" that, he suggests, induces journalists to cover the story; indeed, the analysis discussed in Chapter 1 points to how often this peg becomes the rhetorical driving force of health news stories.

A visit to the doctor and dentist

In October 2009, Charles visited his doctor, Dave Richards, an affable fellow in his early sixties who had studied complementary and alternative medicine as well as training as a general practitioner. A good diagnostician and a listener, he also took patients on a pro bono basis. After reviewing lab results and addressing standard questions, Richards asked whether or not I wanted periodic PSA tests for prostate cancer, given the problems with false positives and unnecessary procedures. Attempting to construct myself as an expert patient (Dumit 2012), I shot back: "I know the literature. I know the pros and cons. But if it were your body, what would *you* do?" "Oh, no," Richards, responded, "I never give my patients advice: I simply help them sort through all the information that comes their way." Shifting from patient to researcher I asked: "Could I come back on a different day and interview you?"

We met in his office, where I produced a small digital tape-recorder and ran through the same sort of consent protocol that he would negotiate if he recruited patients for clinic trials (he refuses). His response to my standard question about "daily routine" was depressing—he sees 35–40 patients, reviews 100–200 charts, and receives/makes an equivalent number of telephone calls and faxes. "I don't even have time to pee, let alone to eat lunch," he announced. I had expected resistance to my questions about "information" that patients brought from "the media" to the examining room, but Richards is the quintessential neoliberal physician—in biocommunicable terms. "I encourage my patients to bring in all the information they can. It enhances our conversation." Though he embraced the active patient-consumer model, I nevertheless detected a trace of biomedical authority: "I like to see my patients come in with ideas and not demands." "Ah," I followed up, "then what about when they enter the examining room asking for a medication they just saw advertised on television?" Slipping out of my trap: "That's fine with me, it just makes for a more informed patient." The idea that patients might appear with a printout from the Internet in order to query him about a new diagnosis, test, or treatment elicited a fascinating comparison of patient populations.

> I wish I got more of that! Some do come in and want my advice on something they have seen. But lots of my patients are poor or elderly—they are the last people who will get information over the Internet. I don't have many people who come in asking for something available online.

Not all clinicians have moved away from the biomedical authority model, thereby forfeiting some of the power it affords them as health professionals, as I learned when I interviewed my dentist, Rodney Powell. In his mid-sixties, Powell is a third-generation health professional and one of the leading African American dentists in the area. Richards and Powell clearly occupied opposite ends of the biocommunicable spectrum. Powell interrupted me as I formulated a question regarding his patients' reception of mediatized health material:

> Yes, that's a problem, that's a real problem! Much of what my patients get from the news, advertisements, and the Internet frightens them—and they get 50 percent of it wrong! I have to educate them, and it takes more time because of what they think they have learned from the media.

In nearly a decade as his patient, I never once saw Powell depart from biomedical authority biocommunicability. His focus on whether I understood and would comply with his treatment recommendations left no room for questions that exceeded this narrow range, let alone for suggestions.

The mediatization of health entered into the daily life and practice of all of the clinicians we interviewed. They all subscribed to medical journals and most to services that filter articles and offer summaries. All reported reading newspapers and watching television news; some listened to the radio driving to work. All spent time discussing with their patients the materials extracted from media sources. But from there, it was heterogeneity all the way down. Some reported being intrigued with how medical issues were presented in health news, while others viewed such discussions with disdain. Although some, like Richards and Powell, clung either to biomedical authority or patient-consumer models, others—like the physician assistant who worked in Richards' office—moved between them. Some clinicians shifted between one model and another depending on how "well-informed" the patient in question appeared to be, pointing to the relevance of race and class here. One plastic surgeon provided an excellent example of how different models intersect. He noted that the popularity of plastic surgery had prompted extensive media coverage but had instilled high expectations in his patients and too little awareness of risks. "The role of the doctor," he suggested, "is to educate and inform patients of the reality behind procedures." Nevertheless, he saw press coverage as free advertising, boosting incomes by bringing more patients to plastic surgeons. Clinicians, in short, were all over the map in terms of biocommunicable models and the ways that biomediatization entered into their practice.

Public health officials

At the same time that public health officials and spokespersons in local, state, national, and international public health agencies hold a wide range of views of health media and engage in a variety of biomediatization practices, it would be hard to find individuals who are more focused on health news. Institutional hierarchies differentially allocate rights to interact with journalists; generally, only the senior administrative officer, official spokesperson, or an individual that he or she designates can respond to or initiate contacts with other institutions or "the public," including journalists. Many regard biomediatization with ambivalence, seen as a necessary part of the job and an opportunity "to get our messages out there," and perhaps the most acute arena of discomfort and vulnerability.

Here we focus on San Diego County, which had a population of almost 3.1 million in 2010 located on the Mexico–United States border and boasting a sizeable Latino/a population. Entering a "Mission style" county building, a tall, slender woman wearing a professional-looking dark jacket and blouse greeted us with a smile and introduced herself as Dr. Susan Norris.[2] Norris has both a medical degree and a Master's of Public Health from a prestigious California public university. Confident and poised, she gained substantial experience with the press in her nearly three years as the county's Public Health Officer. Within the county government, the Department of Health and Human Services Agency (HHSA) splits the state-mandated obligation to disseminate public health information with the Department of Environmental Health (DEH); the former handles clinical issues and the latter vector control and food safety. We had previously interviewed DEH Director Dr. George Murdoch, along with the directors of DEH's food safety and vector-borne disease programs, Judy Evans and Art Smith.[3]

Interacting with journalists was a big part of Norris's job, but the amount of time she spent varied. "When there was something happening," Norris noted, "I spend all my time, really, at least the majority . . . dealing with the press."

Norris distinguished two modes of interaction with journalists: responding to inquiries from reporters *versus* attempts by county health agencies "to get our message out"; Murdoch referred to these as "pull" versus "push." Most "push" efforts involved producing press releases, holding press conferences, and staging events aimed at engaging journalists' attention. "Campaigns" are organized by staff members with journalism and/or public relations experience or contracted to specialized commercial agencies.

County biomediatization practices gained further clarity through an interview with Traci McCollum, Media Specialist in the Office of Media and Public Affairs (OMPA), who coordinates press relations for HHSA.[4] McCollum previously worked for 14 years as a reporter. She noted that press inquiries were sorted according to a four-fold classification. Agency staff members were instructed to refer all "cold calls" from reporters to McCollum, who screened them "to figure out who it's going to." Questions should never be answered on the spot, "cold," but only after they had been sorted and replies designed. McCollum worked down the hall from Norris, having been assigned full-time to work with her agency. McCollum herself often responded to requests that were classified as routine, non-controversial, and relatively non-technical. Otherwise, she took a message and consulted with Norris and her staff in sorting them into one of three additional categories.

One type consisted of questions deemed non-controversial that had been previously addressed but were too "technical" for McCollum. In order to reduce time spent with reporters, Norris often assigned these to the deputy public health officer, a physician with public health experience. A second category consisted of issues not previously addressed and potentially controversial. Then, Norris suggested, "I need to be the one to respond." She tried to find "somebody who's the expert . . . who really understands the issues, is really on the ball" to interact with reporters. Expertise alone was not sufficient here; Norris looked for articulate people trained "to deal with the media." The "expert," Norris, and McCallum then discussed whether to return the reporter's call, issue a press release, hold a press conference, or stage some other sort of event, and thus constructed "a message" to guide what designated persons would say to journalists; they sometimes assembled visual or other materials in advance. Our review of television footage and newspaper photographs suggests that in initial presentations at least, Norris usually introduced "experts" and then stood by their side during interactions with journalists.

Finally, the most potentially explosive issues were discussed, before responding to reporters, with the "county-level public affairs office." Norris:

> I will go down there, tell them what the problem is and talk it through with them about what is the most appropriate vehicle. . . . Talk through what's the purpose? Teasing out the content. Who will be the contact person? The timing for the media? What are their deadlines?

When the issue might result in negative coverage for PHS or the county as a whole, the HHSA director and other high officials sometimes participated.

These officials saw reporters as both crucial and problematic. Norris also noted that she reads the *SDU-T* before leaving home and listens to radio: "I'm a radio addict!" She uses an electronic service that searchers stories about HSSA and the San Diego area. Thus, public health officials are some of the most avid *receivers* of health news, just as they are key sources. News coverage, in their view, also provided crucial opportunities. Murdoch suggested that "this county's culture," meaning the county government, centered on a media partnership: "We need to work with the media to the maximum extent possible to get our message out, no matter what program it is." He added that compared to health education "campaigns," the news media is "much more effective" in reaching "the population." When asked whom they wished to reach, Murdoch responded "my neighbors" and Evans added "family, friends, public." Note that these officials were white, middle-class, US-born professionals. Norris suggested that her audience also consisted of "providers," that is health professionals and health-oriented organizations; in other words, they sometimes try to use journalists to contact other health professionals, evoking the elite public sphere biocommunicability we explored in Chapter 1.

Nevertheless, these health professionals described media interactions as one of their deepest professional anxieties, frequently invoking the "two cultures" take on media/medical relations. They contrasted their own orientation with reporters' goals, characterized as selling newspapers or television advertising; in Norris's words, "their main thing is to get customers to read their stuff, to do the sensational stuff." She acknowledged that journalists often see such statements as cynical or jaded. Murdoch defined his job as "trying to educate the uninformed reporter. So I'm going to go a little bit further to educate them, to get my message across." Given that reporters are, Smith told us, "more effective when they really know what they're talking about," health reporters rank above journalists who only occasionally report health. Similarly, they deemed print reporters more likely to "spend some time on an article"; television journalists are "superficial," focused on soundbites.

The biomedical authority model invoked by such statements and its projection of the opposition between public health and media organizations does not, however, capture the complex biomediatization practices in which public health officials engage on a daily basis, the majority of which, according to Norris, are initiated by journalists. Projecting a linear relationship between opposing professional logics is complicated by the presence of McCollum, a former reporter embedded in the county government, who probably interacted with Norris more than anyone else, and PHS's employment of "marketing-type firms," like Harrison's, for "push" campaigns. We wonder if Norris and her colleagues ever worked with ABC's multi-credentialed Richard Besser while he was employed as a television health reporter in San Diego in the 1990s. Similarly, do Murdoch and Norris still fit neatly into a biomedical slot, given their media training and the degree to which biomediatization was finely woven into their everyday work? Their daily practices were closely shaped by the temporal and technological requirements of health journalists.

Norris also invoked the biomedical authority model in reference to "evidence-based" medicine. Vincanne Adams (2013a) has traced the migration of the logics and practices of "evidence-based medicine" into global health, transforming the sort of experimental metrics produced by clinical trials into the measure of truth, authority, and cost-effectiveness. Norris suggested that her media involvement was similarly "data driven." In keeping with the weighting of research over the experience of clinicians and public health practitioners (Dumit 2012; Petryna 2009), Norris positioned "experts," specialists on a given topic, as ideally determining the content of "push" campaigns and of responses to reporters' inquiries. As she talked in detail about the county's health campaigns, however, it was clear that more was going on than a simple translation of scientific knowledge into public communication. Norris acknowledged that "push" efforts are often "funding driven." The funds provided by the tobacco settlement had enabled PHS to buy substantial amounts of air time and newspaper space; although they had pretty well evaporated by 2005, funds earmarked for HIV/AIDS and particularly for "bioterrorism" were still available—examples of issues that were "driven by the funding." Norris noted specifically that biomediatization practices changed "because of all the risk communication training we've gotten in the last few years, because of bioterrorism preparedness money," a topic to which we return in Chapter 4. Norris stressed one aspect of how the 9/11-induced "risk communication training" had shaped biomediatization strategies in her office—"we're learning to put out more . . . being first on the spot with bad news."

One major media focus of Norris's office at the time was West Nile Virus, generally transmitted by Culex mosquitoes. First documented in California in July 2003 (Reisen *et al.* 2004), by the end of 2004, the virus was reported in all California counties (at least in mosquitoes or animals), 830 people had been infected, and 28 people died (CDHS 2004). That campaign was driven by a mandate from the California Department of Health Services. Norris complained that journalists were reluctant to cover a story that, much of the time, involved nothing but the "dead bird thing" and no human cases, though our monitoring of media content suggested that the county was fairly successful at getting reporters to pass along advice about vector control. Despite heavy public attention, few cases materialized: 73 human cases and no deaths (between 2004 and 2014).[5] If biomediatization efforts were guided primarily by epidemiological evidence, San Diego County health officials might have focused more on the leading causes of deaths in the county that year (coronary diseases, cancer, etc.).[6]

Norris also noted that elected officials sometimes affected biomediatization. I presented Norris with a clipping from a "push" in which she made a case to journalists that low-income patients were over-utilizing emergency rooms. A confident professional, she suddenly seemed embarrassed. "It's a very touchy issue. And there was a politician who wanted us to do something about it. . . . There were a lot of issues around it. It was very, very debatable." This exchange provided one of those fascinating moments when a poised and cautious interviewee opens up, exposing a personal and professional dilemma and the difficulties in neatly fitting complex biomediatization practices within biocommunicable models.

Reporting along the border with *El Hispano*

Interviewing Graciela López, one of only two reporters employed by *El Hispano,* involved finding a few rented rooms in a small, nondescript office building in south San Diego County, a contrast to large, sleek buildings of "mainstream" media.[7] A very fit 25-year-old with long brown hair and expressive almond-shaped eyes, López was born in Mexico City and moved to Tijuana as a child. Initially drawn to medicine, she studied communication in Mexico, tried creative writing, worked as a freelancer, reported for a weekly, then landed the *El Hispano* job, doubling her income but imposing the demands of working at a daily paper.[8]

López was assigned the full range of news stories, except for areas covered by her colleague: entertainment and sports. She had to write three to four articles and translate three more daily, totaling around 5,000 words. Health was one of her two preferred focuses. Her mother was trained as a dentist, and López believes that growing up in a household where medical terminology and perspectives emerged at the dinner table and her early work in biology enabled her to go beyond the "really basic" way that other journalists handle health topics and their lack of attention to prevention. *El Hispano* was directed to "Spanish-speaking immigrants," whom she projected as having "approximately eight years of formal education." Accordingly, with respect to her health reporting, "the information must be very clear and very simple" and devoid of technical terms.[9] Nevertheless, López did not have a concrete set of individuals in mind: "I don't know if I am writing for the old woman who came here and didn't learn English and her only contact with the outside world is a newspaper" or the Latino/a university student who wants to read the news in Spanish as part of an ethno-political commitment.

López wrestled with the problem of sorting through mountains of press releases and inquiries to avoid merely doing "publicity-reporting" (*publireportajes*) and gauge whether a "new discovery" by a San Diego biotech firm is really years away from FDA approval—and therefore not yet "news." Finding "local angles" involved, for López, focusing more on ethnicity than geography. Beyond the material she translated into Spanish, she spent a great deal of time finding stories in other papers, the Internet or news services "that I can expand and I can give a Latino angle." Laws, programs, or other things "that are going to affect low-income people immediately become Latino themes" due to the number of Latinos/as, especially immigrants, in this socio-economic category. She preferred to find material in English and translate it herself. Translations of studies, reports, and policy statements are often much less sophisticated and only a fifth as long as the English text. Moreover, Spanish-speaking spokespersons tend not to be the higher-ranking officials or the "experts." Indeed, none of the county officials we interviewed spoke Spanish. County Health Officer Norris admitted that "I don't really have somebody at my level that's Spanish speaking, so that's a deficit."

López rejected the biomedical authority model's relegation of journalists to a passive role in the process of health communication. She projected health authorities as trying to interpellate journalists vis-à-vis the linear model in an uncritical role as circulators, asking them to act "like sheep," suggesting: "we often become disseminators (*multipicadores*) of the official sources." She argued that her work is not reproducing medical facts "like an encyclopedia" but helping immigrants exercise their health rights. There is a strong element of service journalism here, with an activist twist. The issue is not just providing information about free prenatal care or mammograms but identifying facilities where low-income Latino/a patients will be treated with respect. Imagining a biocommunicable circuit that extends beyond the article, López suggested that "my editor always asks me to include a telephone and address at the end of each story."

López also distanced herself from patient-consumer models. She did draw attention to contradictory recommendations that health professionals give to reporters, thus "driving people in multiple directions simultaneously (*como manejar a alguien a chorros de agua en direcciones opuestas*) and the reduction of physicians' authority through the rise of HMOs. But López does not project herself as providing resources to enable readers to make rational decisions about which health services to consume. How López characterized her work would seem to line up most closely with the "public sphere" model of biocommunicability. She stressed that many of her readers' lives were shaped by inequities of access to services and health outcomes, the struggle to survive economically, restrictions on the use of Spanish as a language of healthcare and public communication, stereotypes of the Latino community, and ways that issues of migration and citizenship structure access to public debate. Nevertheless, López did not project her readers as active participants in producing health knowledge or debating policies: "We're talking about a population that is not accustomed to going to the doctor, . . . that often lives on remedies, not medications." She described a woman who received her first pap smear at age 46 as "dressed very humbly, she had indigenous features, I don't know if she spoke English, she had worked her entire life as a maid." This woman, López suggested, had no idea about available health services, had been too fearful of doctors, dying, and "bad news" to ever realize before that "'wow, we do have rights, we do have access.'" Accordingly López herself claimed the role of actively scrutinizing and contesting health and rights issues.

Shortly after our interview, López left *El Hispano*, graduated with honors from a prestigious US school of journalism, and won several awards. She returned to work as a freelancer in Tijuana, by then a precarious site for journalists. By 2013, her attention centered more on immigration, the environment, smuggling, and drug dealing.

A health reporter for the *New York Times*

In approaching López, Charles simply rang *El Hispano*, spoke briefly with her, and appeared at the appointed time. Getting past the row of guards on the ground floor of the *New York Times* skyscraper in midtown Manhattan, on the other hand, was like assaulting a castle. Charles eventually succeeded in interviewing four *NYT* reporters and one editor, but arranging each interview involved e-mails, telephone calls, and, in one case, crafting detailed replies to critical takes on our published work. Looking up at the *NYT* building's imposing 52 floors before entering to interview veteran health reporter Linda Kelley, Laura Nader's (1972) metaphor of "studying up" came to mind. She used it in urging anthropologists to challenge power relations by studying elites as well as subalterns. Whatever one's view of the *NYT*, it is an imposing presence on the US media landscape. Kelley appeared in the vast, brightly colored lobby area to take me upstairs.[10]

A confessed exercise addict, Kelley's fitness, white teeth, and easy smile seemed to belie her 60 years of age. After majoring in microbiology, she spent a year in graduate school but found lab work less appealing, received a Master's degree in a related field, then decided that her real interest was writing. After working at a leading scientific magazine, she applied to the *NYT,* where she saw great "demand for health news," but thought much of it was "just not such great reporting." By 2008, she had been an *NYT* health and science writer for over two decades. Her health column appears every two weeks and she sometimes writes "dailies," but her preference is for in-depth feature articles.

Kelley reads e-mails that announce articles in leading medical journals and has a large pool of sources that she organizes in terms of biomedical specialties. This might lead to the conclusion that she embraces the linear, hierarchically organized model of biocommunicability, but it would be hard to imagine a clearer rejection of the linear transmission model. When I asked, "What, overall, is the role of the reporter in informing the public about health," she shook her head:

> Well this is not my job. I'm not an educator. I'm an entertainer. It sounds flippant, maybe, but if people can't read past the first paragraph or two then I haven't done my job. I want people to start a story and finish it. That's my job. And that doesn't mean I want to make things up; it doesn't mean I want to exaggerate or hype something, but it's not my job to educate—that's not my role. So if people are not educated, that's their problem. If they read the stories, maybe they would be, but that's not why I wrote them. I wrote them because they're good stories. And they make you think about things in our society and they make you think about how evidence is developed, I don't know. There's something about them that made me interested and made me think that this would make a good dinner-table conversation. . . . I don't care if [people] improve their health. That's their problem, not my problem. It's their doctor's problem.

Kelley similarly denied that "the public" is her audience: "I write for myself. I really don't care who my audience is." Kelley invoked the analogy of painters and poets, arguing that her reporting similarly involved "a lot of creativity," intuition, the capacity to rapidly sense what is important, and the ability to find a story. At the same time she was quick to distance herself from the patient-consumer model:

> People are obsessed with their health, and they think that they can make a huge difference by doing things. . . . They think there's too much power in things like what they eat, which I think has very little power if you are going to get cancer, but they all think that it makes a huge difference. The ideas that have long been discredited just sort of hang around forever.

As with other interviewees, I asked her to explain how she researched and wrote one of her favorite stories. In developing a feature that attempted to debunk common beliefs about heart disease, her research was so extensive that the series required her full-time attention for an entire year.

> But then we had to have a narrative that would just sort of carry you through, so I thought, well, I would hang out at a cardiac intensive care unit and see what happens. And I really lucked out because at the very end of the first day the perfect patient came in, and I mean he was perfect for the story; and he was very articulate and he was pleased to be in this story. . . . I want people to remember it. I want to write a story where it really stays with you, where you say, 'wow!'

This story was part of a series on "six leading killers," written for both the print version and the *NYT* website.

In her work on this series, Kelley, like many journalists we interviewed, belies the "two cultures" dichotomy. She works hard to find a personal story that will help turn facts into a compelling narrative.[11] At the same time, she is deeply immersed in the culture of science. She rejects what she refers to as "the tyranny of the anecdote," providing a single powerful narrative that convinces readers to overlook statistical evidence. Particularly given her belief that laypersons cling to unproven, outdated, or even ridiculous claims about health, her process of discovery starts with "the science." For this series, Kelley "went to the databases of the National Center of Health Statistics" to choose diseases on which to focus. The epidemiology then took her to the medical evidence and only then to the search for an individual case on which to hang the story. Despite her rejection of an instrumental conception of her role, moreover, Kelley expressed pride that these stories had impact. "I've had medical groups say, '. . . we've been trying for twenty-five years to get people to call 911 and finally people are reading your story and doing it,'" she said. "So it's really gratifying to hear that people feel their lives are changed, but also that everybody remembered it." In Kelley's view, it is precisely because she doesn't subordinate journalism to "health education," because she is a writer first and foremost, that she can have this impact.

Scholars have explored issues of what becomes news (Gans 1979) and how stories are framed (Gitlin 1980). The linear, hierarchically organized biocommunicable model would seem to address both of these topics in advance: reporters should turn the problems identified by leading clinicians and epidemiologists into news and translate biomedical frames into terms accessible to lay audiences. For Kelley, this, like the patient-consumer model, is a recipe for ho-hum, run-of-the-mill health journalism. Nor did she seem to see equipping citizens to be active participants in debating health policies as her job. She combined biocommunicable models in complex and selective ways, but her approach could perhaps best be described as a distinctively journalistic version of the public sphere model. Finding a story and developing an interesting angle on it involved identifying "a real important issue that's not being paid attention to"; a perceived break in biocommunicable circuits thus provides a key criterion for turning facts into memorable stories. Good journalism, for her, springs from a model of artistic creativity, albeit one that respects scientific evidence. Its goal is to produce stories and ideas that circulate for their own sake, because they are interesting, and any instrumental purposes they may serve are secondary.

Kelley suggested that for reporters on local papers, it's "a lot easier because you don't have to worry. You don't have to do much. It's like you go there and you write it down and then you interview one person maybe and that's it. It's just the news." Here she positioned the *NYT* in journalistic hierarchies as setting "an amazing standard" to which other journalists can aspire but cannot easily attain. She articulated a conception of health journalism that revolves around a more central, active role for reporters than passive transmission of biomedical knowledge. One dimension of this role relates to perceived errors in reporting, which prompt immediate reactions from "readers all over the world." More significant, however, is the way that readers require the *NYT* "to find the important stories. So if we write about something, they think it must be important. So if we write something that is really stupid, you know, we are going to hear from them—and the whole world." The *NYT*, in short, plays a central role in determining what will count as "important" in the field of health and medicine, not just reflecting the agendas of health professionals. "It's a very creative thing at the *Times*, what I do. But, like I said, I don't think many people have this kind of a job."

Managing clinics, managing "the media"

Just the second person we interviewed for this project, in September 2004, Jim Montoya remains, for Charles, one of the most impressive and one of the people who taught him the most. In his fifties with slightly graying black hair, glasses, and wearing a dark blue suit with a blue dress shirt and red tie, Montoya clearly filled the CEO role. Having received his BA in public administration, his MPH was from a distinguished Ivy League university. Montoya led a series of community-based clinics along the border, nearly 90 percent of whose patients self-identified as Latino/a. Federal funding and the voluntary participation of health professionals enabled the organization to provide healthcare, much of it free of charge, primarily to uninsured and underserved patients. Created nearly four decades earlier through a community, university, and medical association partnership, Montoya summarized it as "about as indigenous, grass-roots a program as you can find." He is remarkably visible in health news, regionally and nationally, regularly appearing as a source in stories on Latino/a health, healthcare reform, pediatric oral health, and access to care. He reads the professional and popular literature on these issues and regularly writes op-ed pieces and articles for newsletters and magazines. This media engagement is unusual for community-based clinics, he suggests, which generally "can't afford it. They live on scraps, almost. They go from grant to grant . . . and [they] don't have the time to do it—they're just treading water." Beyond his large network, Montoya benefits from a long-standing relationship with a media consulting firm that creates press releases and helps organize press conferences. He also draws on professional associations, such as the Council of Community Clinics, which works actively with reporters and legislators. His goal is not just to publicize his clinic's activities but to shape health policy.

Montoya's view of journalists is not a great deal more positive than Norris's; like Norris, he invoked something like the "two cultures" view of media and medicine. He views reporters as contacting him generally "because some editor told them to write a story about something." Journalists' basic interest, he says, is "to sell whatever they're selling in their newspapers or advertising things. You have to give them what the buyers are wanting." He contrasted "the sensationalist part of it, the headlines" with "the facts and the true stories, the real solid public health message." The basic problem, he suggested, lay not with reporters but with people who "like to read that stuff." Nevertheless, Montoya felt that he could operate successfully within such constraints. Calls from print reporters were easier, because "they usually have more time to sit down with you and ask questions" than television reporters. Exchanges with journalists during initial contacts enabled him to assess their agendas and figure out how to respond. Television revolved around a politics of urgency: "'we need to do an interview, it's gotta be tomorrow or this afternoon.'" Often he mobilized a staff physician skilled in media contact, who in turn provided a couple of patients for interviews. Health fairs provided another common venue, enabling Montoya to send out press releases and put together "a package" on issues of interest to his organization. Overall, Montoya thought that "the media in San Diego does a good job."

Given his emphasis on increasing awareness of health issues and his active media engagement, Montoya might be expected to endorse the view that media provide a means of health education directed as lay audiences. In fact, at no point did he even hint that he saw "the media" as a means of communicating with "the public." He noted that "the patient population, our patient population, they're not reading—I don't think—the editorial page of the *Union-Tribune*." Although he did project a cultural gap between the clinic's patients and white, middle-class San Diegans, his rejection of the notion that the biomediatization of health was about influencing individual behavior was more fundamental. Not only were audiences in general too oriented toward "this sensational thing," but "even people who are educated, they don't take good care of themselves." Health content provided through news media did not produce the sort of behavioral change needed to improve health. In the end, "the ideal situation—there's no better, I think, person to do it than the provider," that is, health education should take place within the walls of the clinic and events undertaken by health professionals elsewhere in "the community." His vision of a "new paradigm for healthcare in the twenty-first century" looked a lot like conceptions of the linear, hierarchically organized model of health communication that predominated before health news entered into the process more centrally in the 1960s, in which health professionals—not journalists—educate patients (see Chapter 1).

Nevertheless, Montoya's op-ed articles and press releases issued by his organization seemed to project a process of using recently published academic studies to inform laypersons. He suggested that invoking this model lay at the core of his strategy for reaching "policymakers," not "the public." When a small group of policymakers, such as the county Board of Supervisors, is about to make a decision on an issue that interests him, Montoya works to create media coverage that will suggest that "the public" is concerned about the issue and feels that a particular course of action—the one he favors—is required. Another key audience is "funding agencies"; when his organization is competing for funds or he wants to draw funding towards an issue he thinks important, press coverage "builds, I think, credibility," suggesting to funders that "'hey, this is interesting, you know, it does apply to us.' And you get your name out there, and then when you apply for a grant, I think it helps, that they know that you gave some thought to the project." Another common audience for Montoya consists of physicians, dentists, and other professionals, among whom he wants to build consensus on "policy-type things." In short, in our interview, Montoya most clearly invoked the elite public sphere model.

How Montoya organizes the complex relationship between biocommunicable models and biomediatization practices is surprisingly similar to that of media/public relations consultant Harrison. Both locate their attempts to catalyze and shape health news as part of larger strategies. Montoya refers to biomediatization strategies as "packaging," and suggests that "packaging is really important, whether we do it for the *Union-Tribune*, or for my own medical staff, or packaging a message to our patients." Both, too, conceive of biomediatization as extending far beyond news coverage, as playing a role in influencing elite actors, be they investors, policymakers, or funders. Their practices remind us that health news and the processes of biomediatization that produce it are complex and multidimensional. We visit Montoya again in Chapter 6.

The physician-correspondent on network TV

Network news divisions are familiar places to me (Dan). I have interviewed journalists there starting in the late 1970s, when I was a graduate student. It was easier then. It took a while to convince network correspondents to talk to us. We were perplexed about this until we found attacks, particularly on websites and social media, leveled against some of these same health journalists for their reporting on such controversial issues as vaccination. As with others in this chapter, we refer to them with pseudonyms, except for Dr. Richard Besser, a former public health official who was willing to be quoted by name. In this case, to maintain anonymity, we randomized the genders of the pseudonyms.

When I arrived at the news division to interview one of the physician/journalists who served as medical editor, I was met at the lobby security desk by an assistant who escorted me through a wonderful labyrinth of little rooms to the newsroom area. I am a bit of an old-school TV news "techie"; though the technology is different now, I was glad to see that there are still plenty of little editing rooms where words and images are polished for broadcast. Led to a small lounge to wait, it was explained that "Dr. Ellen Cumberland" was running late. She apologized upon arriving and explained that she had been doing a medical procedure across town and it had taken longer than expected.[12] Needing a cup of coffee after rushing from the clinic to the newsroom, she led me to the network cafeteria where she greeted the checker in Creole. She explained that she had been going to Haiti since a few months after the 2010 earthquake, both to report and to treat patients, and had learned Creole to be able to relate to Haitians more directly. After we left the cafeteria, she checked in with her producers. The medical unit at her network has three producers, as well as four researchers—medical reporting, she told me, "is highly valued here." They were talking about finding a patient in New York for a story, a standard part of their working routine. Cumberland suggested a doctor they could try, and then we went to her small office to talk.

We argue in a number of contexts in this book that the "two cultures" interpretation of science and medicine as separate and in many ways antagonistic is inadequate. The centrality of the physician-correspondent in television news is a strong illustration of the limitations of this view. All of the major television networks at the time of our research had medical correspondents who, like Cumberland, were also practicing physicians. At ABC it was Dr. Richard Besser, and the network added Dr. Jennifer Ashton, an obstetrician/gynecologist, as "Senior Medical Contributor" in October 2012. CBS featured NYU gastroenterologist Dr. Jon LaPook. At NBC it was Dr. Nancy Snyderman, a head and neck surgeon and faculty member at the University of Pennsylvania School of Medicine with a broadcasting career that began in 1984 in local television news and a stint as vice president of consumer education for Johnson & Johnson. NBC also had a chief science correspondent, Robert Bazell, who left a doctoral program in immunology at UC Berkeley to take up journalism, working for *Science* magazine and the *New York Post* before entering television journalism. CNN had neurosurgeon Dr. Sanjay Gupta, whom President Obama was reported to have considered for the job of Surgeon General; Fox had a "Medical A-Team" of physician contributors; and, early in 2013, Univisión added Dr. Juan José Rivera, director of cardiovascular prevention for Mount Sinai Hospital in Miami Beach.

This kind of career path, combining journalism with another profession, is highly unusual. Journalism's status as a profession is shakier than that of medicine, as journalism does not require specialized training and access to the profession is not legally controlled. But it does have a professional culture that places strong value on its own integrity. Hiring a practicing member of another profession to cover that profession potentially undermines that integrity, raising questions of whether a journalist will lack both critical distance from the actors being covered and commitment to the norms of journalism itself. Some news organizations have had military or legal correspondents with backgrounds in these fields. But the prominence of the hybrid role of physician and correspondent in television news is essentially unique. It is a striking reflection of the convergence of biomedicalization and mediatization as well as one of the factors that is shaping it.

Television production is a collective and not an individual enterprise, and the medical correspondents, or medical editors (their titles vary) work in teams that are also hybrids in terms of the backgrounds of their members. Those teams include producers, who are more firmly rooted in television journalism, though the producers in the medical units often stay on that beat for long periods of time and some have specialized training. Ami Schmitz, for example, the producer for NBC's Snyderman, graduated from a degree program in Health Communication run jointly by Tufts Medical School and Emerson College, intended mainly to train public health personnel in communication skills. They also include researchers, who may have scientific or journalistic training or both. At ABC, at the time I visited there, the medical unit included four medical residents, MDs whose residency focused on researching stories and writing for ABC.com; at other times ABC's staff has included a medical researcher with a Ph.D.

Although their titles vary, all the network medical correspondents report across many platforms: evening news, morning news, prime time magazine programs, the "dot.com" (that is, the website of their news organization), their own blogs and twitter feeds, and sometimes radio. They also work with local affiliates and owned and operated stations, talking live, for example, with local anchors. Kathy Knight, a producer for one of the correspondents, explained that her job included

> guiding my colleagues across platforms: so we got [together] our dot.com writer, medical writer, . . . our news channel, affiliate medical producers [at local TV stations], and we all got on the same page and guided the ship of [network] news so we had consistent messaging from top to bottom.[13]

Cumberland is also a guest blogger for a "net native" news organization.

The fact that they have these two statuses, as doctor and journalist simultaneously, makes the network medical correspondents different in important ways from traditional journalists. One interesting manifestation of their dual role is the fact that correspondents in the field covering a story are sometimes needed to help treat patients. This happened, for example, with in the aftermath of the Haiti earthquake in 2010. This is a doubling of roles that most correspondents worry about. Cumberland told us:

> What I said to my producers was, if I click into doctor mode, you turn your cameras off. . . . I didn't want anything to creep into my head that there's any other motive for me taking care of this patient, other than I should take care of this patient because I'm a doctor.

Here Cumberland, both in her negotiations with media colleagues and her own self-representation, projected boundary-work as required by clinical practice as primordial, even as she skillfully crossed these boundaries in her reporting.

Physician-correspondents address their audiences differently than other journalists. While journalists in general—as *NYT* journalist Kelley articulated in a strong way—usually see their role as entertaining and informing, not educating or shaping people's behavior, ABC's Besser, not only a doctor but a former public health official, was particularly explicit in stating that his goal was different:

> Every week I find ways to practice public health in front of the camera. . . . Many of the health problems we face in this country and around the world require behavior change. And if you're looking at changing behavior, you have to be looking at communication. . . . [T]hat's what I'm trying to do at ABC.[14]

Besser went on to observe that this made him different from other journalists in an important way:

> I serve two roles—I cover a story and I also give my opinion on the story. And there's some friction with traditional journalism, and I've been criticized on this. . . . They want my opinion here—I am not just reporting. I am ABC's doctor, and the doctor for our audience, and so if I'm doing a story on the next diet drug, they want to know not just what did the FDA do today, but what's my take on that.

Lacking Besser's prior visibility as a public health official, the other medical correspondents constructed their roles differently. They also, however, expressed both continuity between their roles—the fact that they spoke to the audience just like they spoke to patients—and the potential tensions this involved. The authority of journalism, the right of the journalist to mediate public communication, is based traditionally on the journalist's claim to keep their personal opinions out of the news. There have always been exceptions to this, based partly on the expertise beat reporters acquire or their status as eyewitnesses. And of course the rise of new forms of journalism is creating journalistic subject-positions that do not require the separation of news and opinion. The network evening news still represents that traditional model, however, and the freedom that physician-correspondents have to give their opinions is clearly derived from the cultural authority of medicine and is different in kind from that of journalism.

It is "a unique position for Robert [Barnes] to have," said Knight, a producer working with him:

> As a doctor-journalist, . . . a lot of times we're approached by senior staff here for [the correspondent] to offer an opinion, so it's not just, you know, 'here's the story,' which we present, but also, you know, Robert, so, what should people do?'

As Besser suggests, however, this hybrid character of the medical journalist's role, much as it may be desired by the network, is potentially problematic. Medicine is not a relativistic culture, and these medical correspondents have strong and clear views on certain subjects. They often described tensions they felt between the desire to speak strongly from the position they believed medical science showed, reflecting the power of evidence-based medicine, and the concern that this position would violate the norms of journalism, and stressed the importance of separating the two parts of their role.

Cumberland, for example, described the strong outrage she felt about persistent shortages of cancer drugs, which all the networks reported on in 2011–13. "I cannot be a political activist," Cumberland reflected.

> I'm balancing. . . . I'm a doctor, I'm a journalist, I'm a human being. . . . I'm very conscious about that line that I'm walking. . . . Now, but I'm a journalist, you know, so how do I—am I crossing the line by saying I'm personally [outraged]? And . . . the advice I got was just, 'communicate who you are talking as.'

Recalling conversations with his producer, Barnes noted:

> Over the years we realized that my being an active physician in the trenches gave me more credibility in the field. And while I learned to be a journalist, it gave me skills speaking to the patients. . . . [W]hether I'm sitting at a patient's bedside talking one-to-one, or whether I'm speaking to 11 million people at night, . . . the skill set is the same. I take complicated information and I distill it—not in a condescending way but in a way that I'm a conduit and sometimes an advocate. . . . There are some things we've done where I say to the public, 'I want you to know I'm a pro-vaccine doctor. I believe in the power and the benefit of vaccines.' But, it's an opinion; it's not my general role of just reporting "just the facts, ma'am." And when I do that, I separate it for the audience, because I think it's dangerous when people throw opinion and fact and observation into the same report.[15]

In general, as we will see when we look at the content of network health reporting in Chapter 3, this mixing of roles is handled through a two-part structure which characterizes most health stories on network TV, with the correspondent playing the more traditional role of "objective journalism" in the film report and then speaking as a physician—and giving his or her opinion—in conversation with the anchor.

The professional norms of "objectivity" not only enjoin journalists to keep news and opinion separate, but also mandate "balance" between opposing views. This has always been a complex issue for journalists, who often face difficult questions about "balance" and "accuracy" and about the range of views that should be included in the scope of what Hallin (1986:117) calls the sphere of legitimate controversy. If journalists are firmly convinced that Sarah Palin's claims about "death panels" in the Affordable Care Act are false, do they have an obligation to report them (Lawrence and Schafer 2012)? As American politics has become more polarized in recent years, there have been particularly sharp controversies over this sort of issue in science coverage, including charges that journalists fail in their responsibility to inform the public by practicing false balance and allowing the politicization of issues that are widely considered in the scientific community as settled matters of scientific fact (most significantly in the case of climate change).

Medical correspondents are constrained to follow the norms of balance to a significant extent. But they do have more authority than the typical journalist to set the boundaries between the spheres of consensus and legitimate controversy. Barnes, for example, who made clear his view that vaccines do not cause autism, insisted that the network accept that boundary even beyond the bounds of the Evening News:

> So we have said, adamantly, you cannot let these famous people come on and say, 'well, I know,' or 'my child.' No! It's not true. They can come on and talk about their books or their movies, but they cannot come out and say there's a controversy. Because there is no controversy, as the [Morning Show] now agrees.

Other exclusions are a bit more subtle. Another network correspondent, James Levine, for example, talking about a story about freezing human eggs, characterized it as one that didn't involve any controversy, then added, "I mean you can make some controversy, I guess about religious stuff, but we don't touch any of that."[16] In our analysis of network coverage, we often found stories that involved sharp partisan controversies, which the network correspondents almost totally ignored.

Many of the comments quoted so far imply that network medical correspondents adhere to something close to the biomedical authority model of biocommunicability. And indeed many of their comments suggested exactly this. Talking about hormone replacement therapy (HRT), Barnes told us, "I believe I'm a scientist. So I tell the science." He felt that the evidence against HRT indicated "a price to be paid down the line" that audiences didn't want to hear about. "So, especially in parts of the country . . . where people are more affluent and believe their own science, there is sometimes room for self-treatment. But I would have said it doesn't necessarily mean it's healthy and smart."

Both in their coverage and in our interviews with them, however, physician-correspondents reflected complex ideas about biocommunicability. When I asked how she saw her role in relation to the audience, Cumberland said:

> I have gone to medical school and I have been a doctor for 32 years, so that's what I have to bring to the table. But I'm not God yet. . . . I always say to people [in my medical practice], . . . we're communicating with one another, you're going to give me information and I'm going to try to digest

it and put it into perspective. . . . I do think of my audience as a patient. Or at least somebody who might be a patient. And, how can I take this information and not just report it, because people generally get their information from the Internet now, and by the time they come to the [evening news] they may know a lot. But how can I take it and put it in perspective, so that they understand the arc of how we got to this point?

She went on then to describe how she reported on a story about human papillomavirus (HPV), where she had noticed a pattern in the existing research, not noticed by the wider professional community, that indicated it affected men as well as women. Here, then, Cumberland moved in the course of our discussion from the starting point of the medical authority model into something more like the patient-consumer model and finally to something closer to the public sphere model, where her role is less to transmit information to individual patients than to contribute to the shaping of the public agenda. It was also Cumberland who described her efforts to put the issue of cancer drug shortages on the political agenda in Washington. And when I asked Barnes and Knight to talk about the stories they had done that they were most proud of, they pointed to investigative reports they had done, mostly for a prime time magazine show—stories that are more clearly compatible with a public sphere model of biocommunicability.

Issues related to biocommunicability also came up consistently when we turned to the H1N1 pandemic. The correspondents were proud that they had informed the audience honestly about the difficulty of knowing how great the threat really was. "My basic premise," Cumberland said, "is people are smarter than we give them credit for. . . . I'm not looking to filter anything I say to my patients. . . . My idea is they can take it, they are grown-ups." Knight also told me, in connection with H1N1 coverage, "we just don't believe in dumbing things down for our viewers." Journalists, in general, have a bias toward an open flow of information, including disagreements and uncertainty; as we shall see, this orientation often puts them at odds with actors who have a more strictly linear, hierarchical conception of health communication and would prefer not to "confuse" laypersons with complex, conflicting information. In this respect, the network physician-correspondents are not radically different from their lay counterparts who cover health at newspapers and other media.

In addition to the journalistic commitment to neutrality and the medical commitment to scientific truth or to public health goals, another potential tension in the hybrid role of the physician-journalist is between the commercial imperative of television and the scientific point of view. This, of course, is a central focus in the literature on the "two cultures" of science and journalism, and it is often assumed in that literature that commercial pressures lead to substantial "distortion" in medical reporting. We heard versions of it from both Norris and Montoya. The television correspondents we interviewed did not, however, describe that tension as being particularly sharp, and they did not formulate it as an issue for them as strongly as they did the tension over neutrality. Cumberland told me:

> At no time, not one microsecond . . . have I had any pressure whatsoever about ratings, hyping something, about doing something more frequently to get ratings, . . . never. . . . They don't tell us what our ratings are, what they are moment-to-moment, minute-to-minute; 'this is how you did last week.' I never hear any of that. My positive reinforcement here is 'did you get the story right? Did you report it correctly? Did you do it without bias?'

The perceived absence of strong concern about ratings is probably due both to the fact that medical news is in general considered good for ratings and is cheap to produce, and therefore high on the priority list, as well as to the fact that their outside professional authority gives health journalists unusual autonomy to make their own decisions about what stories are worth doing. However, a number of stories came up in our interviews that suggested medical correspondents did have to resist pressures in some ways and that ratings-related factors affected the news agenda.

"I'm the only reporter I know who goes to the two-thirty meeting and explains why I shouldn't be on the air that night," Barnes told us. Knight then added, "It's almost more important what we *don't* do than what we *do* do." The two of them mentioned an incident earlier that day, when the morning show producer asked "if there's any truth to the fact that gel nails are damaging nails, and if the UV lights used to dry them are causing cancer." "So just because the [Morning] Show wants me to do a story," Barnes went on, "I don't necessarily do it. I would say to them, 'Well here's a dermatologist, please feel free to call somebody.'"

On the other hand, some stories that the correspondents consider important may be a hard sell to the executive producer. We asked Cumberland about findings in health communication research that news coverage often didn't match the epidemiology. He replied:

> Absolutely. . . . Nothing would save more lives in the world then clean water for everyone. . . . It's not a story by and large. . . . They want to put health news on these shows . . . because they want people to watch and be interested. So it's far easier to get a story about arthritis than it is to get a story about some rare disease, unless it's a very compelling story about an individual.

I asked Barnes why stories on social and economic factors affecting health and medicine were relatively rare, referring to findings we report in Chapter 3. Signaling agreement, he said that "they're harder stories to tell." He went on to make reference specifically to coverage of the Affordable Care Act, asking, "How do you tell it with pictures?"—a point familiar to scholars of the sociology of news across many areas of content. Another, somewhat different constraint had to do with the breadth of the evening news audience. Cumberland explained to us that some stories, particularly having to do with sex, were "tough to do on the evening news." These stories would be done on the Internet, instead, "away from little kids."

A journalist that Charles interviewed, Donald Schultz, worked for almost two decades for a leading cable news network. He acknowledged important influences of commercial pressures, while at the same time repeating the claim of ultimate independence.[17] He noted that the network had negotiated with one of its most important advertisers, a pharmaceutical company, to provide a minimum of two health news stories each day. The special funding that came with this arrangement turned the health division into "a profit center" and resulted, according to his assessment, in a much greater presence for health there than at any of the national television networks at that time. The advertisements generally appeared immediately before or after the health segments; when the news was negative, however, stories and ads were separated, and they did not count toward the daily minimum. Accordingly, there was an incentive to report positive stories. Producers sometimes dropped a "controversial" story, "even though the news value was higher," despite the fact that it did not count toward the health news quota. Nevertheless, worried that Charles would think that he was confessing to having surrendered journalistic principles to business interests, Schultz was quick to add, speaking of the separation between advertising and news divisions, that "they set it up as being editorially independent. . . . We were never told 'cover this story because the advertiser wants it.'"

Closely related to issues of commercial pressures is that of personalization. This is also central to the "two cultures" perspective, the idea that science deals with the universal and the abstract, journalism with the personal and particular. Critics of health journalism often see personalization as a key source of "distortion" in the transmission of scientific information through the news. Personalization is certainly central to television news production, for medical reporters just as for other journalists. When I asked what were the characteristics that got a health story on the evening news, Knight made an interesting segue, starting out by saying, "Sometimes, you know, the choice is made for us by what's in the medical journal, right?" All the correspondents emphasized the importance of medical journals, which they typically received a week in advance of the "embargo break" when the information was authorized for public release. They also emphasized their thoroughness in judging the quality and significance of the research before deciding to do a story; both Cumberland and Knight told of finding errors in the tables of major medical journals.

After Knight told me about the importance of medical journals in setting the news agenda, she continued: "So, but in general, if there's a formula, it is character-driven. So someone that our viewers can sit home and connect with, and feel their pain, feel their anger, be invested in the right and wrong." Could these two criteria of newsworthiness—significance as medical research and personalization—come into conflict? Of course they could; the kinds of stories cited above by correspondents as "tough" to get on television are challenging to a large extent because they are difficult to produce as character-driven stories. Unspoken in Cumberland's observations about the difficulty of covering clean water issues (despite her engagement with Haiti) is certainly the issue of *who it is* that lacks access to clean water, and whether the network's target audience could "sit home and connect with, and feel" the pain of people quite differently situated.

When Barnes and Knight told me that stories came from major medical journals and that a good story had to be character-driven, I asked whether this was a contradiction, since "the characters are not there in the *New England Journal of Medicine.*" Knight responded:

> Well sometimes they are. I mean sure . . . because somebody has to have subjects in their medical study, and we reach out to them. We always reach out to the researchers first to see if they can talk, right? And if they're articulate enough to put on television, then we say, 'Well, do you have people involved in the study?' 'Yes,' and then . . . our partners, our unofficial partners are the PR at these medical centers around the country. They know what we're going to need.

Knight thus points to a key element of biomediatization: the role of public relations firms in biomedical research and their "partnership," as she puts it, with journalists like herself.

Conclusion

Scholars have introduced us to war correspondents, international reporters, on-line journalists, and others who cover a variety of "beats." Here we wanted to present a new set of actors, who are shaping not only contemporary news coverage but our fundamental understandings of the contemporary world. Placing them in their particular social and professional worlds has, however, largely left them in isolation from one another; now we need to explore the connections.

Health journalists, leading medical researchers, and public health officials constitute a clear elite public sphere. They are constantly listening to and often speaking with one another, even if only some of their conversations appear in the news. They share a largely medicalized view of health, privileging "evidence-based" knowledge—particularly as embodied in articles published in professional journals—as the benchmark for what constitutes knowledge of health, even as some leave complementary spaces for alternative medicines. As Kelley's rejection of "the tyranny of the anecdote"—her declaration of "evidence-based" medicine as biocommunicable ground zero—or Barnes' arguments with the producers of the morning news suggest, they agree that audience ratings or profits should never trump science. For all of them, biomediatization is an important part of their jobs, even if some spend more of their days focused explicitly on it. Such actions as responding to reporters' queries and receiving press releases and invitations to press conferences connect them on a daily basis. Their jobs partially depend on access to one another and how they evaluate one another's reputations; health journalists could not keep their jobs if well-placed health professionals refused to speak with them, just as public health officials are likely to get fired if they are repeatedly portrayed by journalists as incompetent, uninformed, or unresponsive to "the public."

Constantly interacting links them in deeper ways. Media professionals like Harrison and Kelley have science backgrounds and clearly love how their jobs require them to be constantly learning about contemporary research through exchanges with highly regarded scientists and health professionals; they are clearly proud of their fluency in technical vocabularies. Although they may regard their virtuosity more as a necessity than a source of pride, public health officials and preeminent researchers become deeply familiar with media logics and practices. Rather than simply coming together from autonomous positionalities when a story is emerging, these media and health professionals are deeply enmeshed: their jobs are profoundly shaped by how they constantly accommodate each other's daily practices of biomediatization.

They were, nevertheless, all over the map in terms of the biocommunicable models they invoked. As we suggested, Charles' physician and dentist respectively embraced patient-consumer and biomedical authority models. Demographics cannot easily explain this difference: both were in their sixties and well established in their practices, and they served roughly the same racially diverse urban population. Neither López nor Kelley accepted either of those models, but this hardly placed them on the same page. Kelley characterized the content of her reporting as deeply evidence-based and its form as quintessentially journalistic, in keeping with a model of journalism as entertainment-oriented creative labor. Like Montoya, López sought to shape the politics of immigration and race in bi-national public spheres, a focus that became even more explicit in her work subsequently. Besser framed his job as enabling him to "practice public health in front of the camera," even as Cumberland suggested: "I do think of my audience as a patient." Here the role of knowledge producer and circulator seem to collapse in a strong form of the biomedical authority model, not expressed by any US non-physician journalists we interviewed. These professionals depicted laypersons in quite different terms, from patients to readers to, in Montoya's view, relevant mainly as an imaginary presence constructed in order to persuade policymakers or funders.

These people's jobs revolved around making both connections and disconnections. For his clients, Harrison links researchers, investors, science writers, journal editors, patients, and reporters, helping to provide the "angles" and views of each other that will shape their interactions, but he does so in a highly selective, interested fashion. Ironically, making connections quintessentially involves boundary-work. Journalists recruit researchers, public health officials, patients, FDA regulators, politicians, clinicians, and others as sources, but they place them in distinct biocommunicable slots through the way they introduce them. On network television news, for example, professionals are generally identified by name and title in texts that appear below their images. The *NYT* identifies physicians as Dr., but not people with other types of doctoral degrees. Clinicians, researchers, and public health officials frequently distance themselves from journalists as "sensationalist" and "biased," even as media professionals, like McCollum, populate every shape and size of health institution. Boundaries are drawn between print and television journalists, "local" and elite national newspapers.

This intimate dance between connection and disconnection, accommodation and boundary-work has much to tell us about mediatization and biomedicalization. These case studies seem to provide striking evidence of mediatization, in the sense of media practices and logics colonizing other domains. But the seeming invasion of network television news bureaus by physicians and the assimilation of biomedical logics and agendas by journalists—many of whom previously worked other "beats"—suggest that the situation is more complex. Nor is it the case that medical and media logics and practices have merged: producing their seeming separation and autonomy is crucial, not only to biomediatization but to how the roles of clinician, patient, public health official, politician, and journalist are defined. This same caveat applies to biomedicalization: it is not simply the case that biomedicine has merged with all other domains. The market is certainly everywhere here, and neoliberal logics are quintessentially embodied in the rise of patient-consumer bio-communicability. Nevertheless, the heterogeneity and the many contradictions we have encountered cannot be reduced to a single market logic.

Spending time with these and scores of other professionals was crucial to our overall analysis. Much of this heterogeneity and complexity would have slipped away if we had confined ourselves to content analysis alone.

Notes

1 All names in this chapter are pseudonyms, except for Richard Besser, as is Stratton-Domenici.
2 Interviewed by Charles and Clara Mantini-Briggs, 4 Dec. 2004. Italics in words transcribed from interviews and news broadcasts indicates particular emphasis on the italicized word or words, as indicated by increased volume and, sometimes, a change in pitch.
3 Interviewed by Charles and Clara Mantini-Briggs, San Diego, 29 Sep. 2004.
4 Interviewed by Charles Briggs, San Diego, 24 May 2005.
5 Figures are based on annual reports available at http://www.sdcounty.ca.gov/deh/pests/wnv/wnv_activity_update/chd_wnv_casesbyzip.html.
6 See County of San Diego Board of Supervisors (2004). For more detail on the county's West Nile Virus mediatization efforts, see Briggs (2010).
7 Given the size of the news staff, we have changed the name of the newspaper in order to help preserve the reporter's anonymity.
8 Interviewed by Charles Briggs and Rob Donnelly, San Diego, 3 Sep. 2004.
9 Stryker, Emmons, and Viswanath (2007) find that ethnic newspapers use quite simple language in addressing readers in health coverage.
10 Interviewed by Charles Briggs, New York, 3 Feb. 2008.
11 On the use of personal exemplars in health coverage see Hinnant, Len-Ríos, and Young (2012).
12 Interviewed by Dan Hallin, New York, 23 Feb. 2012.
13 Interviewed by Dan Hallin, New York, 5 Mar. 2013.
14 Interviewed by Dan Hallin, New York, 20 Apr. 2012.
15 Interviewed by Dan Hallin, New York, 5 Mar. 2013.
16 Interviewed by Charles Briggs, New York, 19 Oct. 2012.
17 Interviewed by Charles Briggs, 24 Jan. 2007 in a Pacific Northwest city.

3

WHAT DOES THIS MEAN "FOR THE REST OF US?"

Frames, voices, and the journalistic mediation of health and medicine

As Seale (2002: 25) points out, most research on health news focuses on the representation of particular diseases, and surprisingly little attention has been devoted to understanding health news as a whole, its basic genres and conventions, and its relationships with other forms of news. In this chapter, we provide that overview of health news in general.

The analysis here focuses on the daily newspaper and network television news, which stand at the center of news production, originating much of the reporting that then circulates through a wide range of media channels. It relies on three systematic bodies of news content, a compilation of the entire coverage of health in the *San Diego Union-Tribune* from January through July 2002 (1,206 stories); samples of *New York Times* and *Chicago Tribune* coverage from five decades, 1960s–2000s;[1] and a random sample of network television coverage over a period of just over three years, from April 2009 through June 2012, including 357 stories.[2] These samples are supplemented by a large but less systematic body of material we collected since 2002, mostly from our reading of the *New York Times*, *San Diego Union-Tribune*, and *San Francisco Chronicle*, though also including a wide and varied range of other material we encountered in various ways.

The dominant view in much research and public discussion on health news, as we have seen, is based on an "information delivery" model (Seale 2002: 3–5) rooted in what we called the biomedical authority model of biocommunicability. Health knowledge is imagined as being produced by biomedical science, and the role of health journalism is conceived as essentially passive, to transmit science downward to lay audiences who lack adequate health knowledge. We have argued that this conceptualization simplifies what is going on in health reporting. Building on the concept of biomediatization, we have proposed that health journalism should be seen as highly active, mediating among a wide range of actors involved in producing and circulating information about health as well as competing forms of knowledge and culture rooted in the diverse social worlds that intersect with health and medicine—science, business, politics, government, the family, and more. True, much health reporting fits the biomedical authority model up to a point, for example seemingly passive forms of reporting like the little boxes in the Health section that summarize how to "find out your diabetes risk score with the American Diabetes Association's diabetes risk test."[3] Many stories involve essentially rewriting press releases from businesses, healthcare institutions, or universities about new developments in medical technology and practice. But even in the most apparently passive forms of reporting, which project a linear flow of information from biomedical science to publics, the role of journalists in creating this projection needs to be analyzed seriously.

Much health reporting, however, involves highly active forms of journalism. Take, for example, an investigative series published in the *San Francisco Chronicle* based on reporters' analysis of hospital billing data released to the state government and "more than 50 million" Medicare billing records obtained through the Freedom of Information Act.[4] Analysis showed suspiciously high rates of treatment at certain hospitals for rare medical conditions that result in high reimbursements. In this case, reporters are producing, not merely transmitting health information, and they are also clearly operating in a terrain where medical science is one among a number of forms of knowledge relevant to the story. While health news has indeed become increasingly oriented around academic research in biomedicine and biomedical sources and perspectives dominate, much health reporting nevertheless deals simultaneously with issues that involve a long list of different kinds of questions and of knowledge—economics, politics, public policy, human behavior, social values, labor relations, etc. In such stories as "Kids' Medical Service Faces Big Cuts,"[5] or "Eager for Grandchildren, and Wanting Daughters' Eggs in the Freezer,"[6] the central issues are outside the realm of biomedical science. As they bring in social, political, or moral issues, journalists combine and reconcile the different social perspectives and epistemologies, and we explore in this chapter how they negotiate among them.

Genres, sources, and storylines in health news

In 2005, the *San Diego Union-Tribune* began to feature health stories on Tuesdays in their Currents section (called the Living section in some papers). Like the rest of the newspaper, that section is thinner today than it was years ago, mostly written by freelancers rather than staff reporters, and with more sponsored content. As in the past, however, the Health section is a form of service journalism, providing practical advice to consumers—similar in many ways to sections on personal finance, personal technology, food, travel, etc. As the editor who established the Currents health page told us:

> We wanted to make it very accessible and consumer oriented and very useful and practical: 'look, this is what *you* need to know, and this is information

that *you* can use in your life to make a decision.' We wanted to give real practical information that they could take away.[7]

The section gives advice on diet, exercise, and medical care. It is generally upbeat, free of controversy (though not always), and focused on the individual. This represents only one small corner of health news in the *SDU-T*, which, as in other metropolitan papers, spans across every section. In our 2002 sample, 42.5 percent of health stories appeared in the A section (including 4.6 percent on p. A1), 21.0 percent in Local News, 19.6 percent in Currents, 5.9 percent in Business, 5 percent in Editorial and Op-Ed, 2.1 percent in Sports, and 3.2 percent other. It involves forms of journalism that vary from the service journalism of the Health section through human interest features, business reporting, specialist science reporting, and hard news reporting of several kinds. The same broad mix can be found in any major news outlet. The Health rubric on Yahoo News, for example, on 10 March 2015, had stories ranging from "Everything You Should Know about Picking the Right Over-the-Counter Pain Killer" to "Federal Health Insurance Aid in Doubt for Nearly 8 Million," a story on an impending Supreme Court case on the Affordable Care Act.

The range of health news is illustrated in Table 3.1, which shows the subjects of health stories in the *SDU-T* and network television. The reporting is spread widely

TABLE 3.1 Subjects in *San Diego Union-Tribune* and network television coverage of health and medicine

	SDU-T	Network TV
	2002	2009–12
	% (N = 1,187)	% (N = 357)
Medical technology and therapeutics	11.3	23.8
Other stories on clinical practice	3.2	7.8
Healthcare policy, insurance	13.6	17.6
Hospitals and healthcare infrastructure	8.6	2.5
Outbreaks of infectious disease	3.6	6.2
Epidemiological patterns, general background on particular diseases	12.7	4.4
Prevention, support, and awareness programs	8.6	3.7
Human interest	10.1	8.1
Consumer health, product safety	2.7	5.0
Diet, exercise	4.6	3.9
Drug addiction, substance abuse	1.2	2.0
Abortion and stem cell research	3.6	2.0
Alternative medicine	2.1	1.1
Environmental health hazards	3.2	0.6
Bioterrorism	3.2	0.3
Occupational health	1.2	0.3
Other	5.7	10.7

across 18 subject categories and includes many more stories in the "Other" category, ranging from disaster relief to medical marijuana issues and bullying in schools. Despite this range, a great deal of the coverage is concentrated in certain categories. Stories on medical technology and therapeutics account for 11.3 percent of newspaper coverage and 23.8 percent of network television coverage; together with other stories on clinical practice, they come up to 14.5 percent and 31.6 percent of coverage. The next pair of categories, having to do with health policy, funding and insurance issues, and with the healthcare system make up another big block, summing to 22.2 percent in the newspaper and 20.1 percent on TV. Stories on outbreaks of infectious disease, epidemiological patterns, and general background on particular diseases make up a third major block of coverage, 16.3 percent in the newspaper and 10.6 percent on network TV. Other kinds of subjects get limited attention compared with these three major clusters.

In the case of network television, some of the results undoubtedly reflect particular characteristics of the time period involved. Television has limited time and is sharply affected by events that steal the media spotlight; we extended our sample period over a period of several years in order to minimize the effects of particular events. But 2009, the first year we randomly sampled national network news, was characterized by heavy coverage of two ongoing stories, the H1N1 pandemic and the debate over the Affordable Care Act, which clearly inflated the number of stories coded under Health Policy and Outbreaks or Incidents of Infectious Disease for network TV. This means that on a routine basis, the percent of coverage that falls into our three Medical Technologies categories would be even higher than in Table 3.1.

Another important aspect of news content has to do with who is projected as speaking about health and medicine—who are "authorized knowers" or "primary definers" in this domain of discourse (Hall *et al.* 1978; Schudson 2003; Hallin, Manoff, and Weddle 1994). Table 3.2 shows who appeared as newspaper sources and television "soundbites." In the case of the television sample, we have removed 51 stories focused on the debate over the Affordable Care Act. This coverage focused almost exclusively on political strategies and tactics; almost 70 percent of soundbites showed politicians. It is thus not representative of health coverage in general.

Anthropologists and sociologists of medicine have argued that important changes have taken place historically, as researchers in academia and industry have increasingly displaced clinicians as the voices of medical authority. They have also argued, in the words of Clarke *et al.* (2003:177), that there is a "heterogeneity of production, distribution, and access to biomedical knowledges." Our data illustrate these changes, particularly if we put them in historical context. In the 1960s, according to our historical study of *New York Times* and *Chicago Tribune* reporting, individual physicians and the American Medical Association represented the most prevalent voices in health news. Stories like "A.M.A. Attacks U.S. Report on Youth Fitness"[8] or "A.M.A. Bids Doctors Prescribe by Brand"[9] are typical of the era. The *Tribune* even reported on the wife of a new

TABLE 3.2 Sources and soundbites in health coverage

	SDU-T (%)		Network TV[a] (%)	
Biomedical researchers	559	16.5	207	17.7
Ordinary people, patients	517	16.2	413	35.4
Individual healthcare professionals	336	10.5	169	14.5
Public health officials	159	8.3	51	4.4
Other public officials	262	8.1	44	3.8
Business spokespersons, analysts	167	5.2	26	2.2
Civil society, community groups	215	7.2	51	4.4
Health-related NGOs[b]	130	4.1	38	3.3
Representatives of health providers	114	3.6	18	1.5
Industry, professional associations	86	2.7	22	1.9
Alternative practitioners	13	1.3	3	0.0
Other	403	13.5	119	10.2

Notes
a Healthcare reform stories excluded.
b E.g. American Cancer Society, American Lung Association.

A.M.A. President, "A.M.A. Gets New 'First Lady.'"[10] By the 2000s, individual healthcare professionals had declined from 14 percent to 5 percent of sources, and the A.M.A. had virtually disappeared from the news.[11] Biomedical researchers—always important—had increased and substantially led other groups, particularly in the elite *NYT*. Business sources had also increased their role, as had NGOs and civil society organizations, to a more limited extent.

Laypersons had doubled their presence, from 4.5 percent to 9.2 percent of sources. Lay sources—patients, family members, and others—are even more prominent in more popular media, particularly television, where ordinary people are the largest category. Laypersons, however, often appear in different roles than biomedical professionals, describing personal experiences and feelings, rather than transmitting authoritative knowledge. This difference is reflected in the fact that soundbites for ordinary people are shorter than those for elites—6.5 seconds on average, compared with 8.1 for researchers, so their presence is smaller when measured in terms of time rather than numbers. Still, the popular character of television news is evident in the orientation toward the experience and perspectives of ordinary people, although it is simultaneously centered on the expert voice of medical science. We need to understand how journalists combine these voices and perspectives and represent the relations between them.

Observers of journalism have often noted that all news is actually "olds," in the sense that journalists fit events into standard, recurring storylines. We identified a number of such storylines and coded stories in our network sample which fit these patterns. The results appear in Table 3.3. The most common were new health risks, which mostly took two forms: breaking events (the H1N1 outbreak, the Gulf of Mexico oil spill) and research (a new study on radiation exposures from CT scans, a report on health risk from excess salt in restaurant meals). Nearly as

TABLE 3.3 Common storylines in network coverage of health and medicine

	N	Percent of stories
New finding of real or potential health risk	56	30.8
Heroism of patients, laypersons	36	19.8
Triumph of medical science	36	19.8
Problems with public reception (misunderstanding, ignorance)	23	12.6
Conflict over safety or effectiveness of medical technology	16	8.8
Heroism of medical professionals	15	8.2
Conflict of interest	13	8.2

common were stories about lay heroism, which again fell into two main categories: patients who heroically faced medical problems and laypersons who took action to address public health problems. Also common were stories of triumphs of medical science—a man's sight restored with a prosthetic eye, a breakthrough in the fight against cancer. About two-thirds of all stories fell into one of these three categories.

The common frames we identified were divided about evenly between "good news" and "bad news." Commentators on the news media—including health professionals and health communication researchers—tend to assume that journalists have a preference for negative news, for controversy and conflict. That is partly true. Threat and conflict are among the basic criteria of newsworthiness, and much health news is selected because of and structured around these themes. A study revealing that a commonly used medication has previously unknown risks or a sharp division in the recommendation of an FDA panel are stories that health journalists would consider particularly newsworthy. Journalists also place strong value on certain kinds of positive news, however. Good news is considered attractive both to audiences and to advertisers, and to some extent news selection is motivated by a desire to put together a balance of positive and negative news. Health news is appealing, in part, because it helps fill the quota of positive news. Just over 7 percent of the stories in our network sample, for example, were features with such titles as "Making a Difference" or "Person of the Week," upbeat personal narratives that served to end the broadcast on a positive note.

Framing health: biomedical, lifestyle, and social frames

"Who bears responsibility for an impoverished child with a mouthful of rotting teeth?" the *NYT* asks, opening a story on a debate in Portland, Oregon, about fluoridation of the city's water supply. "Parents? Soda companies? The ingrained inequities of capitalism?" The article goes on:

> Dental decay rates, numerous state and federal studies say, are linked to income, education and access to health insurance, but also to lifestyle, diet

and parental choices in insisting on a toothbrush. Such conclusions give fuel to both sides, with supporters of fluoride seeing a social problem to be solved by government, while opponents focus on unhealthy habits and diet that they say will not be affected by chemicals.[12]

Health problems involve complex chains of causality, and competing perspectives are possible on how to interpret and address them. The Introduction outlined how public understandings of health and disease became "medicalized" over the course of the twentieth century as the medical profession came to exercise predominant authority over the understanding of health and disease. These constructions were then "biomedicalized" as a more complex structure emerged around biomedical science and the "medical-industrial complex." The "medical model" for understanding health and disease is complex, but at its core is a perspective that centers on individual biology and, to a lesser extent, behavior, and on technological interventions into biological processes. Jaime Breilh, a proponent of a perspective of "critical epidemiology" that has been developed particularly strongly in Latin America, puts it this way: the dominant biomedical perspective "tends to favor more proximate (and therefore biologic and individual/level) determinants over more distal and society-level ones" (2008:746).

A number of researchers have found that health news is dominated by biomedical models (e.g. Hodgetts *et al.* 2008). Summarizing research mostly done in the 1980s both on news and on fictionalized shows, Signorielli (1993:26) wrote:

> [T]he overall picture of health on television minimizes or ignores the social, political or economic factors of disease, while it focuses on and reinforces the individual nature of disease. . . . Television characters typically do not get sick because they do not have enough food, or live in substandard housing.

Clarke and Everest (2006:2598), looking at cancer coverage in Canadian magazines, conclude:

> Prevention possibilities are . . . framed as if they are entirely within the capability of individual actions . . . and system accountability is, relatively speaking, ignored. Pharmaceutical and other medical solutions are described as interventions directed towards individuals, one at a time. These popular frames individualize the responsibility both for diseases and for their treatment.

Clarke and Everest's conclusions were based on a coding of magazine stories for their use of three broad frames, which they called Medical, Political-Economy, and Lifestyle frames. We carried out a similar analysis of our network television sample, coding each story for its use of Biomedical, Lifestyle, or Social Frames. Consistent with the literature on the analysis of news frames (Gitlin 1980; Entman 1993), we coded for the representation both of causes of health or disease and solutions to health problems. The Biomedical frame was coded when the story placed emphasis on biological causality or (most commonly) on biomedical technology or intervention as a solution; Lifestyle frames were coded when the emphasis was on individual choices as cause or solution; and the Social frame was coded when the emphasis was on causes or solutions, that, as Clarke and Everest put it, "lay outside the individual," in the social structure or (more commonly, as we shall see) in the actions or omissions of various political and economic actors.

News texts are complex, and, as the *NYT* article quoted at the beginning of this section suggests, they are not necessarily structured around a single frame but sometimes incorporate multiple frames and even thematize the existence of competing frames. Negotiating competing frames is an important part of journalists' work of mediation, and stories in which multiple frames coexist are particularly interesting. Therefore, unlike Clarke and Everest, we did not treat these frames as mutually exclusive but allowed for the possibility that they would coexist. We coded the stories in our network television sample for each of the three frames, whether it was dominant in the story, present but not dominant, or absent. Table 3.4 presents the results, again excluding reporting on the Affordable Care Act, which was dominated by a political game frame.

Like Clarke and Everest, we found that Biomedical frames were by a considerable margin the most common. This should come as no surprise, given both the results of prior research and our data showing that stories on medical technology made up the largest share of network coverage. The most typical health stories in television news feature new developments in medical science that promise to solve some health problem, or, somewhat less commonly, raise questions about some commonly used drug, test, or procedure. "Groundbreaking news in the fight against cancer tonight," says anchor Diane Sawyer, introducing one such story.[13] Stories like this recur regularly in health news in all media, producing a powerful representation of the biomedical laboratory as the primary place where health problems are solved.

Clarke and Everest found few Lifestyle frames in the cancer coverage they examined; they also found almost no presence of Political Economy frames. For the specific case of cancer coverage—by far the most frequent focus of network television coverage, if we break it down by disease[14]—our data partially confirm theirs: 65 percent of cancer stories were dominated by Biomedical frames. Lifestyle and Social frames were clearly secondary, dominant in 6.3 percent and 14.6 percent of cancer stories respectively, but they were hardly absent. Given that

TABLE 3.4 Biomedical, lifestyle, and social frames in network television coverage of health and medicine (percent of stories; Affordable Care Act stories excluded)

	Biomedical	*Lifestyle*	*Social*
Frame dominant	39.5	15.5	15.5
Frame present, not dominant	20.4	20.7	16.8
Frame absent	40.1	63.8	67.8

environmental causes of cancer and regulatory responses or individual strategies for avoiding them are a common feature of news coverage, a bit more than a fifth of the cancer stories in our network sample had some reference to Lifestyle frames and more than a third to Social frames. Beyond cancer coverage, Lifestyle and Social frames were each at least present in about one of every three stories. This is consistent with the literature on biomedicalization (Clarke *et al.* 2003), which argues that the scope of biomedical institutions and discourse has been expanded in recent years beyond the transformation of external nature into the transformation of human life and culture.

One key form this broadening of biomedical influence takes is the elaboration of "daily life techniques of self-surveillance," which are manifested in the Lifestyle frames that occur commonly in our stories. Nancy Krieger (2011:148) similarly argues that biomedical and lifestyle perspectives "have synergistically dominated epidemiologic theories of disease distribution in the mid-to-late twentieth century." As these points suggest, it should not be assumed that the stories with Lifestyle and Social frames remain outside the scope of biomedicalization. Most of them remain very much within it, and they demonstrate precisely the complexity and scope of biomedicalization, relying on knowledge produced by biomedical science and on authorities located within state public health agencies, institutions of biomedical research, and other elements of the "medical-industrial complex." Typical of many of the stories in which the Lifestyle frame is dominant is an NBC story from 3 November 2011. Correspondent Anne Thompson begins, "Our car-centered culture, desk-bound workplace, and couch-potato habits make Americans an increasingly sedentary people. But today, from a review of 200 cancer studies, comes a powerful reason to get up and move." The story summarizes research showing that physical activity reduced the risk of many breast cancers, and, Thompson continues, "Putting pep in your step can help lower key risk indicators." Obesity and tobacco stories, which were common in our sample, tended to be dominated by the Lifestyle frame. H1N1 stories regularly included the advice that personal hygiene measures, like hand-washing and covering coughs and sneezes, were the most important means of limiting the spread of the pandemic.

While Lifestyle frames can be comforting and up-beat, as they often are in consumer-oriented newspaper Health sections, they can also be threatening to the extent that they imply that people might need to make major lifestyle changes. In our network sample, journalists sometimes reassured viewers that radical changes were not necessary. These stories are interesting as illustrations of the work journalists do as they negotiate the framing of health news. On 12 July 2009, for example, ABC reported on a widely circulated study that found that monkeys on extremely low-calorie diets lived longer lives. Correspondent Stephanie Sy summarizes the study, interviews one of the scientists, then shifts to Meredith Averill and Paul McGlothlin, authors of *Extreme Dieting*, for whom, she says, the new study "reinforces their life style." Here the broadcast departs from the usual projection of biocommunicability in health reporting, with figures outside the biomedical establishment appearing as authoritative producers of health knowledge. Sy listens deferentially as Averill instructs her, "The hunger hormones have been shown to be very good medicine for both the heart and the brain." She then, however, repositions the story back within the mainstream of both medicine and American culture. "Since the last time they were interviewed by ABC more than four years ago, Paul and Meredith seem barely to have aged. But experts doubt whether humans, unlike caged monkeys, could maintain such a diet." The researcher underscores this point in a soundbite, and Sy goes on—with the visuals shifting to images of medical technology: "Drug companies are very interested in understanding the mechanism behind calorie restriction in hope of building a magic pill that will mimic the benefits." The anchor—who in television stories commonly plays the role of representing the viewers' purported perspective—concludes by saying, "The pill sounds easier."

Social, political economy, or ecological frames in health news

That Social frames occurred in our sample almost exactly as often as Lifestyle frames potentially represents a more significant challenge to the hypothesis of biomedical dominance of health news. We will look in some detail, therefore, at how Social frames got into the news and what forms they took. They appeared in many different kinds of stories. The sample included a long investigative report about the use of antibiotics in agriculture and its role in the evolution of resistant strains of bacteria,[15] a story on school bullying and suicide,[16] and reports on a shortage of primary care physicians in Massachusetts,[17] lax control over the dispensing of prescription pain killers,[18] and the lack of sick days for some workers as a factor in the spread of H1N1.[19] Two stories focused on the effects of the recession on health, and a few others mentioned that theme briefly.

Our sample also included a number of stories on environment disasters, including the Japanese nuclear reactor meltdown in 2011 and the BP oil spill in the Gulf of Mexico in 2010. Reporting on health consequences of these disasters was coded as falling into the Social frame, as were stories on a cholera epidemic in Haiti that attributed the outbreak to failure to rebuild a water and sanitation system after the 2010 earthquake.

What we found with the greatest regularity in network television coverage, however, were stories that focused on consumer protection and product safety. As Cohen (2008) argues, consumerism has played a particularly important role in contemporary American political culture as a rationale for collective action and state intervention. Some of these stories involved initiatives to use the state to accomplish health goals through the regulation of consumer markets. Mayor Bloomberg's proposal to ban the sale of large soft drinks in New York City is an example. Our network television sample included a number of such stories. These often combined Lifestyle and Social frames—as in an NBC story[20] on whether food manufacturers were misleading consumers with a voluntary program that purported to help them make healthy choices—and sometimes posed debates between them, as in the *NYT* article on fluoridation in Portland.

Stories on food-borne illness also occurred regularly and tended to focus on policy responses to protect consumers: five of six such stories in our television sample were coded as having a Social frame. On 19 June 2009, for example, ABC reported on a recall of cookie dough contaminated with *E. coli*. Those who had been sickened were thought to have eaten the dough raw, and the story started out as though it would be organized around a Lifestyle frame. In the first soundbite, an FDA official said that the manufacturer and the FDA both recommend the product be cooked and advised that "consumers would be wise to do so." Correspondent Bob Kerley, however, immediately shifted the frame: "Tonight it's cookie dough. Weeks ago it was pistachios. Before that, peanuts. The number and frequency of food recalls, and 5,000 food-borne deaths last year, has Congress on the brink of taking action." This shifted the story from what Iyengar (1994) calls an "episodic" to a "thematic" frame, which implies social rather than individual responsibility for the problem. Another story by the same reporter two years later (21 Aug. 2011) on an outbreak of salmonella traced to eggs, asked "Why did it take the FDA so long to respond?" It quoted FDA officials as saying, "We need stronger author-ity to hold companies accountable." The story also included a soundbite from a representative of the Center for Science in the Public Interest and undercover video of workers at one of the farms kicking a chicken, which had surfaced in an animal cruelty complaint against the company. In these cases, as in many stories on consumer product safety, institutional and civil society policy advocacy contrib-uted to the policy-oriented framing. Our findings on food-borne illness reporting are consistent with research by Nucci, Cuite, and Hallman (2009) on coverage of a spinach recall in 2006, which found that television news focused more on why the contamination occurred and whether stronger regulation was needed than on health education messages about how individuals could avoid infection.

Social framings of health can be challenging culturally and ideologically, and we can see the journalists struggling at times with the implications of these threats, working to contain them, or simply shifting stories to more familiar and com-fortable discursive terrain, with the result that the Social framings are softened, obscured, or redirected. In May 2010, for example, when a presidential panel released a report concluding that environmental causes of cancer had been under-estimated, CBS was the only major network to cover it. Dr. Jon LaPook seemed apologetic as he wrapped up: "The report authors are not trying to scare people. Their point is, even though the impact of things like cell phone waves is hard to evaluate, we still have to do it." His story emphasized the report's call for additional research and for "lifestyle changes," like avoiding plastic containers and filtering tap water, while ignoring its arguments about lax regulation and its call to the president to "use the power of your office to remove the carcinogens and other toxins from our food, water and air that needlessly increase healthcare costs, cripple our nation's productivity, and devastate American lives" (President's Cancer Panel 2010). Print coverage of the report mentioned its more politi-cal recommendations but also focused on criticism from the American Cancer Society, which favored a health–education approach and worried that the report would detract attention from major lifestyle factors like smoking, obesity, poor nutrition, and lack of exercise.[21]

Something similar happened when NBC reported on an initiative by the Environmental Working Group, which had compiled data from cell phone manufacturers on radiation levels from cell phones.[22] Correspondent Rehema Ellis said the organization was "pushing for more federal regulation," but says nothing more about what kinds of regulation might be pursued. After an American Cancer Society spokesman dismisses the idea that such radiation is a health threat, Ellis goes on:

> Eighty-seven percent of Americans own cell phones. The one thing everyone agrees on if you are concerned about radiation: you can use your phone less or use a hands free device. But even the advocacy group admits, the phones are hard to put down.

In a brief soundbite, the spokesperson for the advocacy groups is then shown saying they were still using cell phones, and Ellis concludes, "A personal decision, and everyone has to make their own call."

A number of stories in our sample reflected this pattern—that is, they involved a fusion of Lifestyle and Social frames[23]—and, in contrast to some of the food-borne illness stories discussed above, they involved a shift of focus that put Lifestyle issues in the foreground and Social framing in the background. On 21 October 2009, for example, on NBC's series called "A Woman's Nation," Nancy Snyderman reported the health consequences of women's role as caregivers. Rather than approach this as an issue of social structure or public policy, however, Snyderman focused on individual management of the problem, concluding, "None of us should wait for a crisis . . . to realign our priorities." On 9 December 2010, Snyderman, who often gives special emphasis to stories on women's health, covered a report by the National Women's Law Center (2010) that looked at the differences among states in achieving policy and health outcome goals for women. It again focused primarily on Lifestyle issues, including a soundbite from an NWLC spokeswoman saying that the worst states failed to run "education campaigns to help women know what they could do to get healthier." Snyderman concludes:

> There are a lot of reasons this report card is so dismal. First of all women take care of everyone else, put themselves on the back burner; there is lack of access to good care in some areas of the country; insurance issues; and now the recession. But among the bad news, a bit of a silver lining, Brian. Women seem to be smoking less.

In the NWLC report itself, the emphasis is rather different, with a strong focus on insurance problems, access to care, and the unequal distribution of the latter.

The tendency in many stories to shift from Social to Lifestyle frames no doubt reflects the individualism of American culture and the desire of journalists to address what their viewers can *do* in response to the story—and of course the assumption that the action they would take would be individual rather than collective. It also reflects a predominant view of the role of the state in the age of neoliberalism that the most appropriate role for the state is to facilitate the assumption of individual responsibility for health by the patient-consumer. Let's look at one more example to illustrate this point. Michelle Obama's campaign against obesity generated substantial news coverage; these stories often introduced Social framings of health. A typical CBS report on 9 February 2010 mentioned the following policy elements of her initiative: working with the food industry to put nutrition information on packaging; making meals offered in schools healthier; finding ways in school to help kids exercise; improving access in poor and underserved communities through government incentives. All of these are public policy initiatives, and they touch on structural causes of obesity; for example, a number of stories during Obama's campaign made reference to the issue of "food deserts," that is, to claims that access to healthy food is often difficult for people living in less affluent neighborhoods. The dominant frame, however, emphasized individual choice rather than social structure. "Her strategy: helping consumers make nutritious choices," says correspondent Seth Doane in introducing the report. And, after summarizing the four policy elements, the report turns to a teenage girl, "who's worked hard to lose 20 pounds," responding to the correspondent's questions about "how tough it is to make changes in your life."[24]

Overall, then, while Social frames for understanding health are clearly secondary to Biomedical frames in network television coverage, they are nonetheless a significant part of the news agenda. American journalists, as Gans (1979) observed, are oriented toward a set of values originating in the Progressive era that centers on a vision of "responsible capitalism" in which individuals will be able to make transparent choices in fair markets. Public policy is seen as an important corrective when defects in these markets threaten individual well-being or undercut the transparency of markets, and journalists are on the lookout for abuses or defects that public policy ought to correct. This is part of the "watchdog role" that has long been central to the legitimating ideology of journalism, and it functions in health coverage as in other areas.

At the same time, Social framing in health and medical coverage is generally narrow, and it rarely focuses on structural issues in the political economy of health. As Karpf (1988) observed, when the media adopt what she terms an "environmental" approach in health reporting, they "focus on single issues and incremental solutions"—as they do, for the most part in other spheres of social life. The *NYT* report on Portland's fluoridation debate illustrates this. When the correspondent writes, "Who bears responsibility for an impoverished child with a mouthful of rotting teeth? Parents? Soda companies? The ingrained inequities of capitalism?" the last phrase is obviously flippant. It signals that we have come perilously close to the edge of the biocommunicable world, and we can be sure the correspondent will not lead us any further in that direction. Stories about the cholera epidemic in Haiti—which attribute it to water and sanitation infrastructure unrepaired after the earthquake—could in principle be framed in the context of the health effects of global inequality of wealth. But this is not what we find. Instead, the stories in our sample focus on the efforts of aid workers, particularly physicians, to treat patients, and of public health officials to educate the population on hygiene.[25] (Visually, these stories also feature images of local people exposing their bodies to contaminated water in various ways that signify a divide between modernity and pre-modernity and a failure of individuals to act as sanitary citizens, rather than the distribution of wealth and power.) In the same way, Snyderman's reports on women's health, while they are provocative in addressing the health effects of women's role as caregivers, do not treat this as a structural but as an individual problem. When the Social frame enters health and medical coverage, it is not in the form of a focus on broad effects of social structure on health. It usually focuses on particular interventions by the state either to curb irresponsible practices by businesses or institutions—through closer regulation of food production, for example—or to encourage and facilitate healthy lifestyle choices by individuals, through health education or better labeling of food products.

One place where the social context of medicine might have been expected to get substantial attention was in the massive coverage given to the debate over President Obama's Affordable Care Act in 2009–10. Coverage of "Obamacare," both before and after it passed, is worthy of a more extended analysis than we can attempt here. We can, however, offer a few observations based on the 51 network television stories on the Obamacare debate in our sample. Marchetti (2010) observes that political reporting dominates the internal hierarchy of journalism; once a story enters the realm of high politics, political reporters usually take over, and it is absorbed into the conventions of political reporting. The medical and science reporters were almost entirely sidelined in coverage of the Obamacare debate, appearing on only three of the 51 stories. One of the basic findings of research on political coverage is that it tends to be dominated by a "Political Game frame," which typically pushes coverage of the substance of public policy issues into the background (Hallin 1994; Lawrence 2000; Aalberg, Strömbäck, and de Vreese 2012). This is exactly what happened with healthcare reform. The coverage focused overwhelmingly on political strategy and tactics, the prospects for success of the different political actors, and the implications of the healthcare battle for their popularity and political standing.

To the extent that substantive issues related to the American healthcare system did make it into the news, how were they covered? Two main underlying issues have motivated the recurring public discussion of healthcare policy. One is access, the fact that many Americans do not have health insurance and therefore may not have access to the care they need. A second is cost: healthcare spending accounts for an increasing share of the economy, and it is much higher per capita in the United States than in other industrialized countries. Coverage of access issues was particularly limited. Only two of the 51 healthcare reform stories in our sample focused centrally on access issues; both were reported by health or science rather than political reporters. Coverage of healthcare costs was more extensive but very narrow. One early report by ABC's medical correspondent raised the broader issue of healthcare costs. But in July 2009 the Congressional Budget office issued an estimate of the costs of Obama's proposal, which was heavily covered. Consistent with what Skocpol (1996) found in an analysis of the failure of healthcare reform in 1994, coverage from that point on focused exclusively on the cost of Obama's plan, not the cost of healthcare in general.

Representing biomedical authority

The physician, and medicine more generally, have enjoyed a highly positive image in popular culture since the mid-twentieth century. Karpf (1988:13) wrote of British medical dramas:

> Programmes using the medical approach . . . address an audience of individuals, potential patients, implicitly telling us, 'this is what medicine can do for you.' They describe a world largely rational and ordered, where science increasingly dominates nature, where medical knowledge is incremental, cumulative, systematic. They invite us to feel confident in a knowable and caring world.

As Turow (2010) recounts, American television portrayals of medicine evolved from the highly idealized television doctors of the 1950s–70s—Ben Casey and Marcus Welby among others—toward more "realistic" portrayals in recent decades. The shift toward "realism" was, however, narrowly based, he argues, reflected mainly in more graphic images of blood and gore, in a focus on the personal problems of doctors, and in diminished personal interaction between doctors and patients. The core of the formula—which coincided closely with Karpf's account—changed little: "It was focused on the care of acute problems; carried out in a modern hospital; using high-tech instruments; sparing no expense; with physicians, especially physician-specialists (typically white males), in control." For the most part, he argues, medical dramas have failed to engage with the "political and economic changes that have been coursing through the medical system for decades," ignoring the scarcity and uneven distribution of medical resources, the realities of markets and bureaucracies, the conflicts of interest they set up, and the structures of power within which physicians and other medical personnel work.

What about the news? Does it, too, present an idealized image of medicine? Does it deal more fully with the political and economic constraints and contradictions that Karpf and Turow see as missing in fictional portrayals? Does it perhaps reflect the "negativity bias" that many analysts see in contemporary media coverage of social and political institutions (Lengauer, Esser, and Berganza 2012)?

Table 3.5 summarizes the results of our coding of news coverage for the tone of its representation of biomedical authorities and institutions, including both our historical sample of *NYT* and *CT* coverage and our sample of network television coverage. The coverage of the 1960s was marked by a strikingly positive tone, dominated by stories like "New Drug Eases Pain of Bursitis. . . Compound Just Daubed Over Sore Areas with Cotton – Action Called Dramatic" (*NYT*, 19 Mar. 1964).

TABLE 3.5 Tone of portrayal of biomedical actors and institutions, *New York Times* and *Chicago Tribune*, 1960s–2000s, and network television[a]

	1960s	1970s	1980s	1990s	2000s	2009–12
Celebratory/positive	27	8	9	11	4	65
	(39.7)[b]	(11.1)	(13.8)	(17.5)	(6.2)	(27.0)
Neutral	25	33	34	27	39	91
	(36.8)	(45.8)	(52.3)	(42.9)	(60.0)	(37.8)
Mixed	12	24	17	20	20	64
	(17.6)	(33.3)	(26.2)	(31.7)	(30.8)	(26.6)
Negative/critical	4	7	5	5	2	21
	(5.9)	(9.7)	(7.7)	(7.9)	(3.1)	(8.7)

Notes

a Includes portrayal of public health authorities, health providers and professionals, professional associations, research scholars and institutions, and health-related industry, including insurers and health maintenance organizations. Excludes portrayals of non-health-related public authorities and health professionals or researchers presented as deviants or dissenters.

b Percent in parentheses.

The highly positive tone faded significantly over the years, but in the 2000s, positive coverage still outweighed negative coverage, particularly on network television.

Many health stories are "sphere of consensus" stories (Hallin 1986) in which journalists, rather than following the stance of "disinterested realism," identify with and celebrate the accomplishments of their subjects. Anchor Diane Sawyer in one typical story reports briefly on a new Pfizer drug for lung cancer, then continues, "In a separate study, researchers reported what one called 'historic results' in tests of another experimental cancer drug, this one used to battle advanced melanoma."[26] In a film report titled "Melanoma Hope," correspondent Cynthia Bowers introduces Sharon Belvin, who was diagnosed with melanoma at age 22, just "two weeks before my wedding." Sharon started chemotherapy, "to no avail," the correspondent tells us. "With hope and time running out," her doctor tried a new drug (Ipilimumab). "Sharon's results were nothing short of miraculous." Under this line of narration, the video shows Sharon giving her physician a warm hug (see Figure 3.1), then the correspondent gives details about the findings (sobering, perhaps, if one thinks about the numbers, but the numbers go by quickly):

> Not everyone in the clinical trial had this kind of result. But on average Ipi did increase terminal patients' lifespan from six to ten months, sixty-seven percent. It's the first drug ever to show a survival benefit for this form of cancer.

After soundbites from the physician and a researcher, the correspondent wraps up: "These days, Sharon Belvin has everything she thought she never would, a husband, a family, a life." Here is the biomedical ideal in its purest and most complete form: science, the clinical physician and the pharmaceutical industry working

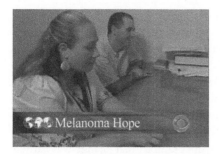 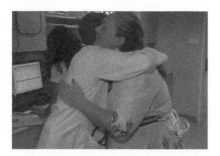

Melanoma Hope

FIGURE 3.1 "Melanoma Hope": Sharon Belvin first pictured with her husband, hugs her doctor. CBS News, 5 June 2010.

together to save a life, no hint of resource limitations or of interests external to those of the patient. These kinds of medical miracle stories accounted for 17.5 percent of our network television sample. One of the standard conventions of this genre is to construct a narrative around a particular patient; in this sense, television news actually represents a return to the patient-centered narratives of early television medical dramas, as described by Turow, in contrast to the doctor-centered narratives that became more common in television fiction from the 1990s.

Television network news is heavily dependent on pharmaceutical advertising. Is it unique in relation to other types of media in its emphasis on medical miracles? Probably not. The same narrative elements that make stories about medical miracles and scientific quests attractive for television news and entertainment make it attractive for other media as well. The "Diagnosis" feature that appears occasionally in the *New York Times Magazine* is entertaining because it presents a medical puzzle, which is then solved by determined, insightful doctors. A story in which the correct diagnosis was never made or the treatment was unsuccessful wouldn't have the same appeal, let alone a story in which the patient lacked health insurance and was never seen by the most knowledgeable specialists.

The flow of medical miracle stories is reinforced by steady streams of press releases from healthcare providers, universities, research institutes, and biotech companies promoting their accomplishments and offering help in the form of access to patients, researchers, and high-tech settings, and we regularly found in the newspapers the same genres of positive stories that appeared in television news. In both the *SDU-T* and the *San Francisco Chronicle* we found dramatic quest narratives about biomedical researchers traveling to Africa. "Deep in the thicket of West Africa," the *SDU-T* story begins, "on a bamboo bridge strung over raging waters, Erica Ollmann Saphire groped through the dark toward a village where pestilence can snuff out life with ruthless efficiency." The biology professor at the Scripps Research institute appeared fashionably dressed and in a sexualized pose in a color photo that filled much of the front page of the Currents section (Figure 3.2 on p. 95). "Awe crept into her voice," the reporter wrote, "'the number and variety and changeability in viruses is almost unknowable. They're outpacing us, and we cannot fight them without the best minds and the best technologies.'"[27] Two common conventions in narratives of disease and science are evident in this story. One is the war metaphor (the subtitle of the article is "biologist wages war against viruses in labs and jungles"), which connects these stories to a different genre of sphere of consensus reporting. The other, closely related, is the dichotomy between culture and nature and the association of the virus enemy with Africa and pre-modernity.

If we look back at Table 3.5, it is clear that there has been a significant historical trend toward more critical portrayals in newspaper coverage of biomedical institutions over the decades. In our newspaper sample, that change was particularly sharp between the 1960s and 1970s, consistent with the argument of Starr (1982) that concerns about Medicare and Medicaid costs, the growth of HMOs, a general climate of skepticism about social institutions, and increasing heterogeneity and disunity in the profession of medicine led to greater controversy beginning in that decade. Even in our television sample 9 percent of stories had a critical or negative tone, and about 26 percent had a mixed tone. Certain patterns are common to many of these stories, and we will explore them in more detail in Chapter 5, where we will look at coverage of pharmaceutical industry scandals. There is typically a representative patient who trusted a drug or medical care institution but ended up being harmed, or one who represents benefits other patients may not be able to get because of increased costs. There are typically physicians or researchers critical of some kind of industry practices who can serve as authoritative sources to legitimate critical reporting. Often the stories refer to members of Congress or advocacy groups that have pushed for action. Many end by quoting the written statements by pharmaceutical or healthcare companies, which seem weak compared with the richer on-camera testimony of victims, physicians, and advocates.

Many of the television stories that have particularly strong scandal or conflict of interest frames are reported not by medical or science correspondents but by national correspondents who report on politics and regulatory and legal issues and who apply standard conventions of "watchdog" reporting to health and medical issues. Although journalists are wary that people with roots in another profession will not have sufficient distance to play a "watchdog" role, there are also circumstances in which television's physician/correspondents take fairly strong critical stances. Marchetti (2010) makes the point in his historical account of French medical reporting that a shift toward having journalists with medical training cover the health beat was associated with a general shift toward more critical reporting that began in the 1980s. Their presence in journalism may represent a penetration of the culture of biomedicine into the news media, but it can be seen simultaneously as an appropriation by the news media of the authority of biomedicine, increasing the power and impact of the news media in the flow of discourse about health and medicine.

On 8 March 2010, for example, ABC led the evening news with a follow-up to an investigative report by ABC's Dr. Richard Besser on Merck's osteoporosis drug Fossamax, reporting evidence that it could weaken rather than strengthen

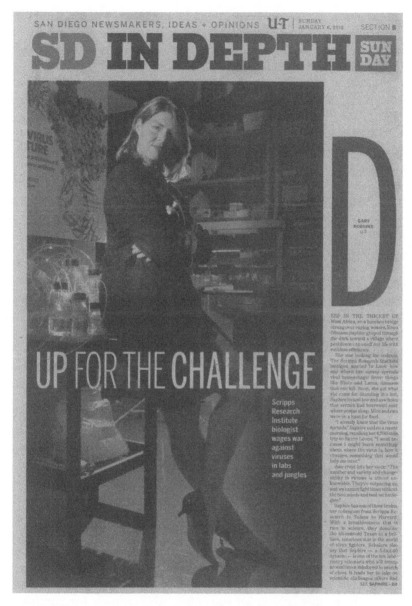

FIGURE 3.2   The biologist as heroine. *San Diego Union-Tribune*, 6 Jan. 2013.

bones in some cases. The following day, "after the flood of responses," as anchor Diane Sawyer said in introducing his report, Besser followed up by grilling the deputy director of the FDA who appeared on a video screen: "Is it time now to send out a notice to physicians to be on the lookout for this?" Besser asks, and after the official says no, Besser persists:

> Given that doctors are telling us they had no idea that these fractures could
> be related to the drug, doesn't it make sense to send something to doctors
> to say, if your patients are having fractures, let us know. We don't know it's
> related, but we are taking this seriously and we want to look at this?'

Following the story Sawyer asks Besser, "Are you surprised that the FDA won't
send word out . . . ?" Besser replies, "I am; I think their threshold is too high. . . ."
Besser, once a senior public health official, clearly considers his own expertise at
least equal to that of the deputy FDA director and has no inhibition in expressing
his own view about what should be done.

Many of the kinds of stories cited here, particularly those with Conflict of
Interest frames (8 percent of the sample), raise questions about the political and
economic context of health and medicine that Turrow sees as missing in fictional representations. At the same time, as with the stories we explored above
that interpreted health and medicine within Social frames, the extent to which
these stories bring into question the authority of biomedical institutions, let alone
biomedicine as a form of knowledge, should not be exaggerated. Few of these
stories involve structural critiques of US health and medicine, of the for-profit
nature of pharmaceutical companies or health-care providers, for example, or
of the fee-for-service system. They involve charges of wrongdoing by particular
actors and calls for particular regulatory responses—taking a drug off the market
or regulating a price. Although they bring in lay voices—those of politicians and
victims—in important ways, they rely primarily on biomedical science as a source
of authority and evidence.

These stories also very typically remain within a Biomedical Miracle frame
rather than questioning it: the scandal, as they report it, is not that the frame is
false but that it has been betrayed. On 29 March 2011, CBS's Wyatt Andrews,
who covers "politics, health care, energy, the environment and foreign affairs,"
reported on a controversy over a synthetic form of progesterone that had recently
been approved by the FDA under the name Makena. The price of the drug
had soared, angering physicians and patients and prompting calls from members
of Congress for an investigation. The report is strongly critical of the particular
pharmaceutical company, and refutes the claim that the costs of research justify
high prices by observing that research on this drug was funded by US taxpayers.
But it begins, "To the Henderson family, it's the drug that produced a miracle"
as we see the mother holding her new infant, who expresses her gratitude that
she had access to this drug." Like many such stories, this one criticizes particular
actors while reaffirming the dominant perspective on biomedical technology as
the solution to health problems.

Repairing disruptions of biocommunicability

There is one more particularly common focus of stories that we coded as negative or
mixed in their portrayal of biomedical authority: many of them focus on confusion

and controversy sparked by changes in or conflicts over medical recommendations. Health news, as we saw in Chapter 1, often tells stories of patient-consumers
forced to take the search for information into their own hands, at least temporar-
ily, when science or health professionals fail to provide reliable knowledge. Such
stories involve disruptions of biocommunicability, and they often provide striking
expansions in the scope of biomediatization: the flow of health information surges
into public channels, with, for example, biomedical professionals debating one
another in the news media and extensive discussion among lay populations, both
face-to-face and through social media. Journalists often play particularly active and
interesting roles in these cases, negotiating the breach of biocommunicability and
mediating between contending perspectives, both lay and professional.

On 21 October 2009, for example, Gina Kolata reported in the *NYT* that the
American Cancer Society, responding in part to an analysis published in the *Journal
of the American Medical Association*, was

> quietly working on a message, to put on its website early next year, to
> emphasize that screening for breast, prostate cancer and certain other cancers
> comes with a real risk of over-treating many small cancers, while missing
> cancers that are deadly.

Immediately after the story ran, Dr. Otis W. Brawly, the chief medical officer
of the American Cancer Society and the main source for Kolata's story, issued a
press release clarifying that the ACS did not intend to revise its guidelines. That
night, NBC's Brian Williams introduced Bazell's report by saying, "Tonight there
is confusion from the experts on how widespread [cancer screening] should really
be." Bazell summarized the science on cancer screening and showed a clip in
which Brawly explained, "Screening technology is complex. What appears to be
simple actually has many layers to it." "These layers lead to controversies," Bazell
concluded, "that, Brian, never seem to end." In the face of this disruption of biocommunicability, with science apparently not providing clear answers for the lay
public, the anchor turns to Bazell, and says, "And now this is where we ask you
to be Bob 'Bottom Line' Bazell. . . . What's the deal?" The standard structure of
health and medical stories on network television follows the film report with a
conversation in which the anchor asks the medical specialist for "the bottom line"
or an explanation of what this means "for the rest of us."[28] Here, Bazell responds:

> The deal is that neither mammograms nor PSAs are as good as anybody
> would like them to be. They can miss deadly cancers, they can see things
> that aren't really there and require unnecessary surgery. We need better tests
> for both of these deadly cancers, and that's the bottom line. Until we have
> better tests, this controversy is going to continue.

The following month, the US Preventive Services Task Force issued revised
recommendations, saying that women without elevated risk for cancer did not

need to start routine mammograms until age 50. That story led the NBC Nightly News (17 Nov. 2009) with a five minute, forty second report—exceptionally long for television—by Chief Medical Editor Dr. Nancy Snyderman. In introducing the report, Brian Williams says of the jump from 40 to 50, "a change that big, that sudden, isn't being taken lightly. Women are surprised, they're angry, they're skeptical. . . . " Snyderman shows reactions from women across the country, summarizes the guidelines, then shows soundbites from one doctor who supports and one who rejects the change. It is followed by a lengthy conversation with the anchor, which includes the following exchange:

> [*Williams:*] And with people currently so suspicious about insurance companies and for that matter a lot of doctors . . . will this wash through the medical community slowly or quickly?
>
> [*Snyderman:*] . . . Slowly, we'll see younger doctors take this on. The doctors who are entrenched and believe they're working off anecdotes and what they see in their offices, how they want to practice medicine, I suspect that these doctors will be a little slower to pick up the recommendations.
>
> [*Williams:*] . . . My e-mail file today, and I imagine yours as well, filled up with so many women between the ages of 40 and 50 saying, "I am a survivor. I wouldn't be a survivor today if my tumor hadn't been caught by a mammogram when I was in my 40s." . . . What do you say to all those women? [*As he asks this, Snyderman looks agitated, perhaps annoyed, anxious to jump in.*]
>
> [*Snyderman:*] Brian that's where we have to be very careful to remember that anecdotes and this big body of science don't necessarily jibe. The anecdotes are important but they're just individual studies, and this big piece of new information in fact looks at all the numbers and takes a lot of the emotion out of it. I think that's one of the hardest messages for today. Whether or not this was a false safety net for most of us, the experts on this panel are saying that the data speaks for itself, in fact it's very strong, Brian.

Williams then concludes, as is also now standard with major medical stories for which a big public reaction is expected, by referring viewers to the NBC website, where they can ask their questions directly to Snyderman.

These kinds of stories involve breaches in the legitimation of medical authority, of expectations, rooted in the biomedical authority model, that medical science will provide clear, unambiguous recommendations. The controversies arise as biomedical actors grapple with the limitations of medical technology and come into conflict over how to respond. These disagreements are not only over science and clinical practice but also over issues of biocommunicability. There is obviously some irony in the fact that the American Cancer Society was "quietly" considering a message on its website to reflect the doubts about cancer screening that specialists were debating, and yet its chief medical officer spoke about this to a reporter for the *NYT*. The controversy that forced him to issue a clarification, as the *Times* story raced around the Internet and increasingly broad forums of popular media, was rooted partly in a disagreement over whether health authorities should try to project the traditional Medical Authority model of biocommunicability and present recommendations as if the science were clear-cut, in order to avoid "confusing" the mass public, or on the contrary should encourage broader discussion and awareness of the limitations of knowledge and the complexity of the decisions involved. The former view is probably unrealistic in the contemporary media environment, and as we saw in Chapter 2, health journalists, by the nature of their structural position, are almost always advocates for some version of the patient-consumer and public sphere models of biocommunicability, with their emphasis on greater openness. The nature of the journalists' mediating role makes it imperative for them to foreground the professional conflicts and doubts that underlie the controversy as well as the strong reactions among laypersons these controversies generate.

These lay reactions are often directed at the media as well as at biomedical institutions: one typical thread of comments on an on-line breast cancer discussion board said of an *NYT* follow-up story on the American Cancer Society guidelines, "Ladies, Have you seen this article in the *New York Times*? Maybe as a stage 4 patient I am oversensitive but it made my blood boil."[29] Journalists feel pressure to acknowledge these strong lay reactions, which in the contemporary media environment circulate through many channels.

Both the Bazell and Snyderman stories cited above were among the 18 we coded Negative/Critical, Bazell's for the emphasis on the limitations of existing screening technologies, Snyderman's for its repeated emphasis on lay frustration and skepticism of medical authorities. Yet the journalists' role here is complex: they are simultaneously playing the watchdog who is subjecting authorities to scrutiny; the voice of the people giving the common woman her say; and the expert, the voice of science. When the anchor asks for their "bottom line" in the face of a breach of biomedical authority, they typically play the role of *restoring* medical authority in their own *performance,* giving audiences the clear, honest answers that seem threatened by conflict of interest or disagreement.

Often the physician/correspondents—and other specialist health journalists—intervene to make the case for "evidence-based" medicine against both lay and professional skeptics. Snyderman's criticism of "entrenched" physicians "who are ... working off anecdotes" is interesting in light of the "two cultures" theory of health journalism and the assumption that media transmission of medical knowledge is distorted by the "personalization bias" inherent in media logic. The conflict between the "anecdotal" and the "scientific" points of view is in fact internal to biomedicine, and is not something introduced from the outside, by journalists. One of very few clear statements of an "anecdotal" point of view in our television sample was expressed by a cardiac electrophysiologist in a story about mandatory screening of athletes.[30] Responding to studies that questioned its value, he says, "If it's your child, I don't think anyone would care what the statistics are, if it saves your child's life, it's priceless." In our interviews, health journalists routinely rejected this kind of reasoning. One *SDU-T* reporter contrasted "qualified sources," on which she relied for information with patients who were often "the last to know" whether a treatment worked or not.[31] Readers, she told us, sometimes urged her to write a story regarding a mode of therapy that helped them, such as chiropractic treatment, and thus purportedly "works for everyone." "Obviously," she concluded, "this is ridiculous." She reported that she had recently spent several weeks "trying to debunk" a claim advanced by mothers of children with aplastic anemia that there was an epidemic of the disease in the region.

Health journalists, like other journalists, see it as their job to deal with controversies and scandals, not just with didactic health education or celebratory stories about triumphs of medical science, and they often do this fairly aggressively. As with other journalists covering controversy and scandal, however (Gans 1979:292–293), their reporting is in a wider sense structured to reaffirm a vision of the correct social order, in this case one structured around biomedical science, which they advocate for, embody, and perform: they appear in the broadcast as idealized representatives of biomedical science who transcend the disagreements and scandals and reassure us that biomedical science can give us the answers. One of the most common patterns in network television medical reporting is simply a closing exhortation from the correspondent to "ask your doctor." For example, when ABC reported on "controversy and confusion about news on multi-vitamins,"[32] generated by a new study that contradicted widespread assumptions about their value, Besser wraps up with the advice, "If your doctor tells you to take a vitamin, take one, because there's many groups for whom they are beneficial." The anchor then says, "All right, Rich Besser, clearing things up." Like his counterparts at the other networks, Besser is attractive and authoritative, a kind of fusion of Dr. Marcus Welby and Walter Cronkite, and his presence represents reassurance that medicine can be trusted after all.

Conclusion

Health news focuses heavily on biomedical technology and intervention, often constructing strong, positive narratives of the miracles of medical science. It is also dominated to a large extent by the voices of biomedical insiders. It might be tempting, therefore, to see health news through the lens of medicalization, as field colonized by biomedical institutions and logics, and serving to extend their cultural influence. Our analysis suggests, however, that the reality is much more complex. Like other forms of news, health news often focuses on issues subject to conflict and controversy, in which competing actors, some inside and some outside of biomedicine, seek to frame the story in conflicting ways, often involving a particularly wide range of perspectives, including those of scientists, business interests, healthcare institutions, activist organization, politicians, patient advocates and other laypersons. Journalists mediate among these different actors and their perspectives, and the resulting stories are often highly complex.

The significant presence of Biomedical, Lifestyle, and Social framings of health in health coverage, often in the same story, is one manifestation of this complexity. While Biomedical framings tend to dominate in the majority of stories, Social framings are often important. In our interviews with journalists, they often stressed that they saw public policy angles as key criteria of newsworthiness, and we have seen here that indeed journalists often steer stories into the realm of public policy, focusing on scandals and breakdowns that, they suggest, ought to be addressed by some form of policy intervention. They tend to be uncomfortable, however, with broad structural understandings of health issues, often raising them briefly only to shift back toward more familiar solutions at either the individual level or the level of specific policy intervention.

Health reporting tends to be positive more often than negative. This sets it apart from most genres of news, and reflects the cultural prestige of biomedicine, the assumption that it stands above controversy and public interest to serve consensual ends of truth and well-being. The kinds of historical transformations described by Clarke *et al.* (2003) and Starr (1982), the increased internal complexity of biomedicine, its blurred boundaries and deep engagements with other social fields, have eroded the more purely deferential coverage of an earlier era; our historical data suggest that these changes probably began in the 1970s, somewhat earlier than Clarke *et al.* suggest.

Much contemporary health coverage focuses on breaches of dominant models of biocommunicability, cases where scandals, conflicts, or shifting messages seem to threaten public trust in science. Journalists, often interacting with a variety of other actors, from conflicting factions of researchers or clinicians to angry or confused laypersons who "flood" their phone lines, e-mail, and websites, often highlight these conflicts, presenting themselves as voices to whom the public can turn for answers. In these cases, they very often take on the role of *repairing* the breach in biocommunicability; this is illustrated most graphically by the role of physician/correspondents on television, typically strong advocates for "evidence-based medicine," who perform and embody the restoration of biomedical authority as they advise viewers how to negotiate shifting or uncertain medical advice. We will see other kinds of examples in Part II, particularly in our discussion of boundary-work in pharma coverage in Chapter 5. Here the intertwining of biomedicalization and mediatization that is at the heart of this book can be seen clearly as the news media take on the role, not of passively transmitting information from biomedical authorities, but of actively negotiating among competing constructions of biomedical knowledge, negotiating the boundaries between biomedical and other forms of knowledge, and representing and advocating for biomedicine with the multiple publics they address.

Notes

1 For a more extended analysis of these historical trends in health reporting, see Hallin, Brandt, and Briggs (2013).

2 The sample was constructed by randomly selecting 12 dates out of each month and then randomly selecting one of the broadcast networks (ABC, CBS, NBC) for each date. If that network was not available for that date in the Vanderbilt Television News Archive, another was substituted. We then scanned the Vanderbilt Index and Abstracts to find stories related to health and medicine, a procedure that produced a wider and fuller sample than would be obtained using key word searches. Stories less than 30 seconds in length were excluded. Stories were coded by a team including undergraduate research assistants at UC Berkeley participating and by the two principal investigators, following a period of training using a sample not included in the final content analysis. Two graduate research assistants at UC San Diego coded later months not available when the Berkeley team did its work, following similar training. Each story was coded by two coders, and discrepancies in coding were discussed and resolved by the research team.

3 "Taking Charge of Diabetes," *SDU-T*, 11 Apr. 2006.

4 Christina Jewett and Stephen K. Doig, "Chain's Billings for Rare Ailments Stand Out," *San Francisco Chronicle*, 14 Oct. 2011:A1, 10; Lance Williams, "Hospital Chain Frequently Bills for Rare Malady," *San Francisco Chronicle*, 21 Dec. 2011:A1, 11.

5 Marisa Lagos, *San Francisco Chronicle*, 28 May 2012:A1.

6 Elissa Goodman, *NYT*, 14 May 2012:A1, 16.

7 Interview by Dan Hallin and Charles Briggs, San Diego, 18 Jun. 2007.

8 *CT*, 27 Jun. 1964.

9 *NYT*, 7 Nov. 1964.

10 30 Jun. 1966.

11 Verhoeven (2008) similarly found that individual physicians had a diminishing presence in the news.

12 Kirk Johnson, "Doubts as Portland Weighs Fluoride and Its Civic Virtues," *New York Times*, 9 Sept. 2012:A17.

13 ABC, 29 Apr. 2010.

14 Cancer stories were 13.5 percent of the total sample; Influenza, due to the H1N1 pandemic, 8.4 percent; Substance Abuse (of all kinds), 5.4 percent; Cardiovascular Disease, 4.8; Other Infectious Diseases (than Influenza and STDs), 3.15 percent; Obesity, 3.1 percent; all others, below 3 percent. Thirty-one percent of stories did not focus on particular diseases.

15 CBS, 9 Feb. 2010.

16 CBS, 16 Sept. 2011.

17 CBS, 18 Aug. 2009.

18 ABC, 14 Dec. 2010.

19 ABC, 7 Oct. 2009.

20 21 Oct. 2009.

21 Denise Grady, "U.S. Panel Criticized as Overstating Cancer Risks," *NYT*, 6 May 2010.

22 10 Sept. 2009.

23 Unlike Clarke and Everest we did not treat the three frames as mutually exclusive, and allowed for the possibility of coding more than one. In fact, the frames co-occurred frequently: 43.0 percent of all the cases for which at least one of these frames was coded, another was also coded. There was, moreover, some tendency for Lifestyle and Social frames to occur together. With Health Reform stories excluded, the gamma coefficient for the association between the two (the appropriate measure because they are ordinal variables with skewed marginals) was .295 ($p<.002$). The Biomedical frame, on the other hand, tended to drive other frames out of the story: the gamma coefficients for the association of Biomedical frame with Lifestyle was -.496 ($p < .001$) and for Biomedical and Social, -.347 ($p < .001$).

24 Lawrence (2004) found a significant shift toward what she called Systemic frames in newspaper and television coverage of obesity from 1985 to 2003.

25 There were two in our sample: ABC, 24 Oct. 2010 and CBS, 25 Oct. 2010.

26 CBS, 5 Jun. 2010.

27 Gary Robbins, "Up for the Challenge," 6 Jan. 2013:B1,4; Kathryn Roethel, "The Virus Hunter – S.F. Scientists Leads the Way to Prevent the Next Pandemic," *S.F. Chronicle*, 19 Feb. 2012:A1, 13.

28 This phrase came from NBC's anchor Brian Williams, when asking Chief Science Correspondent Robert Bazell to explain reports of a potential "swine flu" pandemic on 24 Apr. 2009.

29 https://community.breastcancer.org/forum/109/topic/777002?page=4, posted 25 Oct. 2011.

30 CBS, 10 Mar. 2011.

31 E-mail interview by Dan Hallin, 9 Jul. 2007.

32 12 Oct. 2011.

PART II

Biomediatization up close: three case studies

4

"YOU HAVE TO HIT IT HARD, HIT IT EARLY"

Biomediatizing the 2009 H1N1 epidemic

On 23 April 2009, NBC News reported a press conference at the Centers for Disease Control and Prevention (CDC) that discussed seven US cases of what anchor Brian Williams described as "a strange new kind of swine flu." The story, only eighty seconds long, was sandwiched between segments on credit cards, unemployment, and wildfires. Science correspondent Robert Bazell described officials as "very concerned" about a new virus that combined genetic elements from pig, bird, and human flus, "and it's exactly that kind of virus that officials have been worried about setting off a possible pandemic." He noted that officials stressed "there is no reason for any kind of public panic," as none of the US cases had resulted in serious illness, before mentioning a larger number of cases in Mexico, whose connection to the US cases officials "very, very, very seriously want to find out."

NYT health reporter David Duncan[1] also followed the story; his short article similarly reported the "unusual strain of swine flu," its genetic components, and its person-to-person transmission in Texas, but quoted the low-keyed assessment by CDC briefer Dr. Anne Schuchat of the National Center for Immunization and Respiratory Diseases, who said that "we don't think this is a time for major concern." Duncan mentions that "the agency has been wary of causing panic over influenza cases" since the 1976 fiasco in which President Gerald Ford ordered massive vaccination to prevent an H1N1 epidemic that never materialized (see Neustadt and Fineberg 1978; Fineberg 2008). Duncan, like Bazell, noted "a 'relatively high' fatality rate for people in Mexico." He added an oblique criticism of the CDC, about which we will say more later: "Asked about [the Mexican cases], American officials said they had no information." The story's placement on page 13 suggests its status, like the NBC segment, as routine news.

This chapter focuses on the way that—within 24 hours—these brief reports mushroomed into one of the year's major news stories, globally and across media. Given that leading US health journalists and officials often cite H1N1 coverage both as a model for risk and emergency communication and as demonstrating that "investments" in biosecurity were "successful," we decided to turn that coverage into one of our central case studies of biomediatization.

A day later, "swine flu" led the news on all three broadcast networks, as on CNN. NBC's Bazell again covered the story, a three-minute package that included shots of headlines from Mexico City newspapers highlighting the word "*Emergencia.*" Bazell began, "This much is known: there is an outbreak in Mexico of a new strain of flu that can be deadly." The camera then zooms in on a vial held by a lab worker in protective gear (Figure 4.1). This is a familiar technique in science reporting, one that seems to insert the story's scientific referent directly into the media frame (Manoff 1989), like an illustration in a scientific text (Latour 1987), transforming the virus into a object of scientific knowledge—even if, in this case, it was still largely unknown. Then came another standard visual in representing epidemics—one that health coverage shares with "national security" reporting—a map of the Mexico–US border, situating the new virus geographically. The flu has killed "some 60 people" in Mexico and sickened eight in US border states, Bazell reports. Acting CDC Director Richard Besser then appears in a news conference, speaking from a lectern flanked by flags, with a dark blue background and the CDC's blue logo behind him: "This is something we are worried about, and we are treating very seriously, and I think that it's important that people are paying attention to what's going on" (Figure 4.2).

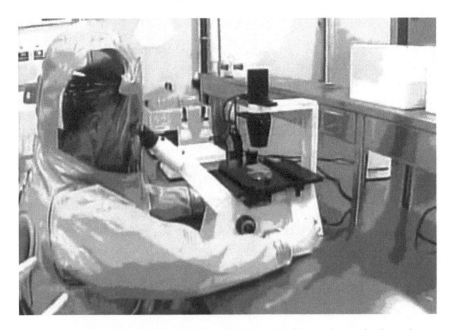

FIGURE 4.1 H1N1 Pandemic, day one, NBC news: a lab worker in biohazard gear works with a vial presumably containing the mysterious and threatening virus. NBC News, 24 Apr. 2009.

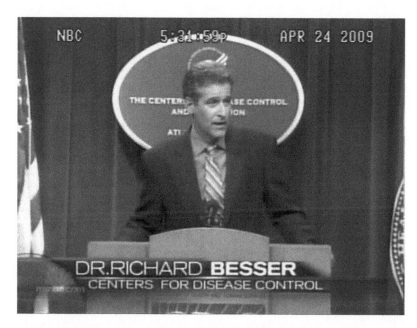

FIGURE 4.2   H1N1 Pandemic, day one, NBC news: Dr. Richard Besser, Acting
Director of the CDC, holds a press briefing. NBC News, 24 Apr. 2009.

Bazell returns to Mexico, reporting that "the Mexican government has closed
schools, museums, libraries, and other public facilities." We then encounter what
would become the iconic visual image of the H1N1 pandemic worldwide, familiar
to audiences from the SARS epidemic: people wearing surgical face masks. Bazell's
introduction promises to tell us what is "known," but implies that much is not;
he soon turns to "the big question now, how much further will the virus spread?"
"We really are in a very difficult position right now," says University of Minnesota
infectious disease specialist Michael Osterholm, a frequent NBC source, "where we
have much more uncertainty than certainty." Osterholm is a significant figure in
the movement to bolster public health "preparedness," an important theme in this
chapter. When he says "we," he seems to mean simultaneously experts and public
health officials who must manage the crisis, and society as a whole, which depends
on those experts. Osterholm continues, "and, unfortunately, that uncertainty all
bodes poorly for the future if we show ongoing transmission."

An image of pigs fills the screen, followed by one of "the virus" itself juxtaposed
with shots of pigs, chickens, and people, visualizing its genetic origin (Figure 4.3).
Bazell notes that experts have long worried that a new virus could have pandemic
potential. The most ominous segment evokes the 1918–20 pandemic that killed
"some 50 million people worldwide." Black and white images, first of a patient in
bed, then of rows of crosses, give way reassuringly to an image of public health:
the ever-calm Besser appears before the blue background and flags saying, "WHO
is not at the point of declaring a pandemic. We are at the point of trying to learn

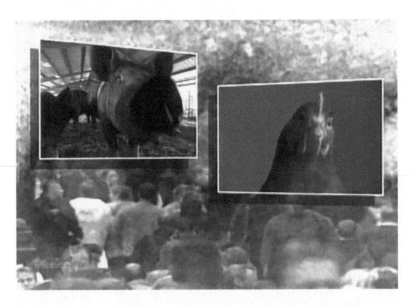

FIGURE 4.3 H1N1 Pandemic, day one, NBC news: "The new virus has genetic elements, not just from pigs, but from humans and birds." NBC News, 24 Apr. 2009.

more about this virus, and understand its transmission and how to control it." Then we see images of scientists donning "space suits," entering a high security lab, and sealing an imposing door.

After Bazell explains that current vaccines don't protect against the new virus, the anchor asks what this means "for the rest of us:" "Is this a case of 'and now we wait?'" Bazell's answer is perhaps more complicated than Williams hoped—indeed, his story as a whole is quite complex. "It's the worst situation for public health, because all you can do is wait, although it would be a very good time for all the communities to review the preparedness plans they were supposed to come up with." Bazell thus includes public health officials among those who must wait; suggesting that the popular medium of television can address multiple audiences, including lay and specialized viewers. Bazell then notes that "we'll see in the next few weeks" if preparedness plans "need to be put in place," closing by transmitting advice to the lay audience: officials have strongly cautioned against hoarding the antiviral Tamiflu.

Duncan published an article in the on-line version of the *NYT* that same day, appearing on the next day's front page as a "refer." The story ran to over a thousand words and included five photographs and a map. Co-authored by Mexico correspondent Jeff Richards,[2] it featured most of the narrative elements contained in the NBC broadcast and expanded the epidemic geography to Canada. Duncan and Richards presented more detail on the genetics of the virus, the 1918–20, 1957 and 1968 H1N1 epidemics, 2003 SARS cases in Canada, and the distribution and lethality of H1, H2, H3, and H5 viruses. They cited WHO's figures of 60 Mexican deaths, 800 cases, and 1,004 possible cases, detailing guidelines issued by Mexican officials (including "refrain from shaking hands or greeting women with a kiss on the right cheek, as is common in Mexico") introducing an element of cultural reasoning. They suggested that the demographic profile of Mexican H1N1 deaths, consisting mainly of "young, healthy adults" was a source of concern, suggesting that a "cytokine storm" in immune systems might cause such deaths. Noting that WHO was considering raising the pandemic flu alert from level 3 to 4, Duncan and Richards quote a "flu virus expert" as projecting the emotional effects of WHO's potential action—this would "really raise the hackles of everyone around the world." They quote Besser as having ruled out imposing border restrictions or warning people not to visit Mexico as "containment measures," echoing Bazell's suggestion that a sense of alarm can lead to public overreaction, including Mexicans rushing "to buy masks or get checkups."

This flu virus did spread around the world; WHO declared it pandemic on 11 June. H1N1 was a major focus of attention among media globally; on US network television it was the second leading news story of 2009, after the debate on healthcare reform. It became a central, if passing element of popular culture, widely discussed among mass publics and entertainment media humor. A major global health policy focus, the US Congress allocated $7.65 billion in June and Britain spent $1.8 billion on H1N1. The H1N1 focus sometimes put other public health activities in the background (Enanoria *et al.* 2013). Not terribly virulent, H1N1 did not become the global catastrophe many experts feared, resulting in 60.8 million estimated US cases, 274,304 hospitalizations, and 12,469 deaths (Shrestha *et al.* 2011). One study estimated global mortality at between 151,7000 and 575,000, very difficult to know, as the range suggests (Dahwood *et al.* 2012). These figures are comparable to annual deaths from seasonal flu.

Here we scrutinize a prime example of the co-production of biomedical objects by journalists, health professionals, and other actors. Although news coverage of the 2009 H1N1 pandemic often strongly invoked the biomedical authority model of communicability of health knowledge flowing downward from the realm of science to the mass public, the reality was much more complex. When H1N1 exploded onto the world stage, scientific knowledge about the virus was in its early stages. Based on research with leading virologists and epidemiologists, anthropologist Theresa MacPhail suggests that they had detected the presence of a new H1N1 strain several weeks earlier and had focused on producing a definitive genetic phylogeny, an account of the virus' past that would—in the view of some—enable them to predict its future (MacPhail 2014:32–33). Nevertheless, she reports, these interlocutors "told me the same thing—that certain key pieces of information about the virus were missing during the first few days and weeks of the 2009 H1N1 outbreak: its virulence, transmissibility, and origins" (2014:38). Viruses are not stable entities and might easily mutate into something quite different. Anthropologist Celia Lowe (2010) suggests that it is best to think of viruses not as species with stable borders but as "viral clouds" that shift rapidly through unstable RNA replication and genetic exchanges with other organisms. Research exploring the genetic makeup of the virus, its means of transmission, its mortality rates and risks for various population segments, would be published only several weeks later, after the story had peaked in the news and key decisions about the public health response had been made. Even then, published papers were peppered with phrases like "judging its pandemic potential is difficult with limited data" (Fraser *et al.* 2009:1557). Still today, much about the virus remains subject to debate. Here, clearly, science did not come first, and biomediatization later; both were produced simultaneously.

News coverage of the H1N1 pandemic was extensive and scholars have devoted so much attention to it that it is possibly the most intensively analyzed epidemic to date. This remarkable proliferation of scholarship emerging from a number of disciplines and addressing a variety of audiences provides a striking example of how research on health news coverage can break out of the small niches in which it is usually contained.[3] We build on this research here by bringing to bear the concept of biomediatization, and looking both at the content of news coverage and at the practices and interactions of key actors involved in the production of that content, particularly journalists and public health officials. As in the rest of this book, we seek to go beyond the question of whether media coverage was "over-hyped," whether it correctly reflected the epidemiology of the pandemic. Our goal was to delve more deeply into biomediatization, to discern the extensive networks and forms of collaboration between health and media professionals and others distributed among numerous sites that resulted in the H1N1 coverage. We argue here that the "viral networks" of epidemiologists and virologists explored by MacPhail (2014) and other STS scholars centrally included journalists. Our understanding of these actor-networks will fall short of grasping the nature of epidemic and other objects, their making and impact, if ideological separations between technoscience and "the media" continue to preclude awareness of how networks extend into press conferences and newsrooms as well as into laboratories, hospitals, and corporate boardrooms. H1N1, particularly when vaccination became the focus, also demonstrated how this alliance encounters resistance from both the right and the left, particularly on social media. There are important parallels between health reporting during a "public health emergency" and "national security" reporting, which we also explore.

In keeping with our multimethod approach, we randomly selected 50 articles from two newspapers with national audiences (*USA Today* and the *New York Times*), two regional ones (the *San Diego Union-Tribune* and *Atlanta Journal-Constitution*), and one local tabloid (the *New York Post*). We analyzed these and a sample of national network news stories quantitatively and qualitatively. We focused on sources, how stories characterized public health officials and how officials framed H1N1, the tone of stories, how they characterized the virus, and the relationship between numbers of stories and of cases in April–July 2009. We used the comments sections of newspaper, radio, and television websites and other sources to track Internet and social media discussions. We also interviewed journalists reporting for media ranging from small, local newspapers and radio and television stations to national network television and the *NYT*. We interviewed city, county, state, and national public health officials as well as epidemiologists and other researchers. We also conducted ethnography whenever possible, including in biosecurity "exercises" that came in the wake of H1N1. This chapter demonstrates why this combination of research strategies makes a difference.

Co-producing H1N1: the first day

On 23 April, H1N1 was a minor story about eight US cases. By the next day the virus had not only become a dominant news story but had jumped to the top of public health agendas and generated major commitments of funds and resources stockpiled for biopreparedness. Bazell's and Duncan's stories presented a complex, coherent representation of this new biomedical object that would prove remarkably persistent. Epidemics typically go through a kind of life cycle of public representation, moving from an emphasis on alarming representations of generalized threats to the "containment" of fear (Ungar 1998). To some extent we see this cycle *within* the reporting of H1N1 on the very first day, and we explore below how it played out over the following weeks. We also see different media frames circulating in the fall, as attention shifted to the H1N1 vaccine.

How was it that such a coherent narrative about a still largely unknown health threat emerged essentially overnight and then went on to dominate most public discourse as the epidemic unfolded? In general, the nature of journalists' work is to create coherent narratives about new social objects that emerge suddenly onto the public agenda. The routines of news work function to make this possible, enabling journalists to fit emerging objects into standard categories and storylines (Rock 1973). What these categories and storylines will be in a particular case, however, is shaped by complex social processes that involve not only journalists but other social actors, including, centrally, their sources. In this case, understanding how these narratives emerged more or less full-blown on 24 April 2009 requires going back over a long history of institutional development and of interaction between journalists and public health officials. We trace that story first by looking at the practices of Duncan at the *NYT* and Besser at the CDC, two key actors in the production of H1N1 news, then we detail the biomediatization practices in which both participated.

"I was brewing that night, thinking—this is a pandemic!": a reporters' story

David Duncan is a reporters' reporter.[4] Graduating with high honors in a humanities discipline from an elite public university, he started at the *NYT* as a copy-boy before landing a job there as a reporter, moving on to other media, then returning to the *NYT*, which stationed him in several foreign countries. Returning to New York, Executive Editor Howell Raines offered him a position reporting culture or science: he chose science. The science editor balked, saying she didn't have room in her budget. "And she said: 'Well, I need a health reporter'. And I said, 'OK, I'll be a health reporter.'" A decade later, he was a leading figure in US health journalism.

Duncan had been following reports of unusual cases of swine flu earlier in the week. On Tuesday 21 April the CDC's *Morbidity and Mortality Weekly Report* (*MMWR*) mentioned one unusual case of swine flu. "Very early on," Duncan said, "I realized that what had been spotted in [California] and Texas was probably connected" to how "Mexico City was in the grip of a mysterious disease."

He participated in a 23 April CDC telephone conference call to reporters, a routine weekly follow-up to the *MMWR*. "I often try to listen to the press conference and then try to ask my questions privately afterwards," Duncan noted, "because I don't want to tip what I'm writing." Nevertheless, he asked Schuchat, according to the official transcript, about "reports that the Mexican authorities informed the Canadian authorities that they were having a particularly bad flu season this year with a high case fatality rate" and asked if the CDC was investigating "a Mexican connection" with US cases.[5] The CDC gave him "a brush-me-off answer"; follow-ups yielded nothing. He surmised that his question may have "tipped off a number of reporters to this [being] a bigger story than they thought." An NBC researcher was also on the call. After filing the story, "I was brewing that night, thinking: this is a pandemic–this is the beginnings of a potential pandemic."

Arriving early the next morning, Duncan emailed the *NYT*'s Mexico correspondent "saying, 'would you work with me on this?' And [Jeff] immediately wrote back to me and said, 'yeah, something's going on here, and I was planning to write about it today." The second "hurdle" facing Duncan was convincing the *NYT*'s editors; although this was "usually not very hard—they are usually fairly cooperative. But in the early days of the story, if you think the story is bigger than they realize, some of that can be difficult." Indeed, pitching flu epidemic stories presents a particular challenge. Duncan's editor told us that

> like SARS and like bird flu, these potential global pandemics are extremely difficult things to cover and difficult things to think about in terms of what kind of space we give it, how much emphasis we give it. It's a tough call.[6]

Readers may become disillusioned if coverage seems overblown. The initial article appeared in print on Saturday the 25th, so the weekend editorial staff was in charge; Duncan worked with an editor who had little experience with health journalism.

The science editor suggested a trip to Texas, but Duncan responded: "It's flu. It will be here before I can get to Texas, it will be in New York soon." Duncan's next story led with the news that officials believed 100 students at a Queens school had "swine flu." Although H1N1 coverage began on the foreign desk, with the local cases "the metro desk got excited," followed by the national desk; "for a while there, . . . the paper was full of flu stories." There were three stories in Monday's edition, more daily by mid-week. In the science editor's words, "It became a worldwide, 24-hour story, and we have the resources here and we threw them at it to figure out what was going on." Duncan said it turned "into a complete fire drill, . . . with me writing the lead story with feeds . . . from reporters all over the world." Soon Duncan was able to leave "the daily mish-mash" to other reporters and focus on "a little more analysis." As is often the case with specialist reporters, Duncan played the role of "expert" within the *NYT*, explaining public health to non-specialist journalists. "You're trying to coordinate your story with the metro reporters," he explained at one point, "and the poor graphics people who are being screamed at to have an exact count of the number of cases and deaths and stuff, and I'm trying to explain to them: there is no exact count." He went on to explain what was involved in confirming a case of H1N1 through laboratory tests, and why it would not make sense from a public health point of view to test everyone who went to the doctor with flu-like symptoms.

Duncan's reporting emerged from a process that began long before H1N1 and beyond his *NYT* cubicle. He stressed that his H1N1 stories were shaped by long experience in reporting on influenza. "The truth is, in the minds of people like me and Keith Bradsher and others, simply having been through H5N1 made us better prepared to know what the big issues are for H1N1."[7] Bradsher has been the *NYT*'s Bureau Chief in Hong Kong since 2002, a city that "has taken its stigmatized reputation as the source of global influenza to its logical and empowering conclusion; if someone wants to understand the virus, then she must do research in the city" (MacPhail 2014:77). MacPhail, who studied the H1N1 research conducted in these labs, suggests that there was "a palpable tension" between what a virologist or epidemiologist "might state openly in the media or in a government report" and "what he might say freely or 'off the record' among his colleagues or to people who had access to similarly contextual information" (2014:5). In saying, "I think we were much less naïve on covering the epidemic than most other reporters," Duncan precisely challenged the notion that he, Bradsher, and other leading health and scientific journalists inhabited a separate sphere of "the media." The constant exchanges of knowledge among leading journalists, researchers, and public health officials, complemented by their reading many of the same journals and blogs and watching influenza-related news globally, linked them in a biomediatization process that emerged not simply in April 2009 but over years.

We turn next to the key role of biosecurity in shaping this "viral network" of epidemiologists, virologists, . . . and journalists.

Practicing public health in front of the camera: the top US public health mediatizer

Acting CDC Director Richard Besser was a key figure in biomediatizing H1N1. Like Duncan, his role was shaped by a deep history of boundary-crossing. We have already encountered Besser in Chapter 2, in his post-H1N1 role as chief health and medical editor for ABC news, where, as he told us, he continues to "practice public health in front of the camera." Besser has crossed multiple boundaries in his career. After a residency in pediatrics, he trained in epidemiology at the CDC before joining U.C. San Diego's pediatrics faculty, simultaneously working as a health reporter for a local television station. Returning to the CDC, he directed its Coordinating Office for Terrorism Preparedness and Emergency Response for four years before being named acting director in January 2009.[8]

When Dan asked him what took place in the CDC at the beginning of the epidemic, Besser recalled: "recognition of the outbreak came fairly quickly. . . . It was a couple of days after putting together what we were seeing in the US with information in Mexico that it looked like it could be the start of the next pandemic." On 23 April, when the outbreak was considered still "kind of small" it made sense to convey information in a routine telephone press conference through a subordinate. "Then as it got bigger it quickly made it to the level of me, as Acting Director, to get people's attention." Beyond the content of Besser's remarks, the very format of a press conference provided a metacommunicative frame designed to shape how H1N1 would be biomediatized from the start: "One of the principles we use in communication is you kind of escalate depending on the response you want to get." Besser was clear that the CDC placed biomediatization at the center of its H1N1 efforts:

> We made a decision on the first day that communication was going to be a critical part of what we did, . . . that we were going to make sure that if any news outlet wanted information about the outbreak they were going to be able to get it from us . . . . That we would practice the principles of emergency risk communication . . . a lot of us had been trained in. So we would tell people what we knew, when we knew it. We would tell them, when we didn't know, what we were doing to find the answers. And by doing so, hopefully to engender trust.

Besser was centrally involved, with much of his time during the pandemic devoted to doing press conferences daily and making himself available to morning and evening television news shows.

Beyond news media, the CDC was

> deliberately communicating in multiple directions—up to the political level, out to the public through . . . press conferences, across our agency, so people at the CDC knew what was going on, across to other departments that had a role.

The CDC placed daily conference calls to state epidemiologists and public health officers, local health officials, and clinician organizations. For Besser, successful risk communication required making sure that "the public trusted you, but also that the political leadership trusted you." Besser and his staff also contacted the "leading voices in public health," making

> a deliberate effort to reach out during this time and call those people who I knew were going to be on the networks . . . and say, 'Here's what we're doing, here's what we see, here's what we think is going on, is there anything we're not thinking of?' You know, 'what do you think?' And the attempt to pull people inside the tent so that they felt part of what was going on and they weren't just lobbing grenades.

The CDC constructed what Besser called "Team B, a group of experts." This group included David Spencer, the former CDC director who lost his job in the wake of the 1976 H1N1 vaccination debacle, and Institute of Medicine President Harvey Fineberg, co-author of a book critical of the 1976 vaccination campaign (Neustadt and Fineberg 1978). Besser thus included "the critics or the second-guessers who might have some good ideas but also might undermine public confidence in what we were doing." He added that "this is something that's done in the military all the time" but infrequently in public health.

This massive communication effort has often been criticized, given that the virus did not prove the major threat officials had initially feared. H1N1 has been described by Barker (2012:708) as "the bureaucratic reflex [that] produced an event that accelerated beyond the present actuality of the socio-biological occurrence of the virus." It was, Barker wrote, "a novel virus" that "sprang the sensitized surveillance trap of global influenza preparedness." When Dan asked Besser whether the emergency communication strategy had been *too* successful, he responded, "You only have one chance to get out ahead of a new outbreak. You have to hit it hard, hit it early, and then you can back off."

Exercising pandemic flu

"Public health," Besser told Dan, ". . . is very data-driven. . . . You want to know the science; you want to know the data; you want to know the information. If there's one study that points to something, you want a second study that confirms it." Like the county public health officer Norris (Chapter 2), Besser constructs health communication, like medicine and public health, as ideally evidence-based, as a linear process in which publics are constructed for statistically verified knowledge already existing in specialized biomedical domains. In a case like H1N1, however, Besser explained that biomediatization could not wait for complete data:

> We went in a different way with this, saying, 'we're going to share what we know when we know it, and some of it's going to be wrong. And when we find out it's wrong, we're going to change it.'

How could Besser help create a coherent narrative about H1N1 so rapidly when so little was known about the virus? His answer stressed that the CDC had been preparing for years for precisely this moment:

> [T]he materials were there. They had to be modified, because we'd been planning for bird flu, and this was pig flu, but that's very different from starting with an unknown infection where you may not have materials. Here we had the messages around the flu. . . . So it was a matter of figuring out and tailoring, rather than starting from scratch.

Explaining this apparent contradiction requires pushing further back in time. US health and media professionals most commonly evaluated the biomediatization of H1N1 in comparison with how officials responded when letters containing anthrax

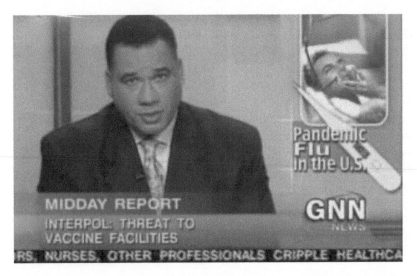

FIGURE 4.4   With video produced by the CDC, a mock news report for a pandemic flu exercise in Idaho on 28 July 2008.

bacteria were sent through the mail weeks after the World Trade Center attacks. That a "newly emerging" strain of an influenza virus would be compared with a "bioterrorism" incident provides an indication of how tightly health communication and security were coupled when Besser "activated" the Division of Emergency Operations, Office of Public Health Preparedness and Response. This unit includes a "large emergency communications unit" headed by Dr. Marsha Vanderford, a Ph.D. in Communication. The "securitization" of H1N1 is reflected in the formal investment of control over H1N1 communication in the Department of Homeland Security, though in this case the CDC, careful, as Besser says to keep the trust of the political leadership, managed to keep effective control. The securitization of health communication was not initiated in April 2009 or even following 9/11 but emerged over years by two massive endeavors in which the CDC played a leading role: the dissemination of techniques of "emergency risk communication" and the proliferation of health-related "exercises" or "scenarios" (Figure 4.4).

Besser noted that "we would practice the principles of emergency risk communication, and a lot of us had been trained in risk communication." These practices were codified in the CDC's (2002) *Crisis and Emergency Risk Communication* manual and associated course; a version focuses specifically on *Pandemic Influenza* (CDC 2007[2006]). An elaborate cultural model of language, these manuals construct pandemic temporalities and risks as much in communicative as in clinical and epidemiological terms. One focus is managing problematic "public" emotions— which "range from terror and shock to blame, anger, and guilt"—by providing information "which restores a sense of control, and by modeling optimistic behavior" while the epidemiology is uncertain (2007[2006]:8). A checklist of "Basic Tenets of Emergency Risk Communication" includes (2007[2006]:15):

- *Don't over reassure.*
- *Acknowledge uncertainty.*
- *Express that a process is in place to learn more.*
- *Give anticipatory guidance [regarding possible negative outcomes].*
- *Acknowledge people's fears.*
- *Express wishes. "I wish we knew more."*
- *Give people things to do.*

The manual stresses the need to "quickly build trust and credibility" by displaying "[e]mpathy, expertise, [and] dedication" (2007[2006]:15), "showing competence and expertise; remaining honest and open" (2007[2006]:11), and repeating information frequently in simple, jargon-free language. This training provides strategies for producing and managing emotions. H1N1 press releases, press conferences, and press reports embodied these principles to a remarkable degree; the terms used in the manual emerged frequently in the words of spokespersons from local officials to Obama himself. The emphasis on "acknowledging uncertainty" is strongly reflected in how journalists, public health officials, and influenza researchers spoke about the epidemic on 24 April and was a key feature of H1N1 coverage globally (Fogarty *et al.* 2011; Liu and Kim 2011; Staniland and Smith 2013) as in "preparedness" discourses in general (Lakoff 2008). Dissemination of "crisis and emergency risk communication" principles across registers and professional domains helped build a biomediatization network that swiftly shaped "the swine flu epidemic."

Health and media professionals frequently referred to a broader, more visible site for creating biomediatization networks, which Bazell invoked in the 24 April broadcast, "In preparation for bird flu, most communities were supposed to develop pandemic preparedness plans." A leading network news health reporter told us,

> I've gone to the CDC and other places or universities and sat in on panels on this stuff. And certainly with respect to H1N1 and the threat of pandemic bird flu, there have been conferences about this and how do we respond, . . . scenarios.

As Besser put it, "we had also been exercising around pandemic flu for years," and the CDC had given "states and locals . . . money to exercise on flu." Moreover, "we had included reporters from some of the major media outlets in our exercises, so we could get a better sense of what things they'd want to know, what questions we might be hearing." These exercises helped the CDC develop ongoing relationships with, as Besser put it, "a cadre of really good public health reporters," ones "that were covering the story really well, and we knew would get it right." From the get-go, "we really worked on them hard."

The more we spoke with public health officials—from local to state and international—and with journalists, the more we grasped the central role of these exercises in everyday practices of biomediatization, particularly in moments of "crisis." Such exercises continued—apparently with increased interest—following the H1N1 epidemic, and Charles participated in several, both on-line and live, including the one in June 2010 that he recounts below. His goal was to assess ethnographically their place in the construction and dissemination of biocommunicable models and biomediatization practices.

The exercise

I (Charles) joined an event in a mid-sized southwestern city; it formed part of the CDC's Cities Readiness Initiative.[9] The result of over three months of planning, it was the city government's second full-scale exercise and included five CDC officials and approximately 120 participants drawn from two city governments, state Health and Homeland Security agencies, numerous city and country departments, several Native American nations, FEMA, and a military base. Why did so many officials and agencies participate in an event that had been long postponed for lack of interest? Many participants repeated the phrase "H1N1 was a wakeup call for a lot of people."

We filed into a room structured like a middle-sized amphitheater, designated as the "Joint Information Center" (JIC), where rising lines of work stations—each fitted with a computer—looked down on a central table at which five officials were seated. The controller, T.M. Ferguson, a calm and friendly man in his mid-forties, spoke from the central table:

> Okay, here's the scenario: [yesterday], during evening rush hour traffic, a crop duster was seen flying over the city spraying an unknown substance before disappearing. The Sheriff's Department found the aircraft but not the suspect. At approximately 6:24 pm, the Civilian Support Team of the National Guard Unit presented a presumptive positive [of anthrax] from the local, state, and unified command. The state requested mobilization of the SNS [Strategic National Stockpile] from the CDC yesterday, and it is expected to arrive at the regional distribution site at 9:30, in approximately one hour. They have a twelve-hour window when they have to deliver this stuff. You're asked to take a role in responding, via your regular roles and responsibilities.

The main focus was transporting SNS medications from a central distribution point to various podsites. The location of the main distribution point was never revealed to us. (A distribution did actually take place at a military base: 10,000 employees received bags of M&M candies.)

The JIC, according to Ferguson, was responsible for "tasking the public, through the media, to go to those sites and receive their medications." It essentially had only one job: putting out press releases for distribution to "the media." The "Emergency Operations Center" (EOC), located next door, was "tasked" with communicating with first responders. One press release confirmed the attack and asked people to "await further information" and a second asked "the public" to go to the nearest high school to receive antibiotics. Press releases were drafted by "experienced news writers," ex-journalists who served as city, county, and state public information officers (PIOs), seated at the central table. Participants seated in the front row of the rising lines of workstations received photocopies of draft releases in order to see "if you're okay with it before we send it out." After discussing their suggestions, the News Manager officially approved the press release and handed it to the JIC chief, who then conveyed it to the EOC (by actually walking to the adjacent building), where it was reviewed by the Situation Analysis Team and the Policy Group before approval by the City Manager and Mayor.

A great deal of energy, both during the exercise and during the subsequent "hotwash" (in which participants were asked for one positive and one negative reflection on what had occurred), focused on policing communication. Efforts to keep discourse moving in a linear fashion through "the chain of command" met with some resistance from participants seated in the back rows, as we had little to do throughout the day. When participants complained of this, a tall man in his forties remarked sarcastically, "Yeah, and they wrote the release *before* the exercise!" People who had called their agencies to check in got harsh criticism from a senior official during the "hotwash": releasing information in this fashion before a press release had been officially approved could have engendered discrepant "messages," leading to chaos, fear, and panic in a "real world event."

Most journalists who were covering the exercise rather than serving as registered participants shot their footage and conducted their interviews at the sites where the virtual events occurred, but some "real life" reporters did interviews at the JIC. A local network television news reporter interviewed Cal DiMaggio, the city's director of emergency operations, who had decades of expertise as a senior law enforcement and Homeland Security official. Skilled in media relations, he let the cameraperson get footage of him holding up bottles of Cipro, the antibiotic being distributed virtually, before opening with a strong soundbite:

> It all boils down to one thing: how do we get this medication into the hands of 800,000 people in 12 hours; all our planning is meant for that. Because if we don't, people get sick, and some could die.

As if on cue, the reporter asked, "how prepared are we?" And, as if he had not himself prompted the question, which lies at the heart of "preparedness" logics and practices (Lakoff and Collier 2008; Briggs 2011b; Caduff 2015), DiMaggio jumped right in:

> Always a good question, always a fair one, 'how prepared are we?' . . . The answer would be: *we're getting there*. We're much better than we were in years past, we have a much more directed effort heading in this direction.

As he continued, the exercise blended into discussion of H1N1:

> H1N1, nationally and global, I think, helped prepare the United States and larger communities, like the metropolitan area here, and the state, much more than we would have been without it. . . . We were able to test our

plans and procedures that allow the state and the municipalities within the state to effectively regulate not only medical supplies but medical care for individuals and to absorb *a lot of unforeseen things.*

What then, we might ask, was the pathogen that effectively prompted the exercise? "Anthrax" was mentioned only in official briefings, but H1N1 seemed to be airborne all day long. The H1N1 "wake-up call" sparked the anxious teleology that underlies preparedness logics and investments, a sense of moving towards a goal that would always remain elusive. As was repeated over and over in the hotwash: we had exercised too little in the past, today's exercise demonstrated both strengths and weakness, and we need to exercise much more in the future. The DiMaggio interview ended with both reassurance and anxiousness: "I feel pretty confident that after today's exercise . . . it won't be long before [the city] will be well prepared— as prepared as we can be—to respond to a major biological event." Paraphrasing Chakrabarty (2000), this classic teleology of preparedness seems to place "us" all in the waiting room of preparedness. In an age in which metrics come increasingly to dominate clinical medicine and public health (see Adams 2013a), the power of preparedness discourse rests, as Carlo Caduff (2015:14) has recently argued, on a lack of metrics: there is no way to know if "we" are really prepared.

My experience in other exercises, including on-line, points to the importance of temporalities. The central term here, as exercise designers and Homeland Security officials frequently emphasized, was "situational awareness," second-by-second knowledge of what was taking place at multiple sites and the ability to position one's own responses perfectly in sync. Like playing a computer game, a tiny delay in sensing and responding to an unfolding action or "interject" resulted in failure to play one's role properly, sure to engender criticism in the hotwash phase. (My experience suggests that fear of being called out in the hotwash, either in the JIC or automated evaluations of on-line performance, generated more anxiety than did simulated biological events.) Having been denied situational awareness of the anthrax-related events, it was our relationship to press release production and circulation that constituted JIC participants' situational awareness. We were expected to be constantly cognizant of which releases had been or were being written, when released, and how long they had been in circulation.

The growing scholarly literature on preparedness points to the proliferation of infrastructures of biosurveillance that track entangled changes in the health of humans, birds, and animals and the genetics of influenza and other pathogens.[10] This fascinating research, however, almost never grants more than passing attention to what are considered communicative infrastructures: PIOs, journalists, press releases, and news reports are seldom analyzed as part of biosecurity actor-networks. Here scholars seem to have missed what Cori Hayden (2010) refers to as the politics of the "proper copy," the policing of boundaries between proper and improper copies, and the capacity of this process to define the "constitutive limits" of emergent biopolitical worlds. Overlooking biomediatization means missing what Michael Taussig (1993) characterizes as mimesis, the power of the copy to produce the original and imbue it with materiality and objectivity.[11] The journalism ex-professionals who dominated the JIC writing project assumed a subordinate role by projecting their work as copying—through press releases—the real action taking place elsewhere. In commenting on how the "artificialities," the make-believe character of the exercise, impeded producing the sense of a "real-world scenario," one official suggested that PIOs should get a chance to see the real locus, the Rapid Deployment System (RDS), in action during the next exercise. Another PIO shifted the locus of the real to the EOC, where elected officials and department heads coordinated infrastructures and first-responder activities. These suggestions reproduced a binary politics of the copy that reduced biomediatization to texts that only represented the circulation of microbes, antibiotics, and personnel.

Ironically, it was not an ex-journalist but Preparedness Area Adviser Roger Strong who used a return to H1N1 to deny this politics of the copy:

> I'm a firefighter. I love being out in the field and all that stuff. But it's important to remember [that] these types of events, similar to H1N1, . . . are *public information emergencies* more than *public health emergencies*. . . . The real work during these kinds of events . . . doesn't happen where I was working in the Emergency Operations Center, it doesn't happen with the guys riding the ambulances, it happens in the timely and accurate release of public information. If you guys can do that quickly and accurately, and even if it's bad news, you've got to give the public, "yeah, 30% of you guys are going to die, but here's what you need to do," it's going to come a long way towards making sure that everything comes out smoothly. . . . You guys just don't know how important this JIC function is. So you guys are worth your weight in gold.

Strong stressed the performative capacity of press releases, their ability to *create* the events to which first-responders must respond. For him, biomediatization lay at the core of the H1N1 pandemic just as much as it did for the day's anthrax exercise.

To extend Strong's critique of the ex-journalists' submissive mimesis further: stories about the exercise were what provided the most tangible product of this massive outlay of time and capital. Frequent references in the initial H1N1 stories to biosecurity exercises and planning provide important reflexive clues to why the "swine flu epidemic" story emerged so rapidly and so closely in keeping with the language of the CDC manual, why the story remained relatively stable for months, and why journalists and health and homeland security officials declared that H1N1 demonstrated the value of all the exercises and training. In short, H1N1 showed the growing power of biomediatization. Perhaps it would be accurate to suggest that the stories of 24 April had already been devised in countless encounters between innumerable media, health, and homeland security professionals and audiences and then assembled—details modified to fit a "novel virus"—in 24 hours. If H1N1 is a success story, at least in the United States, it is due less to the functioning of biosurveillance, which triggered a massive response to a virus that was less virulent than many "normal" influenza viruses, than to the way it converted this colossal rehearsal process into a global performance with associated materialities, masking faces, flooding hands with antibacterials, activating stockpiles of antivirals, and producing millions of units of vaccine.

Crisis and containment: controlling the virtual epidemic

Looking ahead for a moment to 2014–15 Ebola epidemic stories, consider a quotation, attributed to a preventive medicine specialist at Vanderbilt University, in the *NYT* the day after the first US death: "At the moment, we have a much greater outbreak of anxiety than we have of Ebola."[12] It is part of a pattern typical of epidemics in general: one central theme of public discussion invariably focuses on the "outbreak of fear" and the danger that this parallel outbreak will ultimately do more harm than the disease. Producing fear may be attributed to various actors, including public officials and the mass public itself, but it is often blamed on "the media" (Wagner-Egger *et al.* 2011). It thus fits the "media distortion" discourse that, as we have seen, is common in both scholarly and public discussions of health reporting. This was a favorite theme in late-night comedy shows in 2009. Jon Stewart, for example, ran a segment a few days into the crisis titled "Snoutbreak '09: The Last 100 Days"[13] that featured clips of some of the most alarmist coverage from television news. Stewart poked fun at the common practice of using animated maps (Figure 4.5) to show the global spread of the disease—which pandemic coverage borrowed from national security reporting, a biomedical parallel to the domino theory of the spread of Communism.

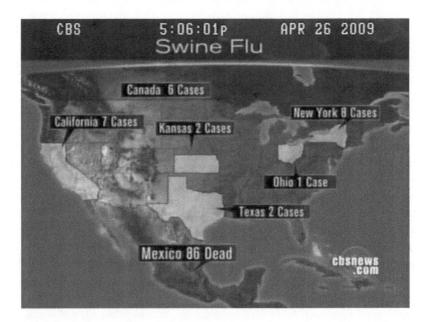

FIGURE 4.5 States and nations turn color as television maps the spread of H1N1. CBS News, 26 Apr. 2009.

After a showing a clip in which Canada is highlighted in red with a graphic showing it had six cases, Stewart quips, "I like a good scare as much as the next guy. But for six mild cases of the flu you're going to turn four million square miles bright red?!" After showing a series of clips of television anchors saying, "We don't want to freak people out," Stewart asks rhetorically, "Do you even watch your own networks? *You're* the only reason we're freaking out!" Even as we appreciate Stewart's humor, we note that it reproduces the same commonsense mode of evaluating health news on the basis of a projected perfect balance between the number and content of news stories vis-à-vis morbidity and mortality statistics.

Discussing coverage of the 1995 Ebola and 2004–5 H5N1 avian flu epidemics, sociologist Sheldon Ungar (1998, 2008) argues that media representations of emerging diseases typically move through three stages, from sounding the alarm to a mixed phase to a phase of containment in which the public is reassured that medicine and the public health system can protect them. These outbreaks began respectively in Zaire and Vietnam, posing a seemingly distant threat to media audiences in Western industrialized countries. Avian flu led to the destruction of poultry in the millions globally but seldom spread between humans. Ungar (1998) argues that the interpretive package characteristic of the alarm phase, which emphasizes the unpredictability and virulence of microbes and the possibility of catastrophic contagion among humans, predominates when the threat remains distant from the media audience. Once understood as close and concrete, the dominant media framing becomes one of reassurance. Ungar implies that these changing "interpretive packages" are patterns of public discourse broadly disseminated by officials, journalists, and experts.

Our sample of stories from five US newspapers, broadcasts that appeared in our national network news sample, and a collection of Internet and social media discussions enabled us to explore how, in the weeks following H1N1's emergence, public health officials attempted both to sound the alarm and to manage the reaction.

Alarm and containment

Was media coverage of the H1N1 story "alarmist"? Certainly, the earliest coverage was dramatic, projecting a tone of alarm. "This sprawling capital was on edge Saturday," the *NYT* reported from Mexico City, "as jittery residents ventured out wearing surgical masks and President Felipe Calderon published an order that would give his government emergency powers. . . . The scene at the airport was alarming."[14] The *NYT* quoted a resident as saying, "The virus could be anywhere. It could be right here"—a typical element of Ungar's contagion–mutation package, the idea that microbes may become ubiquitous. An 28 April *SDU-T* story opened by speaking of "the novel form of swine flu that has gripped the globe" and went on to make a characterization that was common initially:

> It could take a week or more to determine whether the outbreak becomes a pandemic. . . . But epidemiologists are alarmed by the swine flu's ability

to mutate and spread quickly from person to person, combined with a lack of immunity to it in the world population and no knowledge about its long-term effects.

The story contained images of travelers wearing masks and of a woman hugging her daughter at a Tijuana school closed because of the virus—common images depicting threats to ordinary people.

The next day's *SDU-T* reported on a local preparedness document: "If the swine flu crisis reached pandemic proportions in San Diego County, this is what it would look like: nearly 1 million people, or one-third of the county's population, sickened and as many as 3,000 dead." The 1918 comparison was frequently invoked in this period, often with ominous warnings that "millions of people around the world can die."[15] The early tone of alarm was closely tied to official characterizations.[16] "You can tell by the tone of what federal officials are saying," NBC's Brian Williams opened the 24 April broadcast, "that they are concerned about a new strain of flu never seen before." Such statements were also tied to expressions of fear in the general population:

> 'It's one thing to be home with your family, but now I'm out in the street with all these strangers, and you never know who might be infected,' street sweeper Maria Luisa Holguin said [to *USA Today*]. She politely declined to shake a reporter's hand.[17]

Table 4.1 summarizes the dominant tone of H1N1 stories, and shows that "alarming" stories are indeed the largest category.[18] Nevertheless, discourses of reassurance and "containment" were mixed in from the beginning. Taken together, the categories presenting H1N1's threat as uncertain or conveying a mixed message outweigh the alarming stories. US mainstream media coverage of H1N1 never really fit the stereotype of media "hype"; instead, it closely tracked the mixed message of public health officials, and reflected the co-production of the mediatized virus by officials, experts, and journalists that is the focus of this chapter.[19] CBS's 26 April broadcast featured a high-school student at an affected New York City

TABLE 4.1 Tone of H1N1 stories in five newspapers (percent of stories in which threat of virus is represented, $N = 238$)

Negative/alarming	31.5
Positive/reassuring	4.6
Neutral	21.4
Balanced (serious but no need for panic)	11.8
Uncertain (danger not known)	16.0
Skeptical (danger exaggerated, manipulated)	5.9
Humorous	2.5
Other	6.3

school saying, "I think it's really scary, . . . you could die from it," but ended with Medical Correspondent Jon LaPook saying,

> Well clearly there's concern, okay. . . . But to put it in perspective, in the United States, the cases of swine flu so far have been mild. Okay, nobody has died. Officials have been thinking about this for years, . . . they are all over this.

On 29 April, ABC's Medical Correspondent, Dr. Tim Johnson, called WHO Director Margaret Chan's statement that "all humanity is under threat" "a bit excessive," adding, "Most individuals are not at risk. They never will be even under the worst-case scenario. For example, in the big epidemic of 1917–1918 [sic], most people did not get the flu."

In Ungar's (1998, 2008) analyses of Ebola, bird flu, and HIV/AIDS, the shift to "containment" discourse centrally involves "Othering": the disease is asserted to belong to a radically different world, separate from and inapplicable to the reality of "our" lives—in "the West," in the case of Ebola or bird flu, or for middle-class whites and heterosexuals for HIV/AIDS. This kind of framing is typically associated with negative portrayals of the diseased as ignorant and backward. Such "othering" was present to some degree in H1N1 coverage. Stories on Mexico were much more alarming than those on the US and sometimes focused on "the chaos that we're seeing now starting to develop," as Dr. Sanjay Gupta (reporting for CBS in addition to his regular CNN) put it on 27 April. Early coverage often drew a contrast between Mexico's seemingly high case-fatality rate and generally mild US cases. The explanations for this pattern often included stereotypes of poor Mexicans as endangering their health by failing to seek medical treatment promptly. "Experts say some poorer people may be delaying treatment, which could have deadly consequences," reported ABC's Terry McCarthy on 27 April. An extensive elaboration of this theme came in an *NYT* article on 1 May with the subhead, "Culture Plays a Role in High Mortality Rate":

> [O]ne important factor may be the eclectic approach to health care in Mexico, where large numbers of people self-prescribe antibiotics, take only homeopathic medicine, or seek out mysterious vitamin injections. For many, only when all else fails do they go to a doctor, who may or may not be well prepared.
>
> 'I think it has to do with the culture, the idiosyncrasies of Mexicans,' said Dr. Nicolas Padilla, an epidemiologist at the University of Guanajuato. 'The idea is that I don't go to the doctor until I feel very bad.'[20]

We focus on the language of culture in coverage of health inequities in Chapter 6.[21]

Nevertheless, these forms of othering were not central, particularly after the opening days of the epidemic. As US cases increased rapidly, the Mexican focus faded. The vectors for US transmission were generally understood to have been middle-class high-school students who went on spring break trips to Cancun—not people usually subject to stereotyping as threatening, unsanitary subjects. (The *New York Post* had the most colorful origin story, pinpointing a "group of Queens high school students" who "went on a wild spring-break party to Cancun."[22]) Mexicans appearing in television stories seldom fit the stereotype of poor "third world" residents culturally unprepared to act as modern sanitary citizens.[23] Typical is a middle-class resident who appeared on CBS on 26 April saying, "That's why we're all wearing our masks, . . . washing ourselves, drinking lots of water, and if anyone shows *any* symptoms, we'll go straight to a health clinic." References to US Latinos/as as a source of flu risk were mostly absent. "Though the city has neighborhoods with large Mexican populations," the *NYT* reported, "city officials said there was no reason to focus on those communities because the flu spreads quickly" (27 April).

Another kind of "othering" also appeared in H1N1 coverage: historical othering, externalizing the threat of catastrophe temporally. Frequent references to the 1918–20 epidemic quickly incorporated standard qualifications to separate it from the modern era: "However, as experts note, in 1918 there was no Tamiflu, no antibiotics to fight pneumonia, and no powered ventilators."[24]

Another feature of containment involved de-emphasizing phrases like "killer," "deadly," (which mostly disappeared after the first week) and "highly contagious" and stressing the "mild" character of most US cases (Table 4.2), often balanced with warnings not to become complacent: the virus could still mutate into a more dangerous strain. Statistics on deaths from seasonal flu were often included to put H1N1 mortality "in perspective." A 19 May *New York Post* story, "FLU—AND FEAR OF IT," suggested: "After all these weeks, the city's Health Department reports just 178 confirmed cases of swine flu; most victims recovered quickly. Meanwhile, city Health Commissioner Dr. Tom Frieden notes that about 1,000 New Yorkers die every year from flu."

As the *Post* title suggests, journalists frequently foregrounded biocommunicability, warning of panic and overreaction and projecting how officials, laypersons, and reporters could properly manage the circulation of information. "Just as media outlets chose their words carefully in covering the financial crisis last fall—shunning the word 'panic' to avoid runs on banks," the *NYT* reported (28 April), "words and context are crucial in the coverage of a public health threat." As Nerlich and Kateyko

TABLE 4.2 Characterization of H1N1 virus in five newspapers (percent of stories characterizing virus, $N = 119$)

	April	May	June/July
Deadly, killer, lethal	21.4	15.1	0.0
Serious, dangerous	21.4	5.7	20.0
Easily transmitted	26.8	17.0	10.0
Mild, moderate	7.1	49.1	30.0
Changeable, unpredictable	23.2	13.2	40.0

(2012) suggest for Britain, mainstream media and on-line reporting was characterized by a high level of what political communication scholars call metacoverage (Esser and D'Angelo 2006), focusing on media coverage itself.

Some stories paternalistically projected the mass public as over-reacting. Officials—from Obama to local officials—exhorted audiences to inform themselves, not overreact, thereby reproducing the linear biocommunicable model that depicts active lay interventions as pathological or dangerous. *USA Today* quoted a child psychologist: "Parents have to get their own facts straight and calm fears before they approach children." The article continued: "There are plenty of poorly-informed, worried parents. Pediatricians all over the USA have been swamped with calls."[25] A strong version of the biomedical authority model emerged in the *Atlanta Journal-Constitution* (1 May): "The most important thing is to keep up to date with local health authorities and follow their guidance. . . . If you are sick, even just starting to feel sick, consult your physician and stay home." Such assurances that the public could rely on public health authorities for information were common. Recall LaPook's comments that public health officials "have been thinking about this for years" and "are all over this." Collaborative enactment by health and media professionals of the CDC's principle of influenza biomediatization—"*Give people things to do*"—included communicative as much as bodily practices.

H1N1 coverage often echoed Roger Strong's view that communication mattered more in a health emergency than technology. Thus *USA Today* exhorted readers not to rush to pharmacists for antivirals, but to follow official recommendations for prevention:

> . . . President Obama called on Americans Wednesday to help halt the disease's spread by remembering to wash their hands. With so much high-tech medicine available, some may wonder how such a simple step could help. Yet health experts say that basic hygiene is not only more effective, but also more practical.[26]

The "containment package" also emphasized scientific mastery of the virus as an object of knowledge and surveillance. Early characterization of H1N1 as novel, changeable, and unknown never disappeared; health officials and journalists continued warning of future uncertainty. WHO's Chan frequently expressed this in colorful ways. On 11 June she noted: "The virus writes the rules, and this one, like all influenza viruses, can change the rules without any rhyme or reason." Almost simultaneously she reassured the public: "The virus is spreading under a close and careful watch. . . . No previous pandemic has been detected so early or watched so closely."[27] Journalists highlighted efforts by scientists to track and to understand H1N1, often using a metaphor of detective work:

> Things unfolded much like a criminal investigation, with alert epidemiologists cast in the role of the police officer who remembers information on a wanted poster.
>
> (NYT, *27 April, Local*)

It's not exactly the stuff of 'CSI,' but technologies developed by some San Diego life-science companies are playing a helpful role in the real-life swine flu drama that is unfolding worldwide.

(SDU-T, *2 May, Business*)

Public health as national security

"Calm, confidence-inspiring and transmitting compassion even for those who were overtaxing Queens hospitals with mild flu symptoms," an *NYT* columnist wrote about Dr. Thomas R. Frieden, then New York City's health commissioner, "he exhibited evident concern about the situation—but a mild strain of concern, suggesting the current situation was nothing New York's hospitals and leaders couldn't handle."[28] H1N1 coverage portrayed public health officials in a highly favorable manner. This is unusual, given the prevalence of negative portrayals of political leadership, suggesting parallels with the "rally round the flag effect" observed in national security crisis coverage (Zaller and Chiu 1996), where political elites suspend partisan criticism to present political and military leaders as acting in the national interest. Much H1N1 reporting had the feel of national security crisis coverage, like the *SDU-T* on 29 April featuring the headline "Flu fight hits high gear: Nations act to contain, defeat virus." Journalists presented political leaders as making policy through bipartisanship and neutral expertise. "As the administration responds to its first domestic emergency," the *NYT* reported on 28 April, "it is building on concrete preparations made during the administration of President George W. Bush that have won praise from public health experts."

Newspapers quoted politicians relatively rarely; they represented only 12 percent of the source citations versus 51 percent of citations to public health officials, other health professionals and biomedical researchers. Politicians were generally quoted passing on the advice of public health officials. Stories often presented rank-and-file health workers as the equivalent of soldiers at war: "Roach [a public health nurse] and her colleagues at the county Health and Human Services headquarters in downtown San Diego are serving on the front line of the nation's battle against swine flu" (*SDU-T,* 30 April). As Susan Sontag (1990) noted, military metaphors are common in medical discourse.

Marginalized discourses

Containing the virus discursively meant not only controlling the level of response—avoiding "panic" and "complacency"—but also containing competing interpretations. Alternative discourses circulated in blogs, social media, on-line comments, and partisan, activist, and alternative media. One theory that circulated in anti-biomedical/libertarian websites held that H1N1 was created in a government lab, possibly as a biological weapon.[29] Another depicted H1N1 as produced by pharmaceutical companies eager to sell antivirals and vaccines. These theories often focused on the ties Donald Rumsfeld, Bush's secretary of defense, had to Tamiflu developer Gilead Sciences.[30] Neither theory circulated widely in US mainstream media.[31] Pharmaceutical companies' influence on the WHO did, however, become an issue in Europe and other parts of the world. In 2010, the *British Medical Journal* and UK Bureau of Investigative Journalism detailed "conflicts of interest" among WHO advisors who had ties to pharmaceutical companies (Cohen and Carter 2010). That alternative discourses remained confined to narrowly based niche media reflects the "success" of health officials and journalists in structuring H1N1 biomediatization, providing a strong reminder that while the fragmentation of media in the digital age facilitates the spread and persistence of a variety of alternative discourses, mainstream media do still have considerable power to control public discussion.

Some alternative discourses did penetrate the mainstream media agenda, providing challenges to officials' efforts to control framing. Focusing on disease circulation across borders, conservative bloggers, talk show hosts, politicians, and activist groups advanced an argument that H1N1 was a matter of border security (Allison 2009; González and Wingett 2009). "I've blogged for years about the spread of contagious diseases from around the world into the U.S. as a result of uncontrolled immigration," wrote conservative blogger Michelle Malkin. "9/11 didn't convince open-borders zealots to put down their race cards and confront reality. Maybe the threat of their sons and daughters contracting a deadly virus spread from South of the border to their Manhattan prep schools will."[32]

Mainstream media addressed this theme early on. On 27 April, ABC and CBS had reporters at the US–Mexico border. "Border crossings and airports are the new front lines in the battle to halt the flu," reported ABC's David Muir. "While U.S. officials haven't closed the U.S.–Mexico border, they haven't taken their eye off it either." CBS anchor Katie Couric introduced a report from El Paso, saying "it is now potentially the gateway for a deadly virus." Projecting H1N1 as proliferating on the Mexican side had a devastating impact on tourism in the Tijuana area, even though at the time these stories were broadcast there had been confirmed cases in San Diego but not yet in Tijuana. As these stories appeared Duncan at the *NYT* was trying to "spin the story forward," generating new angles and analytical "explainers," including a major story explaining why officials rejected border restrictions. "Everybody at the time was screaming: 'shut the borders, shut the borders!' . . . I wanted to write a story that said . . . when you reach this point in a flu pandemic, . . . when you acknowledge that containment is not possible, it doesn't mean you're saying: 'we give up.'" We were struck in this interview by the similarity between Besser and Duncan in their passion for explaining pandemic flu preparedness plans. After a short time, the border security frame largely disappeared from mainstream coverage.[33]

Another alternative discourse that appeared early and then disappeared characterized H1N1 as a product of industrial pig farming. On 27 April, CBS cited Mexican officials and local residents who suspected that the source was US company Smithfield's pig farm near the town where the first human case was thought to have occurred. That same day, *The Guardian* in the UK published Mike Davis's

article "The Swine Flu Crisis Lays Bare the Meat Industry's Monstrous Influence,"
developing this interpretation.[34] Although this discourse didn't undermine public
health officials' central messages, neither did it contribute to their mitigation goals.
Mainstream media quickly dropped the topic, except for stories debunking the
notion that eating pork products could spread the disease. The pork industry and
health officials called on reporters to drop the term "swine flu," but as Duncan told
us: "'The government calls it technically (S-OIV) H1N1: swine-origin influenza
virus H1N1. Yeah, you know, when that looks good in the headline, we'll adopt
it—that'll be *never.*"[35]

Liberal blogs and public health experts debated whether investment in public
health infrastructure was adequate to deal with a major epidemic, often focusing
on a decision earlier in the year to strip pandemic preparedness funding from the
Obama administration's economic stimulus package in order to win Republican
votes. Little of this discussion made it into mainstream media. Only one story on
this theme appeared in our sample; it was one of the few in which members of
Congress were prominent sources.[36]

Conclusion

Public health professionals often cite H1N1 in 2009 and the October 2001
anthrax deaths as the quintessential US examples of good and bad biomediatization. In 2001, political leaders took control; the CDC was first "muzzled" then
widely derided for botching the response (Winett and Lawrence 2005). In 2009,
the CDC took center stage and was widely praised in the media; politicians were
generally sidelined, appearing mainly to reinforce public health messages. Duncan
said of Besser:

> His movie star good looks aside, . . . he was measured, sensible. . . . There
> was no point at which I said, "God, this guy's a fool, either an alarmist or a
> pooh-pooher." And I thought Obama was exactly the same way, . . . hold-
> ing a press conference to talk about the flu. So the event itself is high drama,
> but his handling of it was calm. And you know, I think it's very impressive
> that the president is willing to get on television and say "Wash your hands."

In the years between the anthrax and H1N1 events, crisis and emergency risk
communication courses and thousands of "exercises," some including officials of
the stature of Richard Besser, Janet Napolitano, and Barack Obama, not to mention
top military and intelligence personnel, and *NYT* journalists, national network and
cable news correspondents, synchronized the registers and discursive practices of
media and health professionals from the smallest local newspaper and public health
office to the centrally visible national news outlets and the CDC. With the possible
exception of the Cold War's focus on civil defense for nuclear war (see Gusterson
1996; Masco 2006), these courses and exercises might possibly constitute the most
extensive and massively funded set of rehearsals in the history of the planet.

"The H1N1 pandemic" merged the processes we explore in this book, mediatization and biomedicalization. Survey data on public opinion confirmed the power of H1N1 biomediatization. Harvard School of Public Health telephone surveys showed, days after the story broke, that 77 percent of US respondents were "following the news very" or "somewhat" closely. High percentages expressed willingness to act on health officials' recommendations; 88 percent reported being very or somewhat pleased with information provided by health officials and 83 percent with how they "have been managing the response" (Harvard Opinion Research Program 2009). Besser at the CDC and the *NYT*'s Duncan were both proud of their roles in managing H1N1. Like Besser, Duncan responded to criticisms that H1N1 coverage might have constituted an "inter-reality distortion" by arguing that news coverage was preventive and that the failure of an epidemic to match worst-case scenarios was a measure of success.

> I think of all those reporters who spent their careers basically covering U.S./ Soviet diplomacy and the Cold War—and World War III never happened. Did that mean they wasted their careers? . . . You know, I think good coverage is part of what kept H5N1 [avian flu] from going pandemic.

H1N1 risk communication reflects deep integration of media logics into institutions of public health and vice versa, foregrounding communicative as much as medical and security "preparedness." Thomas Abraham, a WHO communication officer during the H1N1 pandemic, told us that with "a flu pandemic or any infectious disease outbreak, very often you won't have any other means of response except communication. Because if it's a new disease, there are probably no vaccines, there are no drugs, so all public health people can really do is communicate effectively. . . . There was a huge change from earlier [epidemics], where communication was seen as an adjunct."[37] H1N1 also reflects the incorporation of specialist reporters like Bazell and Duncan into this process and their internalization of modes of understanding and discursive practices on which it is based. Public health officials could never have carried out this response without the active participation of health journalists. Just as media training has taught health professionals to accommodate themselves to temporal and other dimensions of professional practices of journalists, health reporters have become deeply integrated into the forms of knowledge production and circulation of medical and public health professionals. This proximity positions health and media professionals as intimates, particularly during a "crisis."

H1N1 might also be seen as a "success" for legacy media. Though conventional wisdom often assumes that the latter are eclipsed today by digital challengers, it was not the case that H1N1 immediately drove publics to the Internet. The CDC-sponsored Harvard Opinion Research Program surveys reported 59 percent of respondents as following H1N1 in what would normally be called legacy media—local and network TV and newspapers, with TV dominating their attention; only 19 percent favored the Internet and 14 percent cable news. Asked on 6 May, "Have you gotten or shared any information about H1N1 or swine flu online on sites such as Twitter, blogs, Facebook, or discussion boards?" only 6 percent said yes. Analyzing H1N1 tweets, Chew and Eysenbach (2010) found that 23 percent linked to mainstream news sites, 12 percent to news blogs, feeds or niche news, 2 percent to personal blogs, and 2 percent to social networks. Only 1.5 percent linked to government public health sites, underscoring the crucial mediating role of health news. To be sure, media ecologies have changed since then, but they were already shifting in 2009.

H1N1 biomediatization involved a kind of fusion of science, the state, and media, a largely harmonious collaboration between health officials and mainstream journalists, at least until the fall, when controversies over the distribution of the H1N1 vaccine emerged. This stability highlighted biomedical authority biocommunicability, as journalists urged public adherence to advice from public health officials and "experts" and granted them privileged access to the news. Duncan's Cold War analogy evokes the centrality of the securitization of health, not simply to H1N1 in particular but generally to the biomediatization of epidemics. It has parallels to the fusion of media and the state historically characteristic of national security reporting and shifts of news conventions toward what Hallin (1986:117) calls sphere-of-consensus reporting, where officials speak for "the nation" as debate and criticism are minimized.

What are the implications of these communicative practices in "public health emergencies?" In an era when suspicion of the state is central to political discourses and effective state action to address social issues is typically difficult, what Besser called his "little agency in Atlanta" was able to implement a public health response without being immediately undermined by outside critics—including right-wing commentators who deem government agencies incapable of performing any worthwhile role in public health. Certainly if the alternative looked like Ebola in 2014, in which public health responses were thrust into the middle of partisan politics, we might prefer the precedent of H1N1. Besser and Duncan might be right that biomediatization has the potential to mitigate pandemics, and it might have mattered more had H1N1 been more severe.

Nevertheless, there are probably reasons to worry about the eclipsing of debate during "public health emergencies," similar to "national security" crises when journalism and state often become fused (Zaller and Chiu 1996). The Institute of Medicine's Fineberg (2008), a leading figure incorporated by Besser into his "Team B group of experts," drawing lessons from the 1976 swine flu epidemic, put forward two criteria for public health communication: "adequately prepare the media for predictable events" and "deal with contradictory views espoused by contrarian experts." Fineberg argued that in 1976 officials too quickly made decisions based on insufficient evidence, leaving insufficient room for debate and critical reassessment. By his first criterion, H1N1 risk communication was absolutely a success, by the second, less so. Many contradictory views that circulated in 2009 were no doubt legitimately marginalized, but is this true of all of them? Doubts about conflicts of interest at the WHO, for example, were taken seriously by policymakers in much of the world.

Had the virus proved more virulent, issues raised about the adequacy of US public health infrastructures might have been substantiated. H1N1 was a triumph, it could be said, of the low-cost, neoliberal vision of the role of the state in public health as celebrated by George Will (Chapter 1): risk communication is an inexpensive way to protect public health. But it is not clear that it would have been adequate if millions had developed severe complications. Structural issues raised by proponents of social medicine, critical epidemiology, and social epidemiology (Breilh 2003; Krieger 2011; Laurell 1989; Waitzkin 2011) were eclipsed by narrower biomedical perspectives. Researchers suggest that influenza epidemics exacerbate health disparities (Hutchins et al. 2009) and that H1N1 exposure, susceptibility, and access to care were significantly related to race and ethnicity in the United States (Quinn et al. 2011). Widespread perception that the pandemic was much ado about nothing may spring partly from the greater concentration of deaths in poorer regions of Africa and Asia (Dahwood et al. 2012), thus largely invisible to Western audiences. A consensus model of health reporting might limit consideration of social justice issues in pandemic influenza planning by displacing concern with health disparities (DeBruin, Liaschenko, and Marshall 2012). Cartwright (2013) notes that epidemic responses built around models of emerging diseases and health emergencies, subject to short-term saturation media coverage, marginalize long-term chronic health problems like hepatitis C.

The particular harmony achieved in 2009 between health and media professionals is not stable. Thus, we should not imagine biomediatization as a machine that can automatically be set in motion and achieve "successful" results whenever public health crises are declared. H1N1 risk communication reflects particular characteristics of this pandemic and its historical context. If, as Chan said, "the virus writes the rules," public health officials might have lost control over the story if the virus had proved more lethal. It may also have made a difference that the H1N1 pandemic occurred just a few months after Obama's inauguration, when his popularity was high, the next election distant, and partisan conflict somewhat muted.

The CDC's initial success was not repeated in the fall, with the vaccination "rollout." Debates erupted over who was to blame for initial shortages and who should have access to limited supplies. Anti-vaccine forces, whose well-developed alternative networks of health communication include websites like naturalnews.com and nvic.org and extensive listservs, raised safety questions. Chew and Eysenach (2010) found a significant bump in tweets containing "misinformation" in September 2009, as in a naturalnews.com story, "Ten Swine Flu Lies Told by the Mainstream Media" circulated.[38] When NBC's Dr. Nancy Snyderman dismissed the vaccine controversy, anti-vaccine forces circulated mocking videos, showing her in slow motion, sometimes in the guise of a cartoon villain, saying "you know, there's no conspiracy here, folks, just get your damn vaccine! . . . Listen to our government agencies, these guys are telling the truth." This was a moment in which the tensions lurking beneath national network physician/journalists' ability to shift smoothly between roles of reporter, public health spokesperson, and personal physician, that we traced in Chapter 2, were dramatically exposed. Questions about vaccine safety circulated in conservative media outlets. Fox News was divided, with medical contributor Dr. Marc Siegel condemning "fear-mongering" even as vaccine critics got airtime. Mainstream media, as the Snyderman episode suggests, generally backed health officials on vaccination, and early polls showed general public acceptance. Besser interpreted the controversial vaccine roll-out as a misstep in communication: "Had they said that by January we will have vaccine for people, until then you have to do these other measures, and then they had vaccine for people in November—everyone would have said 'Wow! Wow! Incredible!'"

The 2014 Ebola crisis offered a stronger contrast to H1N1 biomediatization. Mainstream media largely cooperated with health officials in disseminating containment-oriented messages, clarifying, for example, that Ebola was not spread by casual contact, but also criticized public health authorities, particularly after the first death in the United States and first US Ebola transmission. A front-page *NYT* article led, "More than six months after an outbreak of Ebola began its rampage through West Africa, local and federal health officials have displayed an uneven and flawed response to the first case diagnosed in the U.S."[39]

The first US transmission of Ebola occurred a month before Congressional elections; Republican politicians and pundits integrated Ebola into a campaign narrative about the failure of the Obama administration to protect the United States from external threats. Calls for strict border controls and claims that officials minimized the danger proliferated on conservative cable, radio, and social media. New Jersey and New York governors repudiated public health recommendations, declaring quarantines on health workers returning from West Africa, who were criticized as endangering public safety. Gossip website TMZ criticized NBC's Snyderman, voluntarily quarantined after she returned from West Africa, for reportedly emerging to go for a cup of coffee.[40] As Joffe (2011) argued, stigmatization and blame during public health emergencies can be directed both downward, toward marginalized groups, and upward, toward government, health professionals, and, we might add, journalists.

Largely absent from US H1N1 coverage, the practice of othering was strongly present during the Ebola outbreak staring in 2014. Conflicting information about Ebola transmission spread widely, as when conservative columnist George Will told Fox News Sunday that Ebola could spread through airborne particles.[41] Exaggerated public fears and stigmatization of victims was extensive, comparable to HIV/AIDS, though more briefly. By October, a Harvard survey showed 38 percent of respondents fearing someone in their immediate family might get Ebola.[42] The difference between Ebola and H1N1 is no doubt rooted in several factors: the different political context, the fact that Ebola proved more transmissible than officials had estimated, the greater familiarity of the flu, typically dismissed as an annoyance more than threat, and the fact that the early coverage from Africa was highly evocative of racialized contagion-mutation frames. Differences in the clinical manifestations of the two diseases, Ebola's higher case-fatality rate, and Ebola's early biomediatization in germ thrillers, including *The Hot Zone* (Preston 1994) and the movie *Outbreak*, are also relevant.

Having analyzed biomediatization at the intersection of biomedicine and the state, we turn to business journalism and the gleaming offices of public relations agencies to explore how the media/biomedicine interface merges with the market in reporting on biotech and "big pharma."

Notes

1 A pseudonym.
2 Also a pseudonym.
3 Researchers have focused on such issues as the frames (Lee and Basnyat 2013; Liu and Kim 2011) and metaphors (Angeli 2012) that dominated coverage, perceptions of risk, uncertainty, and vulnerability (Holland et al. 2012; Stephenson et al. 2014) and associated affective responses (Da Silva Madeiros, Natércia, and Massarani 2010; Mesch, Schwirian, and Kolobov 2013), and how H1N1 compared with other epidemics in terms of a "distancing-blame-stigma pattern" (Joffee 2011). Social media formed a major scholarly focus, including similarities and differences in traditional and social media content (Liu and Kim 2011), the proliferation on social media of conspiracy theories and forms of stigmatization (Atlani-Duault et al. 2015), and the use of on-line comments for gauging lay attitudes and perceptions (Henrich and Holmes 2011). A biosecurity framework treated the circulation of viruses and of information both as "threats" (Caduff 2012; Nerlich and Koteyko 2012). As Caduff (2015) has recently argued, the circulation of scientific knowledge on dangerous viruses in professional journals and news stories is sometimes projected as a greater "threat" than the viruses themselves, given how information can circulate to terrorists. Public discourses about biosecurity can generate, in Lawrence Cohen's (2011:33–34) terms, a type of scandalous publicity that creates a public through the enunciation of a scandal, thereby seeming to require particular forms of redressive actions. Addressing issues of metacommunication and reflexivity (Holland and Blood 2013; Nerlich and Koteyko 2012), researchers explored the question of "over-hyping" (Briggs and Nichter 2009; Hilton and Hunt 2010), the extent to which H1N1 was a "media pandemic" (Lopes et al. 2012) rather than a biological one. Some studies of H1N1 coverage go beyond content analysis, such as Holland et al.'s interviews with scientists and officials who appeared in Australian coverage (2012). Other works are cited elsewhere in the chapter.
4 Interviewed in New York by Charles and Clara Mantini-Briggs 19 Jun. 2009.
5 Press Briefing Transcripts, CDC Briefing on Public Health Investigation of Human Cases of Swine Influenza, 23 Apr. 2009, http://www.cdc.gov/media/transcripts/2009/t090423.htm, accessed 24 Mar. 2012.
6 Interviewed in New York by Charles and Clara Mantini-Briggs 19 Jun. 2009.
7 H5N1 is a strain of avian influenza that had produced considerable concern after outbreaks in 2005 and 2006.
8 Interviewed by Dan in New York on 3 Mar. 2012.
9 http://www.bt.cdc.gov/cri/, accessed 24 Mar. 2015.
10 See for example Caduff (2012), Collier and Lakoff (2015), Lakoff and Collier (2008), Lakoff (2008), Lowe (2010), MacPhail (2014), and Parry (2012).
11 Caduff (2015) suggests that exercises are "para-events," simulating events that haven't quite happened, speech acts that are designed to be infelicitous, in Austin's (1962) terms, to simulate ways of "doing things with words" without performing those actions at all.
12 Manny Fernandez and Dave Phillips, "Ebola Patient Dies in Dallas, Fueling Alarm," New York Times, 9 Oct. 2014:1, 18.
13 http://thedailyshow.cc.com/videos/0v95uj/snoutbreak—09—the-last-100-days, 27 Apr. 2009. Accessed 9 Oct. 2014.
14 Marc Lacey and Elizabeth Malkin, "Mexico Takes Powers to Isolate Swine Flu," 26 Apr. 2009, A1.
15 ABC, 26 Apr. 2009.

16 Vasterman and Ruigrok (2013) similarly found that in Dutch media coverage of H1N1 alarming frames predominated in the early phase, but that these frames originated with official and expert sources on whom the journalists relied.

17 *USA Today*, 28 Apr. 2009.

18 Coders were instructed to code each story for its *dominant* tone, taking into account the headline and lead, as well as the overall balance of assessments presented in the story.

19 There were cases of H1N1 in the United States when the story first broke, so it is consistent with Ungar's framework that containment discourses should be present initially, as Joffe and Haarhoff (2002) found for Ebola in 1995–96. As studies in various countries note, the balance of alarm and containment frame closely tracked statements by public health officials (Vasterman and Ruigrok 2013; Staniland and Smith 2013).

20 Marc Lacey and Elisabeth Malkin, "First Flu Death Provides Clues to Mexico Toll," A1, 10.

21 See Atlani-Duault *et al.* 2015, Wagner-Egger *et al.* 2011, and McCauley, Minsky, and Viswanath 2013 on Othering in H1N1 coverage.

22 Angela Montefinise and Michael Blaustein, "QNS School Fear," 26 Apr. 2009:7.

23 On the distinction between unsanitary subjects and sanitary citizens, see Briggs and Mantini-Briggs (2003).

24 *NYT*, 26 Apr.

25 "Kids Can Be Fearful of Scary, 'Invisible' Illness—Parents Can Help by Staying Informed," 29 Apr.

26 "Stay Safe from Swine Flu with Three Simple Steps," *USA Today*, 30 Apr. 2009.

27 Nick Cumming-Bruce and Andrew Jacobs, "WHO Raises Alert Level as Flu Spreads to 74 Countries," *NYT*, 11 Jun. 2009.

28 Susan Dominus, "It's No Time for Hysteria over New Flu," *NYT*, 26 Apr. 2009: A16.

29 E.g. Mike Adams, "As Swine Flu Spreads, Conspiracy Theories of Laboratory Origins Spread," *Natural News*, 27 Apr. 2009 (http://www.naturalnews.com/026141_flu_swine_virus.html).

30 E.g., owendebanks, "Tamiflu, Rumsfeld and Cheney," *Daily Kos*, 27 Apr. 2009 (http://www.dailykos.com/story/2009/04/27/725102/-Tamiflu-Rumsfeld-and-Cheney#).

31 A content analysis of H1N1 tweets found that only 4.5 percent of English-language tweets contained "misinformation," the category Chew and Eysenach (2010) used for such alternative interpretations of the pandemic. Most came later, beginning in August, as the vaccine campaign ramped up.

32 25 Apr. 2009 http://michellemalkin.com/2009/04/25/hey-maybe-well-finally-get-serious-about-borders-now/.

33 See MacPhail (2014:78) on H1N1 mitigation strategies (hand-washing, social distancing, vaccination, and prophylaxis with antivirals) used by most countries versus China's widely criticized use of containment (including quarantine and border screening).

34 Davis (2005) wrote an avian flu book, *The Monster at Our Door*, using a "mutation-contagion" (Ungar 1998) frame to call for global vigilance against emerging pandemic diseases.

35 The percent of newspaper stories in our sample using "swine flu" rather than H1N1 declined over time, but was still over 60 percent in July. Chew and Eysenbach (2010) found some effect of the pork industry's #oink campaign on the use of the terms in tweets.

36 Fredreka Schouten, "Pandemic Preparedness Money Stripped from Stimulus," 28 Apr. 2009:4A.

37 Interviewed by Dan, Hong Kong, 20 Apr. 2012.

38 Mike Adams, 18 Sept. 2009, http://www.naturalnews.com/027055_vaccine_flu_swine.html (downloaded 12 Feb. 2015).

39 Kevin Sack and Manny Fernandez, "Setbacks on Ebola: Contamination in Dallas, Slow Aid in Liberia," 3 Oct. 2014:A1, 14.

40 http://www.tmz.com/2014/10/13/nbc-dr-nancy-snyderman-ebola-quarantine-restaurant-new-jersey/

41 19 Oct. 2014.

42 Harvard School of Public Health, "Poll: Most Believe Ebola Likely Spread by Multiple Routes, Including Sneezing, Coughing," 15 Oct. 2014 (http://www.hsph.harvard.edu/news/press-releases/poll-finds-most-believe-ebola-spread-by-multiple-routes/).

5

FINDING THE "BUZZ," PATROLLING THE BOUNDARIES

Reporting pharma and biotech

In 2002, the *Wall Street Journal* reported on one facet of biomediatization. Advertising agencies, according to the *Journal*, were increasingly involved in the early stages of drug development, recruiting patients for clinical trials, as "their communication skills help them excel at the task," and in some cases running trials at their own small science and marketing labs.[1] These forms of mediatization, as we shall see, are controversial; but an executive of Omnicon, one of the biggest advertising agencies, defended them to a *Wall Street Journal* reporter:

> All we want to do is speed up the process. . . . [W]e want to . . . look at the molecule in the test tube as a brand. A lot of people don't think a brand is a brand until it has FDA approval. But we are asking, "What is the maximum market potential of this molecule? What will it be when it grows up? What is the message? How should the clinical trial be developed?"

Mr. Harrison's[2] molecule is a "boundary-object" in the original sense of Star and Greisemer (1989; Star 2010): it has "messages" simultaneously in the practices of biomedical science and of marketing. A growing literature has focused in recent years on "pharmaceuticalization," that is, on the power of the drug and medical device industries to transform medicine, culture, and capitalism in such a way as to make human problems seem treatable by drugs. That power is rooted in the capacity of pharma industries to cross social boundaries. Biomediatization is clearly central to it, and in this chapter will explore the shifting and complex relationships between biomediatization and pharmaceuticalization. We will bring to the foreground the role of journalists in constructing pharma as a boundary-object and in both facilitating and policing the flows of knowledge across boundaries that make this form of information capitalism work.

Pharmaceuticalization demonstrates both the power of biomediatization and the need to attend to its specificities: while news coverage of pharmaceutical and bio-technology companies shares many features with other health stories, the networks and practices that give rise to stories of new drugs and devices—and the spectrum of advertisements, Internet sites, medical journal articles, marketing to physicians, and the like—are different in important ways. Going beyond the usual citing of news articles as unanalyzed illustrations to take full analytic account of the role of journalists—including those employed by pharma and biotech companies—in this complex and high-stakes biomediatization process promises to add significantly to our understanding of pharmaceuticalization, not to mention of health, mediatization, and contemporary life more broadly.

In the 1970s, Conrad identified the power and authority of the medical pro-fession, social movements, and interest groups, and the role of organizational and professional activities as the "engines that drive medicalization," which emerges when "a problem is defined in medical terms, described using medical language, understood through the adoption of a medical framework, or 'treated' with a med-ical intervention" (2007:5). Early studies of medicalization seldom devoted much attention to the pharmaceutical industry, but it became a major focus starting in the 2000s (Bell and Figert 2012:779). Three decades later, Conrad suggested that the pharmaceutical industry, genetics, consumers, and managed care had become medicalization's major "engines" (2007). Countering the claim by Clarke *et al.* (2003) that the dominant process has now become one of "biomedicalization," Conrad continues to project a rather reified and stable process even as he seeks to account for these changes. Missing here is how definitions of medicine have shifted in such a way that they have been complexified and transformed by the logics and practices they have colonized.

Relationships between medicine and capitalism are crucial. Scholars have docu-mented the shifting ways that medicine is embedded in capitalism (Navarro 1993; Waitzkin 2000, 2011). Sunder Rajan argues that genomics has significantly trans-formed this relationship, such "that the life sciences represent a new face, and a new phase, of capitalism" (2006:3). Rather than a stable political-economic system that interacts with recent shifts in medicine and public health, he suggests that capi-talism is itself multiple and changing. Pharmaceuticals represent one of the most striking stories of industrial growth in the twentieth century (2006:22), becoming the most profitable US industry (Conrad 2007:15). Sunder Rajan details the het-erogeneous and precarious ways that science and capital are connected through the manufacture and sale of therapeutic molecules and the production of information, the latter involving forms of speculative capitalism that place "vision, hype, and promise" at the center of the production of value (2006:18).

Tracing dynamic relationships between pharmaceuticals and capitalism is what prompted Mark Nichter to coin the term *pharmaceuticalization*. Pointing beyond pharmaceutical agents peddling products or prompting doctors to prescribe expen-sive medicines, Nichter tied pharmaceuticalization to the commodification of health through the assimilation of human problems to medicines (1996[1989]:272).

He argued that "what is being sold to the Indian public today is the notion that health in the short-term can be derived through the consumption of medicines," suggesting that this "ideology" of commodified health "is being swallowed along with the pills that embody it" (1996[1989]:266).

Pharmaceuticalization has been extensively researched in the new millennium. Williams, Martin, and Gabe characterize pharmaceuticalization as transforming "human conditions, capabilities and capacities into opportunities for pharmaceutical intervention" (2011:711). Scholars have described a "pharmaceutical regime," meaning a "heterogeneous socio-technical assemblage" based on

> the close association of medicine with science, the dominance of a science-based pharmaceutical industry with strong links to basic research and the medical profession, and a central role played by government agencies in regulating the process of drug development, production and sale.
>
> (Gabe *et al.* 2015:197)

Das (2015) recently explored a broad ecology of health, disease, and drugs in India, demonstrating how pharmaceuticals enmesh medication, healing, diagnosis, and divination. In Brazil, Biehl (2005) documented how "pharmaceutical governance" joins a reforming state, transnational organizations, and the pharmaceutical industry in framing the right to health as access to pharmaceuticals, resulting in the pharmaceuticalization of public health. Stefan Ecks (2013) suggests that attending to pharmaceuticalization requires questioning standard accounts of the temporality of care as proceeding from lay perceptions of symptoms, attempts to make sense of them, seeking help, receiving a diagnosis and treatment regime; rather, a new illness classification or a new drug may precede and shape the recognition of symptoms (see also Hacking 2007).

Focusing on the United States, Joseph Dumit argued that pharmaceuticalization has eroded space for clinical judgment and "dumbed down and reified" physicians through reliance on statistical logics derived from clinical trials (2012:81). By redefining bodies not as essentially healthy but as inherently ill, creating markets for pharmaceuticals prompts treating not just health problems or risks but also possible future risks. In the end, he suggests, "it is marketers, not scientists or clinicians, who decide what information, knowledge, and facts are worthy" (2012:88–89). Accordingly, "the entire humanistic thrust of medicine is gone," replaced by a pervasive orientation towards creating and expanding markets and maximizing profits. Gagnon and Lexchin (2008) estimated that US expenditures on pharmaceutical marketing and promotion amounted to 24.4 percent of sales, compared with 13.4 percent of sales that went into R&D. Beyond examining news stories and trade publications, Dumit's fieldwork with marketing consultants traced their role in shaping the creation of diseases, research on molecules, clinical trials, professional publications, and appeals to physicians, and advertisements (see also Healy 2004, 2006). In suggesting that pharmaceuticalization is guided pervasively by market logic, he does not capture the dynamism, complexity, and heterogeneity of contemporary capitalisms as elucidated by Sunder Rajan (2006). If pharmaceuticalization is co-produced along with shifting and contradictory logics of capital, it would seem problematic to reduce the production and use of pharmaceuticals to a single logic and a unitary set of affects, motives, and practices.

Dumit draws on news stories about pharmaceuticals but does not document them ethnographically. More generally, in dismissing biotech and pharmaceutical reporters as unpaid advertisers lacking any critical perspective, researchers evince a lack of interest in who these media professionals might be and how they work. Remarkably, scholars who focus on health news seem to have almost no interest in pharmaceutical news, despite its prominence across media venues, perhaps reflecting their predominant focus on individual diseases, perhaps also an assumption that business news in general is uninteresting, merely transmitting information to investors. Health stories that appear in business sections intimately connect complex technoscientific detail, clinical practice, consumer aspirations, demands by patient advocacy groups, investments and stock prices, and an emphasis on the scientific, humanistic, and market reputations of companies and their CEOs. If relationships between capitalism and medicine are mediated by "vision, hype, and promise," then analyzing this genre of health stories might add greatly to our understanding of pharmaceuticalization. This chapter analyzes stories focusing on drugs and devices and draws on our ethnographic work with scientists, marketers, clinicians, journalists, and audiences in opening up this line of research. We are particularly interested in the role of journalists in performing forms of "boundary-work" that regulate the complex relations between multiple, shifting logics of science, medicine, capitalism, and—we would add—journalism.

The biotech beat: a *New York Times* example

Richard Campbell, an *NYT* biotech and pharma reporter, has read the *Wall Street Journal*, *Times* of London, and the *NYT* by 6:30 AM; then his day really begins.[3] Evenings, after deadline, are for meetings: "Basically, any CEO or Chief Scientist who wants to come see me or talk to me on the phone can do so, . . . if they're at all relevant to what I'm doing." Campbell decided to pursue science writing in high school. Viewing environmental issues as the most important interface between science and public policy, he earned a bachelor's degree from an Ivy League university and a Master's in engineering from a leading scientific university. After reporting for the *NYT* on areas related to engineering, Campbell had become a leading pharma and biotech reporter by 2007. His opening comment to me, Charles, reflected both a surprising degree of humility and just the sort of boundary-work that makes biotech and pharma journalism so interesting:

> For your project you would probably benefit more from talking with our health reporter than from me because, in fact, I was surprised my name even came up. I'm really a business reporter, I do write for the science and health sections, but a lot of what I do is kind of corporate.

As he moved between science, medicine, capitalism, and journalism, the interview with Campbell emerged as one of the most illuminating.

Summarizing journalism's role in the flow of biotech information, Campbell invoked linear, hierarchically organized biocommunicability: "we play a role in making the information widely available, and to a more general audience, and in simplified, understandable terms." In distinguishing his role in the *NYT's* division of labor, Campbell complicated this picture. In our study of the *Chicago Tribune* and *NYT* (Hallin, Brandt, and Briggs 2013) we documented that health and medical reporting can address patient-consumer, citizen, professional, investor, and other audiences—and that many stories interpellate readers in multiple roles. (One of the main changes over time was an increase in reporting addressed to investors, from about 1 percent in the 1960s to 15 percent in the 2000s.) Even as Campbell disclaimed having a sense of his audience, he invoked all of these target audiences. Separating his reporting from health-related service journalism, Campbell characterized his stories as less oriented to "the individual who reads something we write and decides to do something." He explained, "a lot of what I write about, the really techy stuff, is over most people's heads. . . . Some new technique in genomics . . . has probably a much more specialized readership." Campbell continued:

> I still think of my mission mainly as to inform. . . . I think information, shedding light, is valuable in its own right. I think people want to know about the latest medical developments that affect their health, so I try to write about significant developments, new drugs that might really change the way some disease is treated, or problems with some widely used drug which people might want to know about. A lot of the coverage I do, since I'm in the business section, is more corporate; there, I guess, you are mainly trying to inform investors. Even there I look for articles that have some sort of public policy angle or a public health angle. I mean, these articles we did on the anemia drugs, I chose to do them not because they were affecting the stock of Amgen, . . . but largely because these drugs are used by millions of people.

Campbell clearly rejects the claim that journalists thoroughly embrace a construction of audiences as "sovereign consumers" (Boyer 2013:4).

Campbell did not, however, project stable, sharp, clear borders between "beats." When I asked him how the *NYT* decides who covers which stories, he replied:

> I don't think there are any hard and fast rules; often it's whichever reporter wants to do a story. Sometimes more than one does and you just negotiate. Sometimes no one wants to do a story; we realize it should be done, and we're pushing it off on the other guy.

Similarly,

as far as where [a story] runs in the paper, that's also a decision that's made by consultation. Some clearly are Business, some clearly are for the Science or the Health section. But there are a lot that are in the middle, sometimes the same kind of subject can end up in one place one week and the other another week.

Campbell's attraction to biotech reporting springs from his sense that "it's really on the frontier . . . it's cutting edge science, cutting edge medicine. . . . There are always a lot of things going on." Here he echoes Stratton-Domenici consultant Harrison's words; Rabinow (1996) suggests that a sense of intellectual freedom and creativity also attracts scientists out of universities and into biotechs. Campbell echoes scholarly projections of how "genomic information traverses circuits of exchange . . . at resolutions and speeds inconceivable before," creating a temporality of "breathlessness" (Sunder Rajan 2006:43). Leading biotech/pharma reporters like Campbell receive a daily deluge of press release and pitches, each projecting breaking news of a discovery on the advancing edge of science and medicine. Rather than assimilate this breathlessness, however, Campbell and the other biotech/pharma journalists we interviewed practice the sort of "slowing" advocated by STS scholar Isabelle Stengers (2005), repositioning such claims within the decade or more it takes to bring a molecule through clinical trials to FDA approval and marketing, separating successes from the hundreds of projects that die along the way. It is this temporal politics of slowing that helps print biotech journalists hang on in a digital age. "Spot news is going to the web," Campbell suggested. Unless a story is really big,

> with the web now, there's a presumption that [spot] news is going to be read by the people really interested, they're going to read it on the Internet. So we're being encouraged now to do less routine news that can be covered by the wires.

Most days, nothing happens on his beat that makes him feel compelled to write a story. Rather, Campbell takes notes on "spot news" until a pattern emerges, then conducts research, does interviews, and writes, often over a period of months or years, until sufficient detail, depth, and analysis emerge. Campbell thus rejects what are projected as the dominant temporalities of on-line journalism—"managing multiple fast-moving flows of information already in circulation" (Boyer 2013:2–3)—and of biotech—"massively compressed R&D time" (Sunder Rajan 2006:43)—by turning his work into *slow journalism*. Indeed, some of his stories seek to put the brakes on particular biotech trajectories themselves, seeing them as too fast, chaotic, and unregulated, leading to misalignments between the scientific/medical and financial trajectories of particular corporations or entire areas of research and development.

As we saw in Chapter 3, health news often contrasts with the "negativity bias" media scholars observe in other genres. Campbell explains:

I think in journalism . . . there might be a little bit of a bias toward negative stories. We're all trying to dig up dirt basically on the pharmaceutical industry, but when it comes to drugs, to drug development, I have a positive bias. . . . [Y]ou have a company that announces that their drug failed . . . and the company pretty much collapses. . . . [T]here's not that much interest among . . . my editors. So I tend to more cover if the drug works; then it goes beyond the investors because then you say, 'Okay, we have a new drug that's going to treat some disease that our readers [have].' The failed drug is not going to treat some disease, not going to affect the medical care of our readers, it just means that investors in one particular obscure company got wiped out.

Campbell simultaneously confirmed the shift toward more critical reporting noted in Chapter 3:

What used to be the best way onto the front page, and it's still a good way, is some great medical breakthrough. But now there's a little more suspicion of the medical breakthrough; now the way onto the front page is mostly 'such and such company hid evidence of problems.'

Why the change? Campbell attributed it to two factors: the rise in healthcare spending and the aftermath of scandals, most notably the Vioxx controversy, examined below. Donald Schultz, the cable news health journalist we discussed in Chapter 2, added that major media venues are now owned by major corporations, which are very interested in holding down skyrocketing health insurance costs for their employees.

Campbell suggested that scandal or conflict of interest is what readers respond to the most. Health stories are popular, often "right near the top" of the 10 most frequently e-mailed articles, but stories attracting the most attention focus on "some scandal about health." He pointed, literally, to a story reporting problems with a sleeping medication posted on the website only a few hours earlier; it had already reached the top-10 on the e-mail charts. Accordingly, he said,

we don't accept things as readily as we used to. We have to always . . . mention . . . if a researcher we're quoting has some financial conflict of interest; and if we don't, there's someone who's reading us who's going to ding us on that and say 'you lazy or irresponsible reporter'. . . . And sometimes we go further and try to report that so and so's opinion is not reliable because of such a conflict.[4]

In many ways, his comments are reminiscent of how political reporters characterize their role after Watergate: "How reporters make their mark is finding some evidence of corruption in the pharmaceutical industry or conflicts of interest or fraudulent data or something, unnecessary expenditures, so there's kind of this whole frenzy to find things like that." This "watchdog orientation" in pharma coverage is clearly connected with Campbell's emphasis on public policy. He cited his articles on potentially lethal side effects not disclosed by corporations or researchers that forced a reluctant FDA to act. The purpose of this kind of watchdog reporting, as Campbell's describes it, is less to push citizens to engage actively in debates than to push elites—particularly manufacturers and government agencies—to act. These two sides of pharma reporting—the orientation toward finding the winners and the hunt for contradictions—are manifested in the two types of "boundary-work" that form the focus of this chapter.

Boundary-Work I: modeling relationships between patient subjectivities, technoscience, and business

In what we call *Boundary-Work I*, journalists chart relationships among technoscience, medicine and capitalism positively. They project interactions that connect these fields at specified, bounded points, such as public releases of scientific and clinical information. The integrity of each is not compromised, and diverse actors and social values—profit, scientific progress, the preservation of human life—are in harmony. Some stories present this merging of social fields as automatic and effortless. In Chapter 3, we considered a television story on a new melanoma drug, Ipilimumab, built around a young woman diagnosed with cancer weeks before her wedding. The story, set primarily in the doctor's office, segued abruptly to a meeting of the American Society of Clinical Oncology—where the story actually originated—and the correspondent noted: "For drug makers it's a crucial opportunity to find investors. For oncologists it's a one-stop shop to learn about landmark drugs like 'Ipi' that, if approved, might one day save their patients." Here, business, medicine, science, and journalism merge, as though their relationships are natural. Pharma coverage sometimes tells a much more complex story in which all players, their interests and forms of knowledge, are in some way blocked from connecting. The stories' heroes find a way to bring them together, and journalists often portray themselves as assisting this process. Despite the variation in content and focus, the emphasis, to draw again on Rabinow (1996:180), is on the novelty of the forms/ events generated, which is what is offered to investors. Biocommunicable cartographies are divided—if the story is positive—into parallel but distinct mappings of "science models" and "business models," even as the events reported are largely events of biocommunicability.

Boundary-work is often understood more narrowly as *separating* fields; Gieryn's (1983) interpretation of the efforts of scientists to distinguish their work from non-scientific types of knowledge production takes this form. The sort of journalistic boundary-work we discuss here is different. As Star (2010: 602–603) writes, "Often a boundary implies something like an edge or periphery," but it can also be understood "to mean a shared space, where exactly that sense of here and there are confounded." Journalists' boundary-work involves drawing lines: they construct the world of science and of business as necessarily requiring separate domains with distinct cultures, mapping proper channels. But the specific parameters of the *flow between domains* is central to their stories, which are often precisely about how barriers between domains are *overcome*. Journalists see themselves as interacting with other actors in mediating pharmaceutical biocommunicability, producing pharma as a boundary-object that is not between but, ideally, *fully in* the worlds of science, business, and medicine, harmonizing them.

Perhaps the most usual type of Boundary-Work I story features upbeat reports on "discoveries" or "breakthroughs." ABC World News Anchor Diane Sawyer and reporter David Muir provided a "package" on 29 April 2010 that announced "groundbreaking news in the fight against cancer." The "hook," the event projected as occasioning the report, was FDA approval of the drug Provenge (sipuleucel-T) produced by biotech Dendreon for patients with advanced prostate cancer. Smiling physicians and patients reinforce the emotional framing, summarized by Muir as "real hope." Two common features of these stories stand out. First, Sawyer and Muir project the trajectories of science and discourses as advancing swiftly: "a *real first*" for science. Scientific pasts have headed toward this precise moment: a cancer specialist declares: "this is something investigators have been trying *decades* to accomplish." The story then projects hopeful futures, scientific and biocommunicable—physicians "predict that within five years time there could be other announcements: same kind of treatment, different cancers." A second feature is the projection of a broad consensus regarding scientific/communicable trajectories. Sawyer frames Muir's words as "the latest reaction from the medical community," uniting all physicians into a single voice: "Doctors today said . . ." Muir cites studies published in medical journals and FDA approval. The consensus is confirmed visually by smiling patients and physicians. A boundary separates research and clinical testing from the business of biotech research and pharmaceutical sales as Muir warns, "But the drug will be very expensive, at least a $50,000 price tag." Muir is thus watching out for possible conflicts or misalignments between business and science.

In television news, on the air and on-line, most pharma coverage is oriented toward patient-consumers. In the newspaper, it is more varied and often appears in the business section or is covered by business reporters. In the *SDU-T*, as in other regional newspapers, it often focuses on local biotechs. Sunder Rajan (2006) emphasizes the distinct relationships between science, medicine, and capitalism in biotech and pharmaceutical corporations. The former tend to be smaller, focusing on selling patents and "information" rather than vast quantities of drugs. Accordingly, reporting on Pfizer versus a small biotech company is not the same. Biotech coverage mixes scientific, medical, and financial trajectories with the personal profiles of CEOs and leading scientists and projections of an ethos of daring and discovery, of breathlessness. Some appear in the *SDU-T* in the weekly series that profiles business leaders. When reporter Thomas Kupper interviewed, Tina Nova, the CEO of Genoptix, which provided laboratory analysis and diagnostic testing for physicians, he focused on the scientific and technological base of the company's services, its business model, and how it distinguishes itself from competitors, as well as on Nova herself.[5] Kupper's biotech insider's perspective projects Nova's career trajectory in relationship to how the San Diego biotech sector has changed through time. Nova characterizes the company's niche in biocommunicable terms—as centering on a "culture" that preserves "intimate" relations with customers, such that physician/salespersons cultivate first-name relations with physician/customers.

Patients sometimes enter biotech stories, producing forms of biocommunicable border-crossing. Recruited and prepped by consultants like Harrison, working with physicians referred to them by the pharma company, their appearance in profiles, quotes, and photographs introduces another subject position and projects the positive effects that accrue when boundaries between scientific research, technology, clinical practice, and business are brought into proper alignment. In "Personal Touch in War on Cancer," *SDU-T* biotech reporter Bradley Fikes introduces ovarian cancer patient Jan Amato and a biotech executive, Dr. Laura Shawver. A PhD in pharmacology who herself faced ovarian cancer, Shawver established the Clearity Foundation to provide genetic profiles of tumors. Fikes frames her decision in biocommunicable terms, as responding to problems of knowledge that she encountered in moving between roles of patient and scientist and overcoming biocommunicable barriers. "'The numbers are against us, and there's not enough of us, and we don't make a lot of noise, and therefore we don't get a lot of attention for a very difficult problem,' Shawver said." The story closes as Amato projects herself as the model active patient-consumer: "'The information's out there, and always ask questions. If I had given up right then and there, you wouldn't be talking to me now.'" Patients, physicians, scientists, administrators, and, implicitly, journalists all play distinct roles that can afford happy endings.

"Brothers Develop New Device to Halt Allergy Attacks," appearing on the *NYT* Business Section's front page on 1 February 2013, projected positive connections between technoscience and capitalism. Reporter Katie Thomas follows the "single-minded quest" of twins Evan and Eric Edwards to construct a simpler device than the one they carried everywhere as children to deliver epinephrine to treat effects of their severe food allergies. "Evan Edwards said the device [he invented] was special because it was designed by people who were intimately familiar with patients' needs. . . . 'This was something that I knew I was going to carry with me every single day.'" Linear constructions of time, knowledge production, and business merge in the fifteen-year trajectory from an idea born from two patients' experience to marketing the device.

Some Boundary-Work I stories provide as much space for lay agency and knowledge production as found in any health news story. Campbell reported FDA approval of a treatment for a rare inherited renal (kidney) disease. He leads with a biocommunicable event, a young patient's appeal: "Reluctant to say it aloud . . . she wrote her 12th birthday wish on a restaurant napkin: 'To have my disease go away forever.'" Constituting a "disability narrative," the story charts the transformation of familial ties into "mediated spaces of public intimacy" for "the body politic as a whole" (Rapp and Ginsburg 2001:550, 545). Such stories portray pharma as bridging barriers between science, business, and broader life-worlds. Confronted shortly after their daughter's birth with the likelihood that she would die prematurely, the napkin-borne wish moved the parents to create a foundation. Invoking the story's biocommunicable "peg," patient and mother are pictured in Washington, "where they awaited word about federal approval." Launched by a press release, conference call, and preceding PR/media "pitch," Campbell told Charles, the story merges subjectivities and daily illness experiences of patients and their families, clinical research, and information on the company's finances. The foundation's website presented the press release, news stories, and a video. Although Campbell positions the story as "yet another example of the important role that determined parents and disease foundations can play in supporting drug development, particularly for rare diseases," he also introduces a discordant element. The new drug would increase the annual cost of treatment from $8,000 to $250,000, raising "troubling questions about whether society can afford to pay extremely high prices for drugs that treat rare diseases."

How "buzz" crosses boundaries: a case study

Our *SDU-T* sample included a profile of a local company, which we will call Venus Pharmaceuticals, and its founder and CEO, Dr. Barney Smith. Charles interviewed Janet Hughes, the reporter, and John Kraus, Venus's media/public relations chief.[6] Telling a heroic story, Hughes' lead uses popular culture to position Venus within a biotech biocommunicable community: "Venus Pharmaceuticals has been the reluctant Rodney Dangerfield of the biotechnology community: it couldn't get no respect." The next paragraph anticipates a happy ending and the boundary-work it requires, linking a new molecule, a "pioneering" class of drugs, and "several new, lucrative corporate partnerships." The following lines, citing CEO Smith, project the notion that a biotech's scientific evolution is identical with its biocommunicable contours, charting a path of "a novel idea" through "initial wild enthusiasm, tremendous disappointment, skepticism turning to bias, bias turning to grudging acceptance, acceptance, and, the final stage, 'Oh, yeah, it was my idea to begin with.'"

The next two paragraphs shift to a scientific register, detailing the drugs' mechanism for delivering its genetic "message." The article summarizes the scientific focus of Venus' work:

> In the lab, RNA molecules could be inactivated by complementary RNA molecules that bind to that specific RNA sequence, blocking their effects. In a person, the technology might stop any disease involving RNA, which could be nearly any disease. And because the blocking RNA molecules, called 'antisense,' could be precisely targeted, the drugs could avoid many side effects.

Hughes then lays out the boundaries between science, technology, and capital, understood here as creating hurdles to be overcome: "Antisense is an elegant idea, beautiful to behold on paper. But putting it into practice has been a nightmare for researchers—and for investors." After two major failures and a "bleak" period, stock "plunged 65 percent on news of the Crohn's disease trial results." Venus researchers went back to the science, producing a new antisense-based technology

for automating discovery of genes and their functions, creating "a second genera-
tion of more powerful drugs." Hughes praises Venus for displaying what it takes to
cross these boundaries: perseverance, innovation, confidence, and "buzz," a sense
of excitement.

Largely a story about Venus's progress toward "the creation of an entirely new
kind of medicine," the plot's twists and turns, its tragic and heroic periods, emerge
from biocommunicable problems. Honest biotechs report clinical results, but
competitors and naysayers reframe statements unpredictably and unfairly, creating
volatile reception frameworks. "Buzz" is mediated by business analysts' recircula-
tions of public announcements as performative statements that can cause stocks
and reputations to soar or plunge. Hughes does not point out that biotech news
stories are very much part of this process. Smith models the ethical posture that
is demonstrated in corporate biocommunicable terms: "'All of us here became
convinced that antisense would be even bigger than we thought. . . . We were
sitting with the data, . . . but no one was paying attention.' Smith said. 'Then all
of a sudden . . . half a dozen major companies were quietly knocking at [Venus's]
door. . . . The buzz had begun – somewhat to [Venus'] surprise.'"

This story depicts a transition from misalignments between science, technology,
health, capital, and biocommunicability to the emergence of a perfect fit. As the
story closes, Smith voices this teleology: "'I'm personally amazed that I live in a
time when someone can say, 'Hey, I got an idea, don't know if it's going to work,
but I know it will take 10 to 15 years and probably a billion dollars or so—would
you mind giving me some of that?' And they did.'" The heroism and positive teleology culminate in a human-interest angle as a lung cancer patient thanks Venus
for the experimental drug that extended his life.

Biotech buzz itself can threaten boundary-work. "Jaded" participants can divert
biotech biocommunicability away from accurate statements made by scientists
and clinicians and assessments of companies' finances afforded by Chief Financial
Officers (CFOs), analysts, and investors. Biotech buzz is a label for a purportedly pervasive form of biocommunicability—an economy of rumors circulated by
unauthorized parties, particularly competitors—that creates communicative chaos.
Self-interest and malfeasance fuse science and capital in ways that can turn a biotech hero into a "reluctant Rodney Dangerfield." Hughes indicates that restoring
biocommunicable order requires scientists like Smith to keep doing the research
and accurately announcing results and CFOs to keep balancing the books and
making fiscal information available. Specialized biotech journalists carefully monitor biotech buzz, which helps them develop story ideas and angles, but they also
accord themselves a crucial role in restoring biocommunicable order by going to
the proper sources and making sure that boundaries are in place. If "hype" is a fundamental part of biotech and pharma, as journalists and social scientists insist, then
specialized reporters like Hughes and Campbell crucially police biomediatization.

Our interviews detailed how the story emerged. For Hughes, writing a profile
"about once every two months" was challenging.[7] It involved choosing "someone
who's interesting and who's in the news and sometimes it's difficult to do. I might

find them interesting, but are they going to be interesting to the broader audience of the *Union-Tribune*?"

Charles also visited Venus, located in a biotech cluster north of San Diego, and interviewed Corporate Communications Executive Director John Kraus.[8] He met Kraus at one of the company's two low, modernist white buildings set in a semi-desert landscape. In his mid-fifties, Kraus, who has a strong jaw, short, graying hair, and a confident air, was dressed informally. Holding an Ivy League humanities degree and an MBA, with 10 years experience at San Diego and San Francisco Bay Area biotechs, he handled communication with investors, potential customers, and journalists as well as speechwriting. He also contracted with "suppliers," firms like Stratton-Domenici, to develop overall public and media relations strategies organized around major events, particularly reporting scientific or clinical results or FDA decisions. Kraus's job involved convincing corporate officials and scientists to meet with journalists, training them on media strategies, writing soundbites, and prepping them on particular reporters and story angles. Another PR/media consultant we interviewed, Johanna Rice, said that her portfolio includes preparing physicians for questioning by FDA advisory committees as research moves from Phase II to III clinical trials, "making sure that all the physicians are on board to support the findings." In the case of questionable findings, she wants "to make sure they're all . . . delivering the same message," adding that "typically you're going to know what the FDA is going to question about your data." She added to her list sponsoring health fairs and organizing disease awareness events with "screenings, free testing, and face painting for the kiddos, and all this is all brought to you by Johnson & Johnson."[9]

Kraus's account of how he develops a "wonderful symbiotic relationship" with biotech journalists paralleled Campbell's emphasis on how a slow temporality separates biotech reporting from "spot news." The temporalities he projected were multiple, involving years of building relationships with biotech journalists, months of build-up to a major news event, and a six-hour turnaround at critical moments. Here we see the other side of biomediatization: Stratton-Domenici's Harrison emphasized the power of mediatization in shaping the production of diseases and molecules, structuring clinical trials, and disseminating clinical results; here, it is the temporalities of technoscientific research and testing—along with those of FDA oversight—that structure the temporal contours of biotech/journalist interactions. Kraus laid out a hierarchy of media and biotech journalists: "The *Wall Street Journal* is God. If you get covered there, unless it's a really bad story, any ink is, more or less, good ink." National media venues like the *NYT* and national network and cable news are in the middle, with "local" reporters on the bottom. Kraus likes journalists who are "in tune with biotech," entailing training in a scientific field, long-term involvement with biotechs, and an understanding of "the biotech business model," i.e., losses for many years in anticipation of huge future profits. Kraus sought to shape, not just react to, this hierarchy: "You build up the trust, you dole the embargos in some way, and dole out the exclusives."

Despite the bias against "local" media and anger over previous *SDU-T* articles, Kraus convinced his boss, Smith, to grant the interview, arguing that the profile format would facilitate the "big picture" story that Venus needed. Kraus asserted that biotech journalists are only interested in "scientific breakthroughs" and dramatic changes in stock prices or revenues, in effect that they are enamored by the biotech "breathlessness" highlighted by Sunder Rajan (2006:43). (Note here the gap between Kraus's perception of biotech reporters and the way our journalist interviewees described themselves.) A profile, on the other hand, would show that Venus's strength was in their "technology platform," generating patents on an "incremental" basis. Kraus "pitched" the "hook" that became the narrative core of the story, the recent transformation of biotech buzz from skepticism to acclaim. He then briefed Smith and the chief scientific officer, talking to them about Hughes's "strengths and weaknesses," the angle that Kraus and Hughes had negotiated, and what Venus wanted to accomplish. The three men gathered, Hughes phoned, and the interview lasted nearly an hour.

We do not read this example through the simplistic narrative that positions biotech/pharma journalists as handmaidens to the industries they report. It rather provides a parallel—*mutatis mutandis*—to the way crisis and emergency risk communication training and biosecurity exercises gradually enmeshed media and health professionals. Biotech reporters construct themselves as uniquely able to operate in all of the spheres that make up this industry, including those of the affected patients and consumers, as capable of understanding the specialized registers that constitute them and crossing boundaries on a daily basis. By virtue of their role in selecting companies and biocommunicable events that evince larger patterns, biotech reporters position their individual stories as allegories, as enabling them to regulate the buzz and hype that excites scientists as much as investors. These stories are thus crucial boundary-objects (Star and Griesemer 1989) that construct an overall sense of what constitutes "the biotech community."

Biotech/pharma journalism has its own complicated relations with capital. Most reporters work in for-profit media corporations, though some work in such organizations as the Kaiser Family Foundation or non-profit activist groups. We related in Chapter 2 the insights that emerged from an interview with Donald Schultz, the founding health journalist at a major national cable news network. He noted that one of the networks' original and major advertisers, a pharmaceutical corporation, made its advertising revenue contingent on producing two health news stories daily. Although Schultz asserted that a policy of editorial independence shielded correspondents and producers from influence by the advertiser, he admitted that conflicts sometimes emerged and lines could get a bit fuzzy: "in practice . . . some things were covered in ways they might not have been if they didn't have that pharmaceutical financing." Direct-to-consumer pharmaceutical advertising, the rise of the Internet and digital media, and many other changes in both healthcare and media deepened and complexified the relationship between health news and advertising. Watch what happens when you click on a health story on the on-line version of a major newspaper: health-related advertisements often pop up next to it. Even as they claim a special, disinterested role in policing boundaries between technoscience/medicine and capital, some of the boundaries between journalism and capital can get messy too.

Boundary-Work I plays a crucial role in mediating contradictions between bio-medicine, public health, and capital. "Big pharma," we hear, is the corporate sector that US residents love to hate; in 2013, Gallup found that the pharmaceutical industry had a net negative rating of ten percentage points among their respond-ents, tied with the banking industry and ahead, among major industries, only of oil and gas.[10] Another poll, however, found 73 percent of respondents saying that prescription drugs have made the lives of people better.[11] We are more medi-cated than ever, and big pharma is making huge profits. How can we explain this apparent combination of fascination and ambivalence? Given skepticism regarding science, biotechnology, clinical medicine, and business elites, many doubt that medicine and capitalism can happily co-exist, at least in ways that enhance the health and well-being of "the 99 percent." Boundary-Work I presents a reassur-ing message: science, technology, clinical medicine, and business can, in Rodney King's famous words, all just get along, producing knowledge for science, health for patients, and profits for investors. When we hear the voices of patients saved by newly discovered drugs or granted access to a "normal life," we can all participate actively in a humanitarian reason (Fassin 2012) that enables us to imagine complex and powerful processes as carried out—at least ideally—by individuals who might one day be standing at our side.

Boundary-Work II: villainous hybrids threaten biocommunicabilities and consumers

Boundary-Work II stories, on the other hand, project journalists' work of policing the technoscience/medicine and capital boundary through cases in which bounda-ries are seen as crossed and interests conflated in ways that are unethical and endanger patients, investors, governmental budgets, or corporate bottom lines. In our inter-view, *SDU-T* reporter Hughes used a metaphor for Boundary-Work II: "the smell factor." In examining articles in medical journals or press releases, she looked out for something "that smells," that is, for "b.s." emerging from a precarious scientific or financial element, a misfit between different domains, or the corruption of the logics and practices in one sphere by pressure from another. The most serious abuses spring from the corruption by capital of the integrity of scientific, technological, or clinical work. Boundary-Work II articles sometimes focus on biotechs, but big pharma has received the most extensive attention and scathing criticism.

Biotech reporting has been transformed, as political reporting was in an earlier era, by scandals emerging at the beginning of the twenty-first century. Thalidomide in the early 1960s and the Dalkon Shield in the 1970s generated substantial cov-erage and public debate regarding how patients are harmed when faulty clinical trials or withholding negative data lead to marketing unsafe products. Anemia and diabetes drugs have both sparked controversy since 2004. But it was the scandal that unfolded after Merck voluntarily withdrew its Cox-2 inhibitor, Vioxx, on 30 September 2004 that dramatically reshaped health news narratives, journalistic practices, and popular views of the US pharmaceutical industry and biomedicine. Anger against Merck and distrust of the pharmaceutical industry were exacerbated by perceptions that, to protect some $2.5 billion in annual sales, the company withheld data suggesting that Vioxx increased the risk of heart attack and stroke.

Though controversies over Vioxx had surfaced in the media from time to time for years, such as in a 12 June 2001 *NYT* "Personal Health" column by Jane Brody, the drug's main media presence before 2004 was its massive visibility in direct-to-consumer advertising. Television news was blanketed with soft-focus ads, reminiscent of 1980s Pepsi campaigns. Featuring parents or grandparents interacting happily with children, they began and ended with the slogan, "Vioxx: for everyday victories." Here in its purest form was the ideal of boundaries overcome, science and capitalism together making it possible for ordinary people to bridge the life obstacles created by pain.

On the day of the recall announcement, each major television network featured someone who believed Merck's promises and felt betrayed. On ABC, Vioxx user Sue Anne Humphries (Figure 5.1) declared, "The majority of people that take Vioxx are senior citizens. And we *trust* our companies. We *trust* our doctors. And then something comes along like this. No more trust."[12] On NBC, Dr. Jack Lock, looking like an icon of the private practice physician of previous generations, suggested

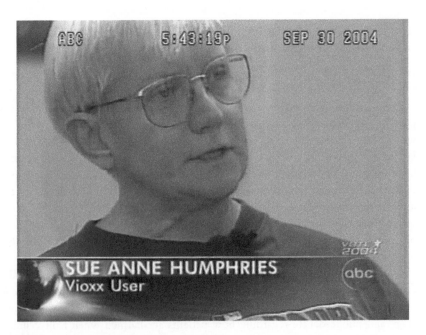

FIGURE 5.1 "We *trust* our companies. We *trust* our doctors. And then something comes along like this." ABC News, 30 Sept. 2004.

that Merck is "pretty high on our list for reliability, so for this to happen is a kind of shock to me and I'm sure to my patients." Conflicts between marketing imperatives and science became a central theme of subsequent coverage. "Researchers have issued repeated warnings," correspondent John McKenzie says. A whistleblowing clinician/scientist who had sounded the alarm recounts how Merck aggressively refuted him. Showing a clip of a Merck ad, McKenzie continues, "And [Merck] continued to promote Vioxx heavily. What many patients never knew: Vioxx was no more effective than cheaper, over-the counter pain pills."

Initial coverage of the recall lacked a consistent scandal frame. On NBC's 30 September story, Bazell did not present economic and scientific spheres as affecting one another. Rather, he cast the rupture of trust as a source of disappointment at the failure of biocommunicability—bewilderment that what was previously understood to be safe was found not to be—not as a cause for outrage. On CBS (30 Sept. 2004), Medical Correspondent Elizabeth Kaledin emphasized the usual advice to the patient-consumer, "Patients should consult their doctors about what to do next. . . . There are options that are cheaper, and, for the time being, safer." A few days later, NBC[13] followed up with a report on drug safety. Anchor Tom Brokaw says:

> When the pharmaceutical giant Merck announced it was taking Vioxx off the market, that was very big news to the medical community, those suffering from arthritis, Wall Street, and public health officials. And it left us wondering, what else is out there? Prescription and over-the-counter drugs that may help many, but also do irreversible damage.

Bazell's report centered on the standard patient-consumer model of biocommunicability, emphasizing consumer responsibility, and lacked a scandal frame. He noted: "Most Americans take over-the counter pain relievers without considering side effects." To the extent that outrage emerged in early reporting, it was mainly directed at the FDA. "Vioxx is one of a number of drugs recalled in recent years after the FDA approved them as, quote, safe and effective," Dan Rather reported, "and critics say the FDA is part of the problem, allegedly too cozy with drug companies."

The story broadened and deepened on 1 November, over a month after it first broke, with the *Wall Street Journal (WSJ)* story "Warning Signs: E-mails Suggest Merck Knew Vioxx's Dangers at Early Stage."[14] It began:

> When Merck & Co. pulled its big-selling painkiller Vioxx off the market in September, Chief Executive Raymond Gilmartin said the company was "really putting patient safety first." He said the study findings prompting the withdrawal, which tied Vioxx to heart-attack and stroke risk, were "unexpected."
>
> But internal Merck e-mail and marketing documents, as well as interviews with outside scientists show that the company fought forcefully for years to keep safety concerns from destroying the drug's prospects.

British medical journal *The Lancet* published what CBS news called a "scathing" editorial criticizing Merck and the FDA. On 12 November, Bazell interviewed Merck CEO Gilmartin. Anchor Tom Brokaw introduced the story with an allusion to Watergate—"What did Merck know, and when did it know it?"—and Bazell asked whether the company put "profits over patient safety." The Vioxx story was now a "moral disorder" story (Gans 1979) centering on the pollution of science and medicine by the search for profits, though with interesting twists suggesting how thoroughly the two are actually entwined in contemporary biomedicine. Near the story's end, after Merck's CEO denied that his company had long known Vioxx's dangers, Bazell countered, "But the charges Merck should have known of the danger have knocked $40 billion off the value of the company's stock, hurting many pension and mutual funds." Television reports commonly presented the scandal as a betrayal of patients, doctors, and *also* investors.

The Vioxx scandal was centrally a scandal of biocommunicability, of projections regarding how medical knowledge was produced and circulated. Beyond the question of what Merck knew and when, a host of biocommunicable problems emerged: What did Merck *not* know and why did it not know it? What did Merck know and not reveal? What did others know that Merck sought to suppress? On 14 November, four leading *NYT* health and biotech reporters published an article based on internal documents provided by "people associated with lawsuits against Merck."[15] *WSJ* and *NYT* reporting was lengthy and complex, ranging across many issues, but revelations about breaches of norms of biocommunicability were highlighted:

- Research on Vioxx clinical trials, written by scientists who received contracts or research grants from Merck or by Merck employees, left out potentially important information.
- Merck played "hardball" (as the *WSJ* put it), with researchers who questioned Vioxx's safety, canceling presentations by one Stanford physician it had agreed to sponsor, calling to threaten Stanford with "consequences," and suing a researcher in Spain.
- Merck marketers were instructed to avoid questions that might hurt sales, colorfully called "Dodge Ball Vioxx" in a training document.
- After results from one clinical trial, conducted for other reasons, suggested that Vioxx might increase the risk of heart attack and stroke, Merck discussed and rejected the idea of conducting a trial specifically to assess whether Vioxx posed cardiovascular risks. Treated as most newsworthy was the revelation that marketing executives were part of the discussion on whether to conduct this trial.

Marketers and PR/media professionals, we learned in interviews, are involved in pharma and biotech research and development from the beginning; scientific knowledge is not created first, in a realm untouched by media logic, only later to be transmitted to publics through the media. This fact contradicts the biomedical authority/passive patient and patient-consumer models of biocommunicability as well as the separation of scientific/medical and capitalist domains.

By drawing attention to the intimate relationship between science and marketing in pharma, coverage of the Vioxx scandal seemed to threaten the fundamental premise of Boundary-Work I, the notion that medicine and capitalism can ethically co-exist, and it complicated journalists' position as enforcing the boundaries between them.

As congressional hearings and legal proceedings continued, the scandal expanded to involve increasingly wider biocommunicable dimensions. In February, the *Times* published another article using documents provided by lawyers and federal and state officials on Merck's strategies to "neutralize" potentially critical doctors, often by paying them to give speeches or to do clinical trials or by subsidizing educational retreats they organized.[16] In April, the *Journal of the American Medical Association (JAMA)* published an article based on internal Merck documents, detailing how Merck hired ghostwriters to draft medical journal articles. "In some cases," the *NYT* reported, summarizing the *JAMA* article, "Merck's marketing department was involved in developing plans for manuscripts," raising "broad questions about the validity of much of the drug industry's published research."[17] In May, the *WSJ* used internal e-mails from the *New England Journal of Medicine (NEJM)* showing that the *NEJM*'s

> expression of concern was timed to divert attention from a deposition in which Executive Editor Gregory Curfman made potentially damaging admissions about the journal's handling of the Vioxx study. . . . Curfman acknowledged that lax editing might have helped the authors make misleading claims. He said the *[NEJM]* sold more than 900,000 reprints, bringing in at least $697,000 in revenue. Merck says it bought most of the reprints.

The *WSJ* went on to express the significance of the revelations this way: "Many articles" in leading medical journals "lend an academic imprimatur to messages hatched by drug companies as part of publicity campaigns. Sometimes they fail to disclose authors' financial ties to companies or the involvement of company-hired ghostwriters."[18]

The scandal focused harsh scrutiny on the FDA. Journalists shift into their "watchdog" mode most readily when dealing with government agencies; scandal frames were applied to the FDA long before Merck. The FDA is seen as primarily responsible for patrolling the boundary between science and business and upholding the primacy of the former. On-going critical focus on the FDA was driven to a significant extent by congressional hearings. David Graham, an FDA epidemiologist who had prepared a report estimating the magnitude of Vioxx side effects, testified that FDA officials had attempted to suppress his findings. CBS's Dan Rather commented, "The Food and Drug Administration insisted today that it is doing what it called a 'good' job of protecting Americans from dangerous prescription drugs. But even some of the FDA's own scientists say the record shows otherwise." The story then placed Vioxx in a series of "regulatory failures" represented by drugs approved and later pulled from the market. This story, like many others, articulated what is often referred to as the theory of "regulatory capture," the charge that "drug companies and regulators have gotten too cozy," and cited corporate funding of FDA research and pharma contributions to congressional campaigns.

The Vioxx scandal illustrates multiple dimensions of biomediatization. It was rooted in the increased centrality of advertising, marketing, and public relations in biomedicine. Despite the embeddedness of many journalists in corporate media, reporters portrayed Vioxx as violating science/medicine versus capitalism boundaries through marketing—which included massive direct-to-consumer advertising. While the scandal brought these forms of biomediatization into the public eye and into question, it also represented an intensification of a very different kind of biomediatization: practices and discussions internal to the biomedical field were forced into the arena of news and public debate. Insiders became subject to the scrutiny and judgment of the mass public and were obligated to enter a discursive space of dialogue with a wide range of actors, including journalists, politicians, and civil society organizations. It is important to look carefully, however, at what biomediatization actually entailed here, to understand the specific role of journalists. Vioxx was not primarily a media-driven scandal; investigative reporting played little role. Like many scandals, including Watergate, beyond its beginning phase (Schudson 1993) most revelations were compelled by congressional committees and the legal system. It is, in this sense, a strong example of a pattern frequently observed in political communication: journalists largely define issues in response to debates among key elites, acting as interpreters and critics primarily when elites are divided.[19] Many prominent stories were pegged to critical reports in medical journals. For congress members, lawyers for plaintiffs suing Merck, dissident officials, scientists who came into conflict with Merck, and critics of big pharma, the surge of media attention provided opportunities to be heard and achieve their ends; Merck corporate officials and scientists, the FDA, and medical journals entered defensively.

What then was the role of journalists in the Vioxx scandal? Ettema and Glasser (1998) show that although journalists conceive of what they do primarily in terms of the verification of facts, a kind of "moral craftwork" is central to investigative reporting and, we could add, to scandal reporting in general. The craft of investigative journalism involves not only verifying that certain actions took place, but establishing that these actions were indeed an "outrage," establishing the story's newsworthiness. This moral craftwork, they argue, plays an important role in reproducing and sometimes reshaping social values. It involves a number of standard techniques, evident in Vioxx coverage, including irony ("Vioxx is one of a number of drugs recalled in recent years after the FDA approved them as, quote, safe and effective"); locating victims the news audience can identify as innocent; and the kinds of juxtapositions that establish hypocrisy or deceit, as in Vioxx television stories shifting from clips of upbeat ads to soundbites about the suppression of information about side effects. This kind of moral craftwork took the form of Boundary-Work II: journalists establish the Vioxx scandal as a violation of moral order by invoking the idea of a necessary boundary separating science and medicine from marketing, profit, and politics.

Before the scandal erupted, journalists had already begun to question "Drug Companies' Wine and Dine Ways," to use the title of a 2002 *SDU-T* article,[20] portraying doctors as consumers of "glorified sales pitches" proffered by drug companies in exchange for free meals, tickets for events, travel, and cash payments. Vioxx intensified such portrayals of biomedical professionals. When Merck's CEO resigned in May 2005, ABC ran a special segment based on Merck marketing documents. "Congress has been looking into how Merck sold *so much* Vioxx," anchor Elizabeth Vargas announced, over the graphic "Pushing Drugs." Correspondent Jake Tapper reports:

> Documents show that Merck instructed its sales representatives on how to shake hands with doctors, cozy up to them. . . . Everything, members of Congress charged today, except the honest way to discuss the serious heart attack and stroke risk posed by Vioxx.

Tapper invokes the boundary between science and marketing, both in words and with his body. "Merck's three thousand salespeople were given this pamphlet promoting Vioxx and allegedly told not to deviate from it," he says, holding a marketing document in one hand. He then says of another document he displays in his other hand, "Not even to discuss Merck's own study indicating health problems among Vioxx users"; the document is quoted in text as saying "Do not initiate discussions," appearing beside Merck's name and logo (Figure 5.2). Before a backdrop of footage of Dr. Martin Luther King he reported: "After a Food and Drug Administration advisory committee recommended doctors be informed about that study, internal documents show Merck advised its sales staff, 'Do not initiate discussions' on the topic. They were told to focus on what they called Martin Luther King's 'goal focus' to inspire greater sales." Then, in a soundbite, Rep. Elijah Cummings expresses disgust: "And then when I see things like this— Martin Luther King? My God. How far will we go?" Using Dr. King's place in the sacred realm of civic life for the profane goal of increasing sales imparts to its other marketing practices the same sense of sacrilege. The next soundbite invokes

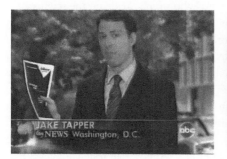 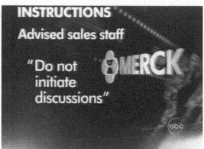

FIGURE 5.2 ABC's Jake Tapper reports on Merck sales documents which instruct representatives not to discuss troubling research findings. ABC News, 6 May 2005.

the traditional image of the autonomous biomedicine with a doctor saying, "We have our own sources of independent information. We should not be relying on a skewed group of *salesmen* to tell us what drugs to use."

Vioxx was followed by smaller but still significant controversies, including scandals involving Avandia, a diabetes medicine produced by GlaxoSmithKline found to increase risk of heart attack, leading to its 2010 suspension in Europe and US restrictions, and another later that same year over Johnson & Johnson hip implants. Avandia debates also expanded transparency at the FDA, among the important effects on biomedical institutions. Reporting on a split vote in the FDA advisory panel, the *NYT* noted, "The agency allowed competing visions to spill out in the advisory hearing—something unheard of just a few years ago."[21] One important element of Boundary-Work II is advocacy for transparency, and it is possible that greater journalistic scrutiny in the Vioxx and post-Vioxx era added to the impetus for this change.[22] Health journalists repeatedly told us in interviews how they had learned to read carefully the sections in journal articles disclosing funding, authors' contributions, declarations of interests, and acknowledgments.

In the Vioxx case, we have emphasized that investigative reporting was limited and public controversy not primarily media-driven. In other Boundary-Work II cases, investigative journalism is more central. *SDU-T* reporter Hughes described one story where "the smell factor" led her to discover an extreme if far less extensive violation. She led a June 2006 story, "A San Diego company said yesterday that it had created the world's first cat that's free of the allergy-causing proteins that afflict many feline lovers." A follow-up article revealed that its "San Diego headquarters" was actually the CEO's apartment—and that she had been evicted for non-payment of rent. Hughes lists companies started by the same CEO that reportedly engaged in fraud, misrepresentation, and violation of intellectual property rights. Hughes told Charles that it all started when her editor, seemingly impressed, passed along a press release and asked her to do a story. When Hughes' "smell" indicator went off, she did research on the CEO, found a long history of lawsuits and disgruntled customers and business partners, called cat experts, then arranged the interview. Rather than take a press release at face value and write a positive story, her boundary-work revealed $3,500 "deposits" on the future delivery of each "sneeze-free cat" and a capitalist who simply made up the science.

At the national level, the kind of slow journalism described by Campbell often gave rise to high-profile Boundary-Work II stories. On 14 December 2013, the *NYT* published a long analytical article by Alan Schwarz, "The Selling of Attention Deficit Disorder," which documented "a remarkably successful two-decade campaign by pharmaceutical companies to publicize the syndrome to doctors, educators and parents." It included an analysis of pharma advertising, illustrated on the *NYT* website with video clips, and results of an *NYT* poll that recruited 1,106 respondents to take a short quiz commonly found on websites sponsored by drug companies, asking, "Could you have A.D.H.D.?" Almost half tested at a level that indicated ADHD was possible or likely. It also included numerous interviews with researchers and pharma insiders, including Adderall salesman Brian Lutz, whose words were central to Schwartz' boundary-work: "What he regrets, he said, 'is how we sold these pills like they were cars, when we knew they weren't just cars.'"

Boundary-Work I and Boundary-Work II stories are similarly organized around a vision of distinct domains of medical knowledge and the pursuit of profit, which both cooperate and remain distinct through flows of information that maintain the primacy and integrity of science and medicine. Both invoke heroes who believe that they are producing something that is, in the words of another dissident bio-medical insider quoted in the *NYT*, "not the same as buying widgets,"[23] who work diligently to keep science, medicine, and capitalism on their separate linear trajectories or, with Boundary-Work II, are identified as dissenters in conflict with dominant institutional actors. Boundary-Work II stories, like other "watchdog" reporting, can be seen as relegitimizing biomedicine, affirming that it is indeed possible for medical science to coexist with the commercial logic of the pharma and healthcare industries without being corrupted by them. But the growth of this kind of reporting in recent years has certainly introduced an important degree of ambivalence into representing the subjects and objects of biomedicine. Health journalists still believe in their policing role, but it is much harder to represent boundaries as ordinarily simple, transparent, effective, and able to ensure the well-being of patients or investors.

Conclusion

Here we have documented the role of media professionals, including those working as reporters, editors, and producers as well as those employed by biotech and pharma corporations and other health institutions. Our contribution to scholarship on pharmaceuticalization goes further than simply filling a gap in knowledge of the actors and practices that enact it. Polls and news stories reflect the contradictions that make pharmaceuticalization so interesting, a vast phenomenon that brings fear, loathing, healing, desire, and infatuation with technoscience together intimately. We would certainly not disagree with scholars who equate pharmaceuticalization with commodification and the power of market logics. Nevertheless, beyond demonstrating the multiplicity, the tremendous complexity and dynamism of relations between technoscience, medicine, and capital, we have pointed to ways that pharmaceuticalization also relies precisely on the denial of this intimacy, on making it seem as if scientists, physicians, and businesspersons can combine forces without conflating goals and logics. Biotech/pharma reporters have a crucial role here. Their stories map networks, projecting the particular scientists, doctors, corporate officials, investors, patients, and activists associated with a specific drug or device and the role each must play in pharmaceuticalization. At the same time, by denouncing the villains, the evil boundary-crossers, journalists open up space for heroes, for the sense that one of the largest and most profitable sectors of capital is fundamentally driven by researchers and doctors who are motivated by the love of scientific discovery and alleviating the suffering of patients, and that they are in turn sustained but not corrupted by people who know how to make money. Our discussion suggests, however, that this illusion has become quite precarious: consuming more and more drugs can now uncomfortably coexist with believing that unethical conflations of boundaries between technoscience, medicine, and capital are now the rule, not the exception. At the same time, the post-humanist counter-narrative, the idea that pharma, if not all of medicine, is driven by a singular and stable logic—the pursuit of even more astronomic profits—is no less a product of these particular forms and histories of biomediatization than narratives of exciting breakthroughs and compassionate scientific geniuses.

The very premise on which both forms of boundary-work rest denies the depth and pervasiveness of biomediatization, even if more skeptical type II stories begin to admit the fundamental imbrication of capital, technoscience, and medicine. If pharma and biotech bring connections between these domains most directly into view, it is in the media-driven practices of marketing, advertising, and public relations that imbrication produces the greater discomfort and the sharpest criticism. We have suggested that the particularities of the complex, shifting, and unpredictable ways that professional logics and practices converge *and* the forms/events that assert their separability are of greater scholarly interest than now commonplace observations about profit motives corrupting science and medicine. Who is doing the conflating and who the boundary-work is not always predictable. PR/media consultant Johanna Rice recounted prepping a doctor as "third person" advocate for a morning news segment featuring a client's treatment for hyperhydrosis—excessive sweating—an example of what is often referred to as a "lifestyle disease." Pharma marketing is much more regulated than other forms, and the FDA had explicitly forbidden marketing it as a "permanent cure:"[24]

> [T]his guy . . . he was calling it, "a permanent [solution] . . . a miracle." And he was offering it to anybody. . . . One of the patients that we wanted to use for a morning news segment, . . . she had the treatment because she was the first to Like his Facebook page. She didn't even suffer from the condition that it's indicated to treat, which really made us nervous. . . . [W]hen he sent us a script or a kind of outline of the segment we just said "no, no, no, you can't. . . you really shouldn't say that." . . . The doctor's response was, "Well, that's what drives sales. This is about marketing, de da da da."

Boundary-work helps order medical and market domains hierarchically; here it is a media professional who is appalled as a physician elevates profit over medicine. Through biotech/pharma biomediatization, doctors and scientists have to a significant extent internalized the logics of marketing and public relations, just as media professionals are integrated into logics of biomedicine.

Research on pharma as a social and cultural influence has focused significantly on advertising and marketing, as Dumit's (2012) work suggests. But news coverage is also central to the cultural reach of pharma, as Rice's efforts to get her client's product on the morning news suggests. The desire of pharma marketers to associate their products with the cultural prestige of biomedicine and present what they do as something more than mere business, as serving humanity, enhances the importance of media interactions. So does the fact that their industry is regulated and in many ways also financed by the state. News coverage is central to how pharma interacts with other social and cultural fields. Reporters' roles are complex, crossing and often merging many genres of reporting—business, consumer, science, political. Journalists have a wide range of different stances, from celebratory to sharply critical.

Our argument against the "two cultures" theory can underscore this point from another angle. Journalism, like science and medicine, sees itself as an autonomous practice that serves the public interest. Its value system is defined to a significant extent in opposition to the values of capital, even as it is embedded in profit-making institutions and to a large extent serves to provide the flows of information and publicity on which capital depends. Journalists champion the autonomy of cultural fields. Here we have traced how journalists position themselves as celebrating those who seek to restore the integrity of technoscience and medicine when capitalism seems to corrupt them and position themselves as the best arbiters of these boundaries. We have also witnessed how they often seem in denial of their deep embeddedness in processes of biomediatization that help to constitute contemporary capitalism, science, and medicine alike, sandwiched between the ads that punctuate and finance their reporting or pop up next to stories in digital versions of newspapers, on Internet sites, and social media.

In covering the Vioxx scandal, journalists seemed reluctant to reflect on whether they themselves had something to do with "how Merck sold *so much* Vioxx." The very ads they scrutinized appeared frequently on their news broadcasts. Journalists reported on Vioxx's FDA approval in May 1999, but they did not pay much attention to Vioxx skeptics. Health journalists did not problematize their own role in making Vioxx into a blockbuster and protecting its aura, not to mention how Merck and other pharmaceutical corporations indirectly finance their reporting through advertising revenue. Bazell noted that public disclosure of Merck's Vioxx cover-up "knocked $40 billion off the value of the company's stock," but mainstream journalists did not scrutinize the role their stories play in building the corporate reputations that help fuel stock prices and investor interest, a key reason that biotech and pharma CEOs and PR/media personnel want to talk to them. In light of our earlier findings about the generally upbeat character of coverage on new medical technologies—much of it facilitated by corporate PR—we could ask whether journalists might have profitably turned the heightened critical scrutiny that they were focusing on their fellow biomediatizers on themselves. This observation does not invite a simplistic handmaiden of biocapital interpretation of biotech/pharma reporting. Rather, it suggests that the central place of health news in biomediatization depends upon the usual denial of biomediatization, the reproduction of a boundary between biomedicine and media.

Notes

1 Vanessa O'Connell, "Ad Agencies Begin to Participate in Development of New Drugs," 13 Mar. 2002.
2 No relation to the Stratton-Domenici's consultant profiled in Chapter 2.
3 Interviewed by Charles 14 Mar. 2007 and again by telephone on 21 Aug. 2013.
4 Pellechia (1997) found a significant increase in the percent of newspaper stories on scientific research (most of which was health-related) that cited critical comments from scientists not involved in the study in question.
5 *SDU-T,* 11 Jan. 2010.
6 All are pseudonyms.
7 Interviewed in San Diego by Charles on 22 Sept. 2006.
8 Interviewed on 22 May 2007.
9 Skype interview by Dan Hallin, 27 Feb. 2014.
10 Jeffrey M. Jones, "U.S. Images of Banking, Real Estate Making Comeback," www.gallup.com/poll 23 Aug. 2013.
11 USA Today/Kaiser Family Foundation/Harvard School of Public Health, *The Public on Prescription Drugs and Pharmaceutical Companies.* Menlo Park, CA: Kaiser Family Foundation 2008. This poll found that 47 percent of respondents had a favorable view of the pharmaceutical industries, and 44 percent a negative view. In 2012, Harris found that 12 percent of the public considered pharmaceutical and drug companies "honest and trustworthy" (http://www.harrisinteractive.com/NewsRoom/HarrisPolls/tabid/447/ctl/ReadCustom percent20Default/mid/1508/ArticleId/1131/Default.aspx).
12 30 Sept. 2004.
13 4 Oct. 2004.
14 Anna Wilde Mathews and Barbara Martinez, A1.
15 Alex Berenson, Gardiner Harris, Barry Meier and Andrew Pollack, "Despite Warnings, Drug Giant Took Long Path to Vioxx Recall."
16 Barry Meier and Stephanie Saul, "Marketing of Vioxx: How Merck Played Game of Catch-Up," 11 Feb. 2005.
17 Stephanie Saul, "Ghostwriters used in Vioxx Studies, Article Says," 15 Apr. 2005.
18 David Armstrong, "Bitter Pill: How the New England Journal Missed Warning Signs on Vioxx," 15 May 2005:A1.
19 The first of these points is known as the indexing hypothesis (Bennett 1990); the second comes from Hallin (1986).
20 Tony Fong, 17 Apr. 2002:C3.
21 Gardiner Harris, "Panel Suggests Limit on Drug for Diabetes," 14 Jul. 2010:A1, 23.
22 Some changes were the product of a 2007 law intended to produce greater transparency (Wood and Perosino 2008)
23 Alex Berenson and Andrew Pollock, "Doctors Reap Billions from Anemia Drug," 9 May 2007, http://www.nytimes.com/2007/05/09/business/09anemia.html?pagewanted=all.
24 As Rice pointed out, the FDA restrictions are binding on the company and advertising or public relations agencies, but clinicians face fewer restrictions, which makes "third person" advocates valuable but potentially problematic.

6

"WE HAVE TO PUT THAT FOUR-LETTER WORD, 'RACE,' ON THE TABLE"

Voicing and silencing race and ethnicity in news coverage of health

As we noted in the Preface, in 1992 Charles made a trip to the Delta Amacuro of Venezuela, where he had done research since 1986, when he stumbled into a major epidemic of cholera, a preventable and treatable bacterial infection. Some five hundred people died there in less than two years. The epidemic was concentrated among communities classified as "indigenous" that lacked potable water, sewage facilities, and more than minimal access to healthcare. When thousands left the rainforest and began living under sheets of plastic in the towns on the mainland, seeking greater access to medical care, they became visible to local and national journalists, thereby opening up public health policies to possible scrutiny. Charles and Clara Mantini-Briggs, a Venezuelan physician who coordinated the public health response in the Delta, documented the subsequent media feeding frenzy in *Stories in a Time of Cholera: Racial Profiling During a Medical Nightmare* (Briggs and Mantini-Briggs 2003).

Media coverage forced the regional health service to send resources into the delta, but at the same time reflected a highly racialized interpretation of the epidemic which deflected blame from public health officials and, more broadly, from "modern" Venezuelan society. It was the culture of the indigenous people, "their" purported rejection of biomedicine in favor of belief in spirits and reliance on healers, that was responsible for an epidemic that challenged Venezuela's image of modernity. Public health officials and politicians collaborated with reporters in portraying "cholera victims" as pitiful, helpless, ignorant, and pre-modern, locked in a world of cultural difference from which they could not escape, which threatened their own health and that of their non-indigenous neighbors.

In Latin America, these sorts of structural inequalities of health have long been a central focus of critical epidemiology and Latin American Social Medicine (see Breilh 2003; Laurell 1989; Menéndez 1981). In the United States, 2002 was a watershed in bringing racial inequities to the attention of health professionals and others. In January, the CDC presented a report focusing on racial differences in health outcomes (Keppel, Pearcy, and Wagener 2002). In April, the Institute of Medicine produced an exhaustive report documenting that, after controlling for socio-economic status and type of health insurance, African Americans and Latinos/ as receive poorer healthcare than whites (Smedley, Stith, and Nelson 2002).

Two bodies of literature point to ways that race is similarly connected to news media. Research suggests that news coverage plays a central role in connecting race and crime. An early study by Stuart Hall *et al.* (1978) focused on widespread perceptions of an epidemic of mugging in the United Kingdom in the 1970s, largely consisting of black-on-white crime. Their study indicated that the phenomenon was created through journalists' everyday practices and the resulting elevation of government officials as "primary definers" of news narratives. Studies of US television news point to the overrepresentation of racialized minorities in crime news and the relative paucity of minority officials (Entman and Rojecki 2000; Gilliam *et al.* 1996; Gray 2004). Moon-Kie Jung (2015) argues that African American unemployment figures are contrastively underreported, reflecting stereotypes that project African Americans out of work as normal. Scholars have also looked at the production, particularly in the 1990s and 2000s, of Latino/a demographics as a threat. Leo Chávez (2001) analyzed covers of weekly news magazines portraying migrants as providing visual images that made these statistical imaginaries seem real and emotionally and politically charged. Chávez (2013) has also examined biopolitical dimensions of what he calls a "Latino Threat Narrative," looking in particular at how Latina bodies are projected as excessively, even pathologically overly fertile, thus posing a threat to the white body politic and public health systems. Otto Santa Ana (2002) examined metaphors in media coverage in creating an image of a threatening "tide" of brown bodies "flooding" the United States.[1] De Genova (2005) argues that producing the image of the "illegal" immigrant is central to reproducing a nativist understanding of a white social body and body politic. The few studies focusing on race and ethnicity in US health news led us to believe that health news might be similarly structured to coverage of crime and immigration and work politically in parallel sorts of ways. Research by Subervi, Vargas, and Brody (1998), Vargas (2000), and Vargas and dePyssler (1999) strengthened this hypothesis. They examined news coverage of Latinos/as, arguing that language, access to particular media, and stigmatizing images contribute to justifying racialized health disparities.

Here, however, it was the limited number of the stories on race that surprised us. If you simply search for news reports on "African American health" or "Latino health" or "race and medicine," the results are somewhat limited. We gathered material on particular diseases we thought might be represented in racialized ways, diabetes and obesity, for example, but did not find pervasive patterns of racialization, that is, of mapping health issues in terms of projected differences between whites, African Americans, Asian Americans, Latinos/as, and Native Americans. We asked U.C. Berkeley student Deirdre Clyde to search a large body of local television health news, looking at who appeared in what roles.[2] The dominant pattern she found was the construction of a generic multiracial visual profile of patients to illustrate each story, but rarely explicit reference to race and ethnicity. We also began to notice stories in which journalists might have been expected to thematize race and ethnicity but did not. The same story could be handled in ways that strikingly foregrounded race and others that avoided it.

One of the most significant US examples of how race, health, and news intersect came in 2003 in widespread coverage of Jesica Santillan, who died after surgeons transplanted a heart and lung of the wrong blood type. As suggested by the contributors to a volume that intensively analyzed the case (Wailoo, Livingston, and Guarnaccia 2006), strong public discourses circulated that connected the Santillan case to a wider narrative about "the Mexican illegal immigrant as a threat" (Chávez 2006:261, 2013). Even as such forums as right-wing, anti-immigrant blogs, websites, and newsletters reanimated alarmist rhetorics in constructing Santillan's body as threatening the bodies of US citizens by usurping organs and illegitimately appropriating biomedical services (Chávez 2006, 2013), we were struck at how often stories in mainstream media avoided these themes, constructing Santillan as a deracialized "underdog fighting the heartless system" and as the victim of rampant medical error. They also largely avoided reference to the social context in which human organs circulate, which involves important patterns of racialization and immigration (Chávez 2013; Lederer 2006; Scheper-Hughes 2000).

We began to realize that patterns of racial and ethnic representation in US health reporting are much more complex than our initial hypothesis proposed. Stigmatization of racialized populations is certainly present. At the same time, when race and ethnicity are foregrounded in health reporting, coverage often centers on activists or mediators from racialized populations trying to focus attention on health issues faced by racialized populations; even positive treatments of the programs they direct may or may not succeed in overturning negative stereotypes. In many ways, however, the dominant pattern in health and medical reporting is *overt deracialization,* the non-representation of race and ethnicity. Health and medicine are generally projected as fields where race is essentially irrelevant, eclipsed by the universalism of biomedical science and technology or by the individualism of the active patient-consumer. Health and medical reporting thus often fits patterns of "post-racial" discourse, deracializing health news either by excluding references to race and ethnicity or by projecting a multicultural image of a health system serving all, across social differences.

Health news coverage, we suggest, is nevertheless a crucial site for constructing racial difference in the United States for three reasons: First, the very process of deracializing health, of suggesting that racial differences should not matter, imbues the stories that do focus on race with particular importance; as racialized figures that stand out from the ground of deracialized health, their particular features play significant roles in shaping contemporary US racial landscapes. Second, deracialization does not render race irrelevant. Looking at which health issues get racialized and deracialized and how, we argue that deracialization pays a key role in the whitening of health, in constructing it as an aspirational state of wellbeing, and associating particular diseases with forms of stigma fostered by racial stereotypes, especially for African Americans and Latinos/as. Finally, deracialization limits and contains attention to racial inequities of access to health services, the quality of those services, and the health outcomes of Latinos/as and African Americans versus other groups. Health inequities thus often get tied to particular populations rather than cast as basic structural features of the US healthcare system. We want to caution, however, that vast generalizations about race and health news are less useful than looking closely at its particular contours. In our view, tracing the differences, contradictions, and heterogeneities that emerge—sometimes in the same story— and paying attention to the complex roles played by persons cast as spokespersons for racialized populations is more fruitful than offering sweeping generalizations or blanket accusations.

Invoking race

While most health news projects the notion that race is largely irrelevant where health is concerned, periodically a story does bring race into the picture, explicitly or implicitly. Using LexisNexis to identify press coverage of racial and ethnic health disparities, Annice Kim et al. (2010) report finding 3,823 articles appearing between 1996 and 2005 in 40 US newspapers (see also Niederdeppe et al. 2013). Through a variety of guises, from the most subtle to the most blatant, from one-word allusions to entire broadcasts or articles, some health stories do indeed invoke race and ethnicity.

Most typically, race enters health news as part of a list of risk factors, usually unobtrusively, in the lower paragraphs of an article. A *New York Times* article on childhood accidents suggests that the types of accidents fatal to children are fairly constant worldwide but that the proportion of accident-related mortality varies widely within countries. Reporter Donald McNeil adds that US "rates were the highest for American Indians, lowest for Asians and about equal for blacks and whites."[3] Another *NYT* article, "Threat Grows From Liver Illness Tied to Obesity" (14 Jun. 2014:A1, 3), invokes race—cautiously—thirteen paragraphs into the story:

> Fatty liver strikes people of all races and ethnicities. But it is particularly widespread among Hispanics because they frequently carry a variant of a gene, known as PNPLA3. . . . That variant is at least twice as common in Hispanic Americans compared with African-Americans and whites.

Further down, the story adds, "People of Asian descent . . . develop the disease at a lower body mass index than others."

Given a common projection documented in this chapter, that health should be located within a post-racial social world, *triggering frames* are often necessary to authorize explicit racial referents. One of these is data on genetics, a frame that, ironically, involves the same sort of biological reasoning that in other cases seems to require erasing race–health connections. Another NBC news story, on low Vitamin D levels, noted that the problem is particularly acute among African American girls due, it asserts, to their black skin. Drawing attention to pharmaco-genetics, the study of how the effects and side-effects of drugs vary in accordance with the patient's genes, opens up an arena that is hugely interesting for biotech and pharma companies due to their interest in expanding and controlling markets through market segmentation. Given the contentious nature of these debates, appeals to genetics are often located alongside other logics. A CNN broadcast thus placed the notion that genetic differences influence disease susceptibility and the effectiveness of medications alongside questions of access to healthcare, culture, communication, and economics.[4]

Some stories project disease and medicine as racially structured—only to explicitly deny the validity of these constructions. Two local television news stories invited health professionals to challenge the identification of anorexia and bulimia with "the stereotypical white, teenage, upper-middle-class, over-achieving girl." Speaking in the first-person plural used by professional experts, who seemingly are not taken in by racial stereotypes, a Fox "medical expert" suggests "we're seeing it in younger kids," including boys, "and we're also seeing it in minorities."[5] A health professional, in another story, also white, female, and seemingly middle-class, comments: "[s]o the stereotype is that eating disorders only afflict young, white, affluent, heterosexual females, but in reality all segments of the population, regardless of age, race, ethnicity, social class can suffer from eating disorders."[6] Here the racial association with anorexia and bulimia is white; in most cases race or ethnicity is not considered relevant unless incidence rates are higher among "minority" populations. These stories, in denying the relevance of race, could be said to restore the generic quality of whiteness, the ability of white bodies to represent the universal body. Particular diseases are also sometimes racialized as white, such as a 2013 *NYT* story on opioid abuse that brings in gender and class:

> For years, drug overdose deaths in the United States were seen as mostly an urban problems that hit blacks hardest. But opioid abuse . . . has been worst among whites. . . . Some researchers say the epidemic has contributed to a sharp decline in life expectancy among the country's least educated white women.[7]

Some stories avoid the word "race" or specific racial labels but portray racially delimited populations, using euphemisms and/or visuals to allow readers/viewers to fill in the blanks. In a local NBC-affiliate report on high HIV-positive rates in Holyoke, Massachusetts, a Latina spokesperson suggests that "it's important to know the population we're working with; a lot of people don't want to know their status, so it's important to get them out here so they know their status before they infect other people."[8] All names and faces seem to be Latino/a, but no racial labels appear. An *NYT* article[9] on government incentives for building supermarkets in inner-city areas where fresh foods are reportedly scarce quotes a source characterizing neighborhoods that are "poorer" or "like this"; a customer purchases collard greens. Racialized terms are absent, even as photographs project only African

American and Latino/a actors. An interesting twist on this pattern occurs in an investigative report in the *San Francisco Chronicle* on high rates of use of particularly expensive heart procedures at a hospital in rural Clearlake, California.[10] A hospital spokesperson tries to explain those rates: "To find this sort of rural community, with this many overlapping health situations, it's kind of like Haiti. You're really dealing with Third World situations here." The population of Clearlake is 73.8 percent white.[11] Its racial makeup is not mentioned in the story, but two white heart patients are pictured. The reference to Haiti and the Third World neverthe-less invokes a racialized image of poor communities with poor health.

Stories that foreground race and ethnicity, while not common (we provide sta-tistics below), do appear from time to time. Some project connections between particular pathologies and social categories. One important example is HIV/AIDS. As Lupton (1997) notes, the racial projection of HIV/AIDS shifted in the late 1980s, as manifested in a 1988 CBS report pegged to a Stockholm HIV/AIDS research summit. The central storyline was that HIV/AIDS had shifted from gay, white pop-ulations to become "a minority disease."[12] Filmed while driving through a Black and Latino area of the Bronx, Columbia University epidemiologist Dr. Ernie Drucker observes, "This is where AIDS is in New York City." Twenty-five years later, "Poor Black and Hispanic Men are the Face of H.I.V." was an *NYT* front-page article.[13] The CBS story interviewed an African American official at the CDC. The *NYT* story included a spokeswoman for Gay Men's Health Crisis and the president of the Black AIDS Institute of Los Angeles. Advocates of various kinds, sometimes in civil society, sometimes in government or from the professional/academic world, often themselves people of color, promote many of the stories and provide key triggering mechanisms for invoking race in health news, as we discuss below.

A long *Los Angeles Times* front-page story, titled, "Seeking to Help Latina Teenagers Avoid Pregnancy" cited statistics showing a decrease in US teenage pregnancies and explored reasons why it remained "stubbornly high" among California Latinas.[14] Written by a Latina reporter, it cited Lucille Royball-Allard, a local congresswoman "involved in efforts to reduce teenage pregnancy," and research funded by the California Wellness Campaign and the Latino Coalition for a Healthy California. The image of the pregnant Latina teen generated suffi-cient moral panic that the California Department of Health Services placed ads on billboards and in magazines in the early 2000s featuring young women and men seemingly trapped by unwanted pregnancies—nearly all of them seemingly Latinos/ as (Tapia 2011). Chávez (2013:71–72) suggests that even as such stories draw atten-tion to what they characterize as sudden, alarming demographic "threats," they draw on a forty-year history of narratives that "have consistently represented the fertility levels of Latinas, especially Mexican and Mexican Americans, as 'danger-ous,' 'pathological,' 'abnormal,' and even a threat to national security."[15]

Statistics figure prominently in many health stories that invoke race and ethnic-ity, a final triggering mechanism. Stories that foreground race and ethnicity often have their origin in research studies highlighting racial and ethnic differences. Many 2000s news stories emphasized African American rates of heart disease. A March

2009 *New England Journal of Medicine* article, along with an editorial on racial disparities in cardiac care, received wide media coverage. "Black adults developed heart
failure at a rate twenty times higher than whites, even dying of it decades earlier
than the condition typically strikes whites" led the *NYT*.[16] CNN cited "physicians"
as concluding that "African-Americans must be screened earlier, more frequently
and with greater sensitivity for high blood pressure." The story cited higher African
American obesity rates as a critical factor.[17] In addition to neglecting questions of
racial differences in access to care and quality of care, stories often overlooked a
robust body of work in public health that relates African American rates of cardiovascular disease and diabetes to the physiological effects of racism.[18] Structural
factors, including racism, are sometimes discussed. "Black adults are more likely than
whites to skimp on sleep," *USA Today* reported, "and the sleep gap is especially
wide for black professionals, a new study shows."[19] The story, pegged to an *American
Journal of Epidemiology* article, addressed possible reasons, including racial discrimination at work. Uses of statistics, as STS scholars have shown (Bowker and Star 1999),
are powerful devices for naturalizing social categories; they do heavy-lifting in the
work of aggregation and disaggregation that constructs racial categories. Health statistics in news stories create (dis)connections with dimensions of class, gender, and
sexuality, creating a sort of light show that can illuminate race and racial inequities
one moment and hide them from view the next.

News stories that focus on race and ethnicity do not simply re-present biomedical research but form crucial dimensions of biomediatization processes that
co-produce research, clinical trials, tests, drugs, and so forth. Biomediatization,
given its role in rearticulating notions of race and health, forms a crucial part of
what Michael Omi and Howard Winant (1986) term "racial projects," pointing to
historically specific ways that racial identities are constructed and infused with social
meaning. As scholars have suggested, race-based health inequities both reflect the
structural effects of discrimination in housing, employment, crime, incarceration
rates, education, and financial services as well as connect and extend them. In this
complex field, we would cite two broad tendencies.

Starting in the late nineteenth century, anthropologist Franz Boas (1965[1911])
challenged reductions of US racial inequalities—especially black and white—to
biological difference, paralleling efforts by sociologist W.E.B. Du Bois (1990[1903])
to scrutinize the role of racism in structuring racial economies and their destructive
effects (see Stocking 1968; Baker 1998; Briggs 2005). Although reducing racial difference to biology in public discourse accordingly came to be widely seen as racist,
conflations of race and biology hardly disappeared from white views of racialized
populations.[20] Chávez (2001, 2006, 2013) documents how news coverage reacti-
vated these connections in turning Latino/a immigrants into a biological "threat";
this biologization of stereotypes is also evident in the Latina teenager pregnancy
coverage we cited. Shifting the locus of fears regarding HIV contamination from
white gays to African Americans and Latinos/as transfers a powerful affective connection, which initially centrally included Haitians (Farmer 1992), from sexual
onto racial economies.[21]

At the same time, these stories participate significantly in what Steven Epstein (2007) refers to as the "difference and inclusion paradigm" that emerged as race-, gender-, and sexuality-based social movements drew on clinical trials and other biomedical research in asserting biological bases for social difference. The role of pharmacogenetics in contemporary pharmaceuticalization connects targeted marketing strategies with social movements. The 2007 scandal surrounding Avandia, a type 2 diabetes drug linked to heart problems, revealed GlaxoSmithKline's focus on marketing to African Americans. "Pharmaceutical companies in general," the *NYT* reported, "have been seeing a higher return on direct-to-consumer advertising to minority groups, because many of the people in those audiences may not otherwise go to a doctor about a problem."[22] This connection has generated controversies, such as over BiDil, an antihypertensive marketed for African Americans. Rodney Hood, president of the National Medical Association (a predominantly African American physicians' organization) praised BiDil in numerous news stories as countering health inequities, while others (e.g., Duster 1990) have criticized such cases as involving "bioethnic conscription" (Montoya 2009), the grafting of social identities and life conditions onto biological explanations of differences and disease causality. As Michael Montoya has suggested, this now-you-see-it, now-you-don't quality is also evident in scientific research in genetics and the development of drugs (such as for diabetes) that it engenders; disclaimers that race is socially constructed fail to preclude "pathologizing the ethnicity of DNA donors" (2011:14).

Racialization beyond US borders: Reporting on Ebola

Reporting in US media on health issues in the global South typically fits the pattern of coverage that makes no explicit reference to race, while images, language, and narrative conventions can unmistakably invoke it. News coverage of the Ebola epidemic that started in 2014 generally exhibits this pattern. Ebola generated enough self-reflexive meta-coverage that racial representation was occasionally foregrounded. This happened most extensively when *Newsweek* published a cover story titled "Smuggled Bushmeat is Ebola's Back Door to America,"[23] picturing a chimpanzee on the cover, which, ironically, also referenced a story on "Post-Racial America." Painting African immigrants in New York who consumed "bushmeat" as a possible scenario for US introduction of the virus, the story, as Laura Seay and Kim Yi Dionne put it, "placed *Newsweek* squarely in the center of a long and ugly tradition of treating Africans as savage animals and the African continent as a dirty, diseased place to be feared."[24]

Newsweek wasn't alone. A Discovery Channel documentary in which "ABC's chief medical correspondent, Dr. Richard Besser, takes us on a harrowing journey to the heart of darkness," warned with music and tabloid-style narration, "Somewhere on the other side of the planet, in a hidden corner of a tropical rainforest, a new virus is surely incubating. A pathological killer that could unleash a deadly plague at any time." This documentary started with an ABC news investigative report about "bushmeat" in New York markets that could "pose a hidden danger here at home." It included footage of an African immigrant who had been convicted of smuggling "bushmeat"; she is described as a "mother of ten," which had no relevance—except to connect stereotypes of Africa as dangerous untamed nature with stereotypes of overly fertile African Americans. The story then shifted to its hero, a white "virus-hunter."

Imagining Africa as a dangerous incubator of viruses that threaten "us" in the West and Africans as culturally backward permeated much Ebola coverage, in blatant and subtle forms. US coverage began in late March 2014 but was sporadic until late July, when two US health workers were infected. It soared in October with the first US Ebola transmission. The first major *NYT* story appeared on 28 July:

> Workers and officials, blamed by panicked populations for spreading the virus, have been threatened with knives, stones and machetes, their vehicles sometimes surrounded by hostile mobs. Log barriers across narrow dirt roads block medical teams from reaching villages where the virus is suspected. Sick and dead villagers, cut off from help, are infecting others.
>
> "This is very unusual, that we are not trusted," said Marc Poncin, the emergency coordinator in Guinea for Doctors Without Borders. . . .
>
> Efforts to monitor [the disease] are grinding to a halt because of "intimidation," he said. People appear to have more confidence in witch doctors.[25]

It continues: "Wariness against outside intervention has deep roots. This part of Guinea, known as the Forest Region, . . . is known for its strong belief in traditional religion." Paul Farmer (1999:23) refers to this pattern of displacing attention from structural inequalities—which would include in this case the lack of adequate health infrastructures in affected West African countries—to culture as an "immodest claim of causality," noting that it uses a single variable to explain complex clinical manifestations and epidemiological patterns.

As is typical both of epidemics (Chapter 4) and of coverage of non-white populations, this article, like most stories of Ebola in Africa, adopts the linear, hierarchically ordered or biomedical-authority model of biocommunicability. The efforts of Médecins Sans Frontières (MSF or Doctors Without Borders) to transmit biomedical knowledge of Ebola prevention to Africans was blocked by logs placed across roads or armed youths at the entrance to "villages"; an MSF physician giving a health education talk "was met with indifference or hostile stares; some turned their backs on him." Here, both Western physicians and journalists project Africans as irrationally equating biocommunicable trajectories with disease transmission and viewing MSF doctors as disease vectors. The MSF coordinator deemed this lack of trust "very unusual," springing from fear and panic. Nevertheless, poor West Africans are not the only ones to view MSF and other medical aid organizations critically. Former MSF President Didier Fassin (2012), now an anthropologist, argues that MSF philanthropy is guided by a "humanitarian reason" that reproduces global inequalities in the name of ameliorating human suffering, thereby providing rationales for maintaining European and American geopolitical dominance (see also Redfield 2013).

Although such portrayals of West Africans diminished as the story was covered more extensively, sometimes replaced by more positive representations, they reemerged periodically. In October, as Ebola fear and stigmatization of those exposed spread in the United States, the *NYT* reported that CDC Director Dr. Tom Frieden "said he expected that type of reaction among uneducated people in developing countries, but not in the U.S."[26] Ebola images typically showed black bodies marked as dangerous by the safety equipment and the distance between them and caregivers (Figure 6.1).

Ebola coverage was, however, complex. Similar to the pattern with H1N1 coverage described in Chapter 4, mainstream media generally criticized calls to restrict travel. Reporters like Besser or NBC's Nancy Snyderman, both of whom traveled to West Africa, emphasized global assistance to West African countries and expressed solidarity with health workers. Snyderman concluded a 3 October 2014 Nightly News report from Liberia saying: "Officials are vigilant" about tracking cases; local officials "want the world's eyes to remain focused on Liberia." NBC partnered with Facebook in promoting attention to the Ebola crisis, with a web-based campaign called "Spread the Story." As the crisis continued, West African health workers became an important focus. They were typically represented, following a pattern

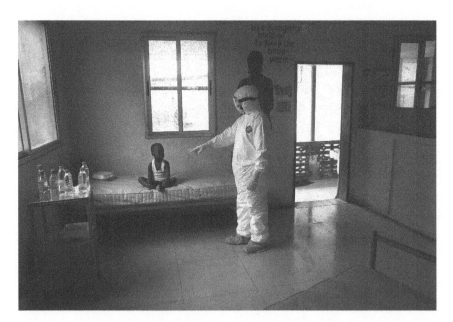

FIGURE 6.1   Cute but dangerous: images of dangerous black bodies appeared in many forms during the Ebola epidemic. We first saw a version of this one, by John Moore of Getty Images, on the Mobile App of the *Huffington Post* on October 5, 2014. Later Ebola images were often less othering, portraying Ebola patients in closer proximity to caregivers, and with more agency.

explored below, as mediators who could repair biocommunicable gaps between racialized populations and the world of biomedicine. A front-page *NYT* story featured US-trained epidemiologist and immunologist Dr. Mosoka Fallah, raised in a poor neighborhood of Monrovia, Liberia. "With his experience straddling vastly different worlds, Dr. Fallah acts as a rare bridge." Photos show him at neighborhood meetings, educating residents.[27]

In conservative social media, Ebola was incorporated into virulently racist anti-Obama discourse. Claims that President Obama is anti-white and anti-American and that he was trying to prompt a massive influx of black bodies into the United States joined, in cartoons, PhotoShopped images, stories, and blogs, with the claim that he was trying to create a massive US Ebola epidemic.[28] Fox News presented a member of their medical staff, Dr. Keith Ablow, as claiming that Obama was actually spreading "Ebolophobia," fear of Ebola, rather than taking the step continually promoted by anti-immigration crusaders: closing US borders to non-whites.[29]

Out of the loop: racialized others, biocommunicable failures

CBS correspondent John Blackstone, in the 1988 CBS story mentioned above, reported:

> Community workers are struggling to spread the word. What once was considered a gay disease is looking more and more like a minority disease. In ghetto schools, students are taught that some 70% of women and heterosexual men with AIDS are black or Hispanic. But, the students say, outside the schools the warning isn't being heard.

In a biocommunicable call-to-arms, a student suggests: "You should bring it to the different communities and bring it more out on television than what you do now." The story, titled "AIDS: Getting the Message," shifts to African American Health and Human Services official Stephanie Lee-Miller, displaying educational materials targeting black and Latino/a drug users:[30] "We have to really communicate with these young men and tell them that they are facing obsolescence as a group." We then accompany Dr. Ernie Drucker through the streets of the Bronx: "This is where the information is needed," Drucker says. "The warnings about AIDS now familiar to most Americans still haven't reached here. . . . There are full-page ads in the *New York Times* . . . but these folks don't read the *New York Times*." "From the Bronx to Watts in Los Angeles," Blackstone says, "the message about AIDS is being missed, and an unprecedented government pamphlet mailed to every household in the nation may not have reached those who need it most." Juxtaposing biocommunicability and epidemiology, Blackstone wraps up: "In the ghettos, many are working to spread the word, but the virus, it seems, is spreading faster."

Save Drucker, the people in this story are African American or Latino/a. Driven by an advocacy agenda, common in health news dealing with race and ethnicity, the story suggests that minority health problems must be addressed by medical and public health authorities. How the problem is understood is standard: it is one of biocommunicability, a failure of information to reach ethno-racially distinct populations. Anchor Susan Spencer, introducing the story from a conference of AIDS researchers in Stockholm says, "The doctors and scientists gathered here will tell you that education is indeed the key to fighting AIDS." Many persons quoted in the CBS story may have understood the problem more complexly, but the story maps a starkly racialized geography of biocommunicable failure, similar in many ways to the Venezuelan cholera epidemic's image of "indigenous" people whose failure to internalize widely disseminated information becomes the principal cause of the spread of disease. The CBS story's visual structure strongly conveys racialized otherness, as we survey the alien landscape of ignorance and disease from the window of the car, until Drucker steps out to approach several young men and "meet the problem face to face." Bronx residents are perceived as failed receivers of biomedical information, certainly not as producing or circulating it.

As we began our research in 2002, fourteen years after that CBS story, we found similar themes recurring in stories on "minority" communities. Sometimes stories had a strong negative tone, often accompanied by themes identifying racialized populations as a threat to the health of the "community at large" or as a burden to the public health system. Even when they did not have a negative tone, stories about racialized populations rarely portrayed their members as active patient-consumers, which, as we saw in Chapter 1, is today the desirable biocommunicable slot. They appear typically as passive patients, and often—like the cholera cases in Venezuelan coverage—depicted as having failed to adequately play their parts. Right through the present, racial and ethnic differences in health outcomes, if not explained as reflecting genetic differences, are typically attributed to failures of such information to reach racialized populations. Racialized populations purportedly overlook biomedical information, suffering from resulting knowledge deficits. Often "they" are seen as listening to the wrong channels, privileging the voices of relatives, friends, or dubious alternative practitioners over those of legitimate biomedical authorities, or hobbled by cultural barriers contrary to ideal projections of modern, self-regulating health citizenship.

This pattern—in its more negative version—is strikingly evident in a 2002 Associated Press article appearing in the *SDU-T* and other US newspapers.[31] Reporter Sandra Marquez frames the death of Salvadoran immigrant Roberto Caceres as caused by a Latina "faith healer," part of a sector of "unlicensed" or "phony" practitioners. Citing how the healer arrested in the case "had been publicized on a nationally syndicated Spanish-language radio show," Marquez reports that "officials have launched a series of Spanish-language television ads informing people that they can instead turn to low-cost medical clinics." The reporter invokes the idea that culture disrupts the proper flow of health information via the voice of Al Aldaz, a Latino Los Angeles Police Department detective investigating the homicide case, who explains that the healers' patients "come from deep Mexico or El Salvador in the hills. . . . They believe in the supernatural." The article constructs two biocommunicable circuits, biomedical knowledge moving through legitimate clinical facilities and mainstream media and a communicative maze in which superstitious health beliefs born in subaltern sectors of immigrant-producing countries are disseminated in other languages through ethnic media and "backroom clinics tucked in bridal shops, bakeries and other stores."

Projecting an insurmountable, lethal, and, here, criminal chasm of cultural and linguistic difference is complicated by the reporter's acknowledgment that Caceres only visited the healer after four dermatologists failed to diagnose or treat an unsightly skin rash. Rather than having been incarcerated on the irrational, anti-biomedical side of a racialized biocommunicable divide, Caceres appears to have embraced a widespread US pattern, one often treated sympathetically in stories on middle-class whites—turning first to allopathic practitioners and then exploring complementary and alternative treatment when the former failed. Indeed, Caceres not only consulted dermatologists first, but only turned to the "faith healer" when threatened with loss of his job—and health coverage. Instead of asking why bio-medical treatment proved unsuccessful, the story attributes his death to a widespread failure of immigrant biocommunicability. This story thus parallels the representa-tion of Jesica Santillan as an organ-stealing menace when her story was positioned within the "citizen/foreigner, legal/illegal, deserving/undeserving" binaries that structure anti-immigrant discourses (Chávez 2006:287, 2013; Morgan et al. 2006).

Stories on Latino/a health, consistent with much immigration coverage in this period (Chávez 2001, 2013; Santa Ana 2002), often combined emphasis on cul-tural barriers and biocommunicable failure with images of a "tide" of unhealthy "brown bodies" threatening U.S citizens. "California's large and rapidly growing Latino population is developing diabetes at an alarming rate," reported another AP story in the *SDU-T*:

> While the report said diabetes is prevalent among the state's black and American Indian populations, their numbers do not rival the Hispanic pres-ence in California. About one in three residents is Latino—11 million people in 2000, a number projected to double by 2005, [thereby posing] new threats to an already-strained public health system.[32]

The *LA Times* teenage pregnancy story similarly dramatizes statistics on projected growth of the Latino/a population, concluding that the "stakes for California and the nation are enormously high."

Reporting a UCLA social scientist's research on high rates of hepatitis A among Latino/a youth, *SDU-T* reporter Leonel Sánchez[33] cites another potential threat:

> The study's principal author, David Hayes-Bautista, said the findings are alarm-ing because of the size of the states' young Latino population and the potential for outbreaks that could spread beyond Latino neighborhoods. . . . Of special concern, the UCLA study pointed out, is the high number of young Latinos who work at restaurants, . . . and the potential for outbreaks due to improper handling of food.

Another Sánchez story,[34] on "high rates of asthma, tuberculosis, diabetes, obesity and other health problems" among Latino/a children, quotes Dr. Glen Flores, chairman of the Latino Consortium of the American Academy of Pediatrics Center for Child Health Research, as warning that "if the disparities continue, it has the potential to affect the health and productivity and well-being of our entire nation." An op-ed piece by Irma Cota, director of community clinics providing low-cost service to thousands of Latino/a patients, was accompanied by a cartoon featuring a white male physician examining an endless line of little brown bodies (Figure 6.2).[35]

These newspaper stories are reported by Latino/a journalists; principal sources are exclusively or mostly Latino/as. These actors draw attention to the problems of populations underserved by the health system and, as we shall see below, typically intend to counter negative stereotypes. How, then, do we explain reproduction of these stereotypes? One important factor is surely the target audience of the metropolitan newspaper. Otis Chandler, then publisher of the *LA Times*, stated in 1979 that "it would not make sense financially for us" to target minority readers because "that audience does not have the purchasing power and is not responsive to the kind of advertising we carry." He asked rhetorically, "how do we get them to read the *Times*? . . . It's too big, it's too stuffy. If you will, it's too complicated" (Gutiérrez and Wilson 1980:53). Mainstream media have shifted as the Latino/a middle class has grown and marketing directed at Latino/as increased (Davila 2001). Nevertheless,

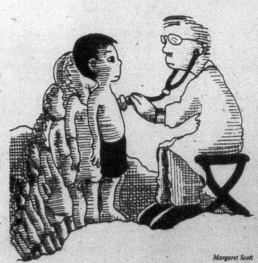

health care for children of migrant

workers and their families each year. Many of these patients are children. Our doctors and nurses see firsthand the profound differences in the health status of migrant children as compared to others. For example, migrant children come in for primary care and preventive services far less frequently. Their families bring them to our centers with aggravated conditions such as chronic asthma, severe oral health problems and tooth decay, advanced ear infections and respiratory disease. Anemia, tuberculosis, and diabetes are also more prevalent among migrant children.

There are several reasons for the health care gap.

Migrant workers most often do not have health insurance. Their jobs do not provide this benefit. Studies consistently find that people who have health insurance are more likely to seek regular primary care. Those who receive regular primary care have their conditions detected and treated in their earliest stages. It's a logical argument to conclude that people who have health insurance are generally healthier than those without.

The state of California has a wonderful program called Healthy Families where parents can pay as little as $4 a

Margaret Scott

FIGURE 6.2   Irma Cota's op-ed "Improving the Health of Migrant Workers" was accompanied by a cartoon depicting a physician treating an endless line of little brown bodies. *San Diego Union-Tribune*, 22 Mar. 2002.

the target audience of a newspaper like the *SDU-T* is largely understood to be middle-class whites; reporters sometimes feel the need to "sell" stories on "minority" health to readers by emphasizing how they will affect readers' *own* health.[36]

These representations also reach deeply into the epistemological roots of whiteness. More than in many other social arenas, blame-the-victim rhetorics can run up against a humanistic impulse in illness stories to express empathy for the sick and suffering. Stories of biocommunicable failure help turn the effects of medical racism—looming differences in access to and quality of care—into widespread health problems that result from individual and collective failures simply to pay attention to what health professionals are saying. A key language for framing biocommunicable failure is what Arjun Appadurai (1988) analyzed as representations of racialized subjects as "incarcerated by culture," purportedly trapped into ways of thinking and acting that contrast with unmarked, seemingly race-free rational and modern modalities. Medical anthropologists have examined the use of cultural reasoning by clinicians and public health practitioners that reify structural inequities as differences of culture (Briggs and Mantini-Briggs 2003; Farmer 1999). Janelle Taylor (2003) critiqued the seductive logic of Anne Fadiman's (1997) *The Spirit Catches You and You Fall Down* for projecting separate and incommensurable social worlds of Hmong shamanism and Western medicine, thereby reading inequalities of race and power as failures of cross-cultural communication.

The invocation of culture is often articulated by actors who are themselves members of racialized populations. It is typically used asymmetrically, however. "Cultural barriers" are identified as existing only on one side of the biocommunicable gap: it is not doctors or public health officials—or media organizations—that are limited by "cultural barriers" from playing their ideal roles in the flow of biomedical information. "Culture" is a characteristic distinct to racialized populations and closely associated—with some exceptions—with projections of biocommunicable failure and negative health outcomes. A 2004 *LA Times* article on teenage pregnancy explains that "traditional Latino households" are so pervaded by sexual taboos and failures of communication between family members that information about sexuality and family planning cannot break in. The executive director of a program seeking to educate young Latino males about sex and contraception is quoted as saying, "Especially in the Latino community, we have so many secrets. 'You don't talk about this, you don't talk about that. God will punish you.'"[37] Cota's op-ed cited above suggests that "primary healthcare is just not part of the Latino culture. We must work to make primary healthcare and prevention part of Latino consciousness." An *SDU-T* "Seniority" column titled "Program tells Latinos about diabetes" cites nurse Ana Perez, who manages a Latino-focused diabetes program: "'Latinos go to doctors just when they feel sick; if they feel OK, they don't go. But sometimes with diabetes there are no symptoms.'" The article goes on: "'there is a tendency to define a disease as God's will, that there is nothing they can do,' [Perez] says."[38] It would seem unlikely that Perez would present *biomedical* explanations of diabetes without scientific evidence. Nevertheless, she only seems to need the cultural knowledge afforded by her status as Latina to elevate *culture* to the status of Farmer's "immodest claim of causality." As their voices emerge in these stories, Latino/a health professionals and social scientists themselves reproduce images of Latinas as incarcerated by tradition, superstition, and Catholic dogma, thereby, in Chávez's (2013:15) words, imbuing features of the "Latino threat narrative" with "organic-like lives of their own. Once given birth, they grow and take on ever more elaborate and refined characteristics until they are able to stand on their own as taken-for-granted 'truths.'"

Patterns of exclusion: health as whiteness

Racialization of health news also emerges in patterns of exclusion or relegation to subaltern status. Members of racialized populations appear relatively infrequently in health news, particularly in elite roles. Table 6.1 shows the composition of people who appeared and spoke on camera in the network television stories in our 2009–12 sample; 61.7 percent of soundbites are from males, 38.2 percent are from females.[39] Gender differences are more striking when the person's role in the story is factored in: 85 percent of physician soundbites are from males and around 70

TABLE 6.1 Race/ethnicity and gender of people appearing in soundbites in network television coverage of health and medicine (Affordable Care Act stories excluded)

	Professionals, health officials, researchers[a]	Business	Public officials	Civil society[b]	Patients, ordinary people	Other[c]
Black/African American	22	2	9	7	57	10
	(4.4)[d]	(6.5)	(20.5)	(14.3)	(14.0)	(10.1)
Latino	5	1	0	0	14	10
	(1.0)	(3.2)	(0.0)	(0.0)	(3.4)	(10.1)
Asian/Asian American	30	0	0	0	2	0
	(6.0)	(0.0)	(0.0)	(0.0)	(0.5)	(0.0)
White	421	28	35	39	321	77
	(84.4)	(90.3)	(79.5)	(79.6)	(78.9)	(77.8)
Other, undetermined	21	0	0	3	13	2
	(4.2)	(0.0)	(0.0)	(6.1)	(3.1)	(2.0)
Female	141	12	14	26	243	52
	(28.5)	(41.4)	(31.8)	(53.1)	(60.8)	(50.5)
Male	354	17	30	23	157	51
	(71.5)	(58.6)	(68.2)	(46.9)	(39.3)	(49.5)

Notes
a Includes health professionals, researchers, public health officials, representatives of healthcare institutions and of health-related NGOs.
b Includes non-health-related civil society organizations, community organizations, activists.
c Includes celebrities and athletes, writers, journalists, cultural figures, attorneys, First Lady, and others.
d Percent in parentheses.

percent of researchers. Laypersons, on the other hand, are predominantly female: 60 percent female to 40 percent male. On television, unlike newspapers, the audience can make identifications of race and/or ethnicity. In important speaking roles, racial diversity is clearly limited. More than 90 percent of health professionals appearing in television news are white or Asian American. Even in the role of patients and ordinary laypersons, whites make up 80 percent of soundbites, and diversity is mainly manifested in the modest inclusion—14 percent—of African Americans. Latinos seldom appear in any category. Asian Americans appear almost exclusively as professionals, rarely as patients. No Native Americans appeared in the 357 stories in the sample.

A significant pattern of racialization also emerged when we looked at the *SDU-T*'s weekly Health section. Like most health sections, it is generally highly positive in tone, providing upbeat advice and celebrating healthy lifestyles and consumer choices. When we asked *SDU-T* editors about the target audience, they stressed that they imagined the readers above all as fit and health-conscious. In 2005–9, as we were developing our ideas about the patient-consumer model of biocommunicability prominently featured in such service journalism, we compiled a sample of 73 Health sections. For the most part, they project a deracialized vision of health, speaking of generic patient-consumers and universalized biomedical knowledge. One issue did focus on "understanding the medical pitfalls associated with your ethnic origin."[40] It listed "health problems that may be more prevalent in some ethnic populations," and explained, "Many of the comparisons are to Caucasians, because they are considered the majority population."

The Health section prominently features photographs, often sizeable, in color and, typically upbeat, showing faces and bodies displaying the discipline, optimism, and *joie de vivre* the texts describe (Figure 6.3). We coded the photographs in those 73 issues for the race/ethnicity of those pictured and their roles and found 53 white non-professionals (75 percent), 10 Latinos/as, 4 African Americans, 4 Asian Americans, and no Native Americans.[41] All Asian Americans accompanied a single article—on martial arts. Given the section's focus on the words and actions of non-professionals, not surprisingly, only 8 professionals appeared—all white. Class is relevant. Nearly all stories mention the occupation of actors—lawyers, marketing specialists, social workers, accountants, and so forth are common. Reporters often match descriptions of their dedication to exercise regimes with mentions of their professional achievements. Occupations such as plumbers, waitresses, and domestics are never represented.

In the preceding discussion of "biocommunicable failures," we saw racialized subjects portrayed as deficient health citizens in need of external health education to correct their failings. In contrast, the individuals featured in the Health section quintessentially embody patient-consumer biocommunicability, performing their status as expert patients (Dumit 2012:35). They know what health professionals recommend, and they mobilize this advice through their own rationality and individual agency—markers of modern, self-governing subjects. Strikingly, this space of ideal health citizenship is strongly associated with *whiteness*—and is largely restricted to

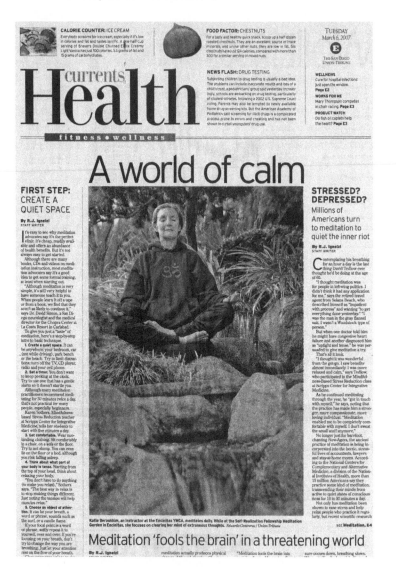

FIGURE 6.3 Fitness, Wellness and Whiteness: in the weekly Health section of the *San Diego Union-Tribune* fit patient-consumers are celebrated—the great majority of them white. 6 Mar. 2007.

middle-class whites. These patterns are not characteristic of all health coverage. But important components of health news do certainly portray a racialized split between aspirational health citizens—projected as white—tuned to the proper channels of information and using that information to achieve the ideal of a healthy life versus deficient subjects—projected as non-white—who remain "out of the loop," suffer the consequences in the form of ill health, and often burden society and the health system. Equating patient-consumer biocommunicability and model patients with whiteness, as much as projecting biocommunicable failure with a black or brown face, forms an important way that health news is racialized. In this fashion, the health privileges bestowed by racial segregation and medical profiling on whites just seem naturally to be theirs. Racial health inequities—even when strikingly revealed—appear to lie beyond the need for any sort of medical affirmative action.

Talking back: viewing health news with Latino/a immigrants

Given the often negative images of racialized minorities and immigrants in health news, we wondered how audiences within these populations responded. Although we do not claim systematic knowledge of how different US populations receive and respond to health news, we conducted focus groups and interviews with individuals and small groups, as indicated in the Introduction. Participants were drawn from working-class and middle-class sectors, Spanish speakers and English speakers. Both by design and reflecting the composition of areas in which we worked, some groups were African American, Latino/a, white, or mixed. Some included only persons under age 25, others 40 and above. We matched interviewers/leaders and participants as closely as possible with respect to age, gender, and ethnicity. Both in interviews and focus groups we asked participants to talk in general about their media consumption and their perceptions of health news; we also provided examples of print and/or television stories for discussion.

One broad generalization emerges. The chosen setting fostered a skeptical attitude, regardless of our attempts to frame the task as openly as possible; the groups seemed to invite participants to adopt a critical attitude regarding health news. Some positioned themselves as attending to health news and using it—along with interactions with health professionals—as a key mechanism for gaining biomedical knowledge, embracing biomedical authority biocommunicability. Others located themselves as neoliberal health knowledge seekers, actively searching print, radio, and television health news, the Internet, social media, magazines and books, and consulting friends and relatives. All focus groups and most interviews also yielded participants who rejected the subject positions in which they were interpellated. White, middle-class participants—those who seemed most directly interpellated by neoliberal patient-consumer stories—often rejected them as free advertising by pharmaceutical and medical-device corporations and physicians. Some, especially Charles's Berkeley neighbors, skeptically claimed that they rejected all health news as mere "advertising"—standing above the mercantilization of health through news coverage.

We are particularly interested here in the critical responses that we heard in interviews and focus groups with Latinos/as conducted in San Diego County. Some discussions took place in clinical sites, others were held in churches or with Latino/a parents' associations for local schools. As in all our focus groups, some participants accepted the positionality of the passive-patient recipient, as receiving health knowledge transmitted by professionals through journalists. These individuals—often middle-class and bilingual—were nevertheless outnumbered by respondents—frequently Spanish-dominant and working class—who distanced themselves from the biocommunicable positions in which they saw themselves as interpellated.

Two focus groups in particular stand out. One took place at a Catholic church in northern San Diego County, a region where recent immigrants live in close proximity to affluent middle-class residents. After attending the church for several weeks, Charles and Clara Mantini-Briggs held a focus group after Mass. As interviews suggested that Spanish-language television was the most popular source of health news among potential participants, the prompts included an Univisión broadcast from San Diego focusing on an information campaign about health services available for children, regardless of immigration status. It had a didactic, paternalistic tone, saying that many Latino/a children were eligible for Medicaid or SCHIP (State Children's Health Insurance Program) "*y los padres no lo saben*" (and the parents don't know it).[42] A Latina professional instructed viewers on the importance of seeing physicians and receiving vaccinations. Introducing an element of meta-coverage, Univisión emphasized its own participation—the story began with an official reading out a number to call for information and saying, "*Gracias, Univisión.*"

A few participants aligned themselves with the proffered subject position. One interjected, "It's true that we do lack information, I think that many families don't have the least idea that there is health coverage for their children." Most, however, reacted skeptically. They recounted, in fascinatingly detailed form, collective processes in which members of their knowledge-production network—family, friends, and co-workers—had acquired information related to these programs. They described how specified individuals visited the offices mentioned in the reports, only to be refused services projected as freely available. Participants accordingly reversed the story's projected knowledge hierarchy: in their estimation, bureaucrats and Latino/a health professionals are ignorant regarding the services their agencies actually provided. The story's projected recipients envisioned themselves as possessing detailed knowledge of the services available for their children.

The social scientific literature on services available to immigrants, documented or undocumented, would question any easy dichotomy between ignorance and knowledge. Indeed, the problems faced both by health professionals and patients in negotiating the labyrinth of complicated and often conflicting regulations, not to mention the transportation costs and lost work days, suggest that these patients might indeed be more knowledgeable.[43] Indeed, research suggests that ignorance and confusion are sometimes hardwired into Medicaid and other health services precisely in order to save money by limiting the extent to which people can overcome forms of "bureaucratic disentitlement" created through "withholding information, providing misinformation, . . . and requiring extraordinary amounts of documentation" (Danz 2000:1006). Participants chillingly noted the differential cost for undocumented immigrants of struggling to find accurate information and demand health rights: fear of deportation. Research underlines the value of their insights here too: fear that a visit to the clinic will lead to an encounter with immigration authorities—along with a social climate shaped by anti-immigrant rhetoric—has been shown to be a barrier that limits undocumented patients from seeking care, even for US-born children (Heyman, Núñez, and Talavera 2009; Horton 2014).

The second focus group that stands out was organized by a Venezuelan immigrant mother, Clara Mantini-Briggs, president of a middle-school Latino/a parents association. Mantini-Briggs invited parents to stay after a meeting for a focus group, led by herself and a Latina student. They showed another Univisión segment picturing a reporter interacting with workers in northern San Diego County fields who seemingly had just discovered that they had been exposed to unacceptable levels of pesticides and complained that they had no idea that their symptoms were due to pesticides. The 40 focus-group participants included some 15 agricultural workers. They quickly rejected the subject-position of the unaware workers, foregrounding their knowledge of the effects of particular pesticides (including those named in the report and several others) and specified which of their relatives and coworkers had been affected, what symptoms they reported, their interactions with physicians and state advocates, and inadequate responses by employers, doctors, and state officials. Rather than lauding journalists for revealing a hidden situation to ignorant Latino/a audiences, they chided reporters for their limited knowledge and interest. One worker, who had been laid off for months due to pesticide exposure said:[44]

> If only they had spent more than a few hours in the fields with us. If they had even stayed an entire day, we could have taught them something. But they just get a little bit and go on to the next story—they aren't really interested, they don't really care.

Thus, some members of these focus groups did their own critical analysis of media projections of hierarchically ordered subject positions, rejecting their interpellation as ignorant, subaltern subjects. They placed the issue of pesticide exposure within an agricultural-medical-industrial complex that produces fresh fruit and vegetables at low cost to consumers, with migrant laborers paying the human costs through, in Seth Holmes' (2013) terms, "broken bodies" whose legacy of disabilities is only minimally addressed through available health services. These participants critically assessed, in short, the intersectionality between structural effects of agricultural labor, medical racism, and biocommunicable projections. It is obvious that the participants in these and other focus groups bore little resemblance to stereotypes of Latinos/as as passive and ignorant, as incarcerated by culture, tradition, and religion (see Chávez 2013). In analyzing why non-Latino anthropologists had reproduced these sorts of stereotypes, Américo Paredes (1977) hypothesized that their Mexican American interlocutors had playfully invoked stereotypes as a means of inviting their interlocutors to join them in critiquing them and constructing alternative narratives (see also Briggs 2012). These focus groups provide flesh-and-blood examples of the sort of critical encounters that Paredes imagined: participants turned them into sites for identifying stereotypes that they saw as lurking within the health news stories, critiquing them, collaboratively constructing alternative biocommunicable models, and positioning themselves complexly in biocommunicable terms.

Surmounting biocommunicable failure: the role of mediators

Clearly, members of racialized minorities are not passive objects either of racialization or of deracialization in health news, but have important roles in voicing race and ethnicity and shaping how it is covered. The central actors and main sources in stories that foreground race and ethnicity are typically professionals from minority racial or ethnic groups—researchers, physicians, teachers, directors of community clinics, and peer educators—often individuals who lead programs addressing health inequities. Thus, paradoxically, stories on health in racialized populations, which often project biocommunicable failure, centrally include and are sometimes initiated by actors of color who epitomize successful biocommunicability.

We have suggested that journalists generally project a post-racial view of health that similarly limits explicit attention to race-based inequities. *El Hispano* reporter Graciela López, profiled in Chapter 2, argued that race and health was a topic that health officials tried to avoid. If you ask them about Latinos/as, "it is as if you had put on the handbrake! They tell you, 'well, I don't know, I can't comment on that.'" López sees such reluctance as going hand-in-hand with a Latino/a stereotype, including its positive and negative dimension:

> On the one hand, the Latino is happy and chubby (*el gordito alegre*), but on the other hand, they tell you that 'they have to eat less fat.' But on the other hand you have to preserve your culture, you should eat tamales.

Here she chuckled, marking the irony. A reluctance to talk about Latino/a health and reliance on stereotypes rather than acquaintance with San Diego's Latino/a population, she observed, went hand-in-hand with a lack of Spanish-language spokespersons. It is in this context that the role of what we call *mediators*, health professionals from minority populations who frequently appear in health news, is particularly significant, given their systematic efforts to draw attention to health inequities. Mediators do not inhabit a pure realm of agency and power but give witness to the particular complexities and contradictions that characterize racialized dimensions of biomediatization.

A typical news story built around mediators appeared on 5 March 2009 on NBC Nightly News. Part of a series on "Hispanics in America," it began with the standard reference to Latinos/as as "the largest and fastest growing minority in the country," which, correspondent Robert Bazell observes, "suffers disproportionately from health problems." University of Illinois, Chicago, Professor Aida Giachello then discusses the problem of jobs with no health insurance. Bazell continues, "but another factor is a cultural divide. That's why a unique program here trains people in the neighborhood, people like Lucy Rosa, to help others stay healthy." Giachello explains: "To be able to treat a population, you need to have understanding of their cultural beliefs." The story details food deserts (without using the term), noting the program's recruitment of store owners to offer more fresh fruits and vegetables. "Food deserts" have been a focus of much health activism and are one of the most common structural factors in health disparities encountered in news coverage. Bazell summarizes, "the store also carries Mexican products, like this cactus, which is also very healthy. Mixing traditions from home countries with best practices here to maintain the health of this rapidly growing slice of America."

This story violates established truths. Although television, we know, is doomed to tell over-simplified stories, this one, like the H1N1 stories we examined in Chapter 4, throws an intricate mélange of complicated discourses at viewers simultaneously, paralleling the complexity of the public health literature on social and economic determinants of health.[45] Racialized subjects, we know, are often reduced to a small range of problematic roles, characterized by simple subject positions, in opposition to the complexity and heterogeneity of white subject positions (see Gordon 1997). In health news, in contrast to the paucity of minority officials in television crime news (Entman and Rojecki 2000), minority health professionals are practically ubiquitous in stories focusing on minority health issues, and they are generally portrayed as sympathetic and authoritative.

We interviewed a range of "mediators," health professionals from racialized communities who frequently appear in health news; here we highlight four individuals in California, all of whom have played this role in regional and national news for decades. Trained as a social scientist, John López[46] directs a health-focused research center at a leading medical school. Darryl Jackson is a physician in private practice who served in high office at the National Medical Association. Jim Montoya, whom we met in Chapter 2, and Gloria Gallegos are both senior executive officers of community clinics and have graduate degrees in public health. Gallegos, Jackson, and Montoya seldom appear in stories not related to health, but López is used as a source in articles and broadcasts that deal with a wide range of Latino/a-related topics.

All four actively monitor news stories relating to race and health. Montoya has worked for years with a media-consulting firm that helps with press releases and contacts; López's medical school has a public relations office that contacts him regularly. They both initiate press contacts to suggest stories on their programs and issues that concern them; Gallegos reports that her organization sends out at least one press release each week, "because we want our name out there." When Montoya holds press conferences at his community clinic, he recruits physicians with strong media skills and they, in turn, enlist patients. The four stay on the lookout for loaded questions from journalists, trying to avoid "walking into a trap" (López) or confirming racialized stereotypes. They have reason to worry; actors like themselves sometimes are principal sources in stories that reproduce stereotypes. They expressed frustration and a touch of anger in describing the stereotypes and overt acts of discrimination they encountered with non-Hispanic white officials and journalists. Gallegos, López, and Montoya work with Spanish and English media outlets. López reports that Spanish-language journalists are more likely to attend his press conferences, and

> it's easier for me if it is a Spanish language [reporter] because [s/he] is not going to out of hand say 'Oh he's just a Mexican, what does he know!' And I do get that from the English language press. 'Oh you're biased, you're Latino.'

They report audience reactions that range from "Finally someone told the truth— that's my story too!" to hate mail. López noted, "There are groups out there that want to pound you down every time you stick your head out."

These individuals did not speak with a single voice, but we see four substantive areas of overlap. First, they framed their media interactions as part of multifaceted efforts to confront racism and health inequities. These included providing accessible healthcare, participating in research, serving on regional and national advisory groups and professional associations, and building relationships with policymakers. López argued that non-Hispanic whites in general have a "pretty negative" view of Latinos/as; the impact he projects for his work is hardly utopian: "I'd like in 20 years to at least have increased that, so at least it would be *neutral*."

Second, each framed media interactions as motivated by the perception that health news—like other media foci—often reproduces racial inequalities, simultaneously perpetuating denigrating stereotypes and creating illusions of a post-racial society. López used research to confront stereotypes with facts, recruiting journalists to respond to anti-immigrant and anti-Latino/a voices. Jackson argued that President Obama's election and his healthcare reform efforts had promoted the sense that racism was a thing of the past and that "all we need to do is get everybody access and that's really going to eliminate health disparities."

Third, rather than attacking stereotypes head-on, they attempted to complicate and recontextualize them by locating minority populations beyond rigid binaries and projections of separate, bounded, and autonomous racialized worlds. López noted how publicity about the "Hispanic health paradox"—the finding that recent Latin American immigrants are generally *healthier* than either non-immigrants or the descendants of immigrants—helped counter stereotypes that all Latinos are "illegal immigrants, teenage pregnant mammas, welfare, gangbangers, or on drugs" (López), therefore threatening the health of whites. They emphasize the heterogeneity of all populations and promote the sense that diversity lies at the core of Californian and US identities. Jackson thus suggested that providing health education and screenings in churches and barbershops (a common focus of news reports on African American health) "has been proven to be a very effective mode [to reach] the African American community," but emphasized that this approach does not mean that African Americans do not also occupy the same biocommunicable circuits as whites.

Finally, none of the four identified with the idea that health reporting is a tool for educating deficient lay populations—the common assumption of the linear transmission model of health communication. Gallegos was particularly clear. The press materials she generates

> are not necessarily designed in a way to compel the reader to make behavioral changes. We do that here at the clinic. Because my background is in public health, because to get the individual or the family to make positive decisions and lifestyle changes . . . you really need the one-on-one.

She used the Spanish language news media—television, the *SDU-T* 's weekly Spanish section, and radio—largely to publicize programs that provide "healthcare for those who don't have insurance or who have limited ability to pay their bills." When she reaches out to the English language media, particularly newspapers, "generally it's for visibility and PR." She wants audiences to know that

> we are comprehensive and that we care about our clients, because you never know when those individuals are going to be reviewing a proposal or when they [will] get a phone call and someone asks, 'tell me what you know' [about my clinics].

Beyond reaching donors, a key audience is small business owners; since many do not offer their employees health insurance, she wants them to tell employees about her clinic's free or low-cost care. Montoya suggested that he sought media attention just before a key set of policymakers was about to decide an issue about which he cares, but Gallegos, Jackson, and López were skeptical about the possibility of shaping policy this way.

Thus, to the extent that these communicators framed their media engagement pedagogically rather than as PR, it was a pedagogical project primarily aimed at displacing racial stereotypes harbored by white audiences. Overcoming post-racial erasures by fostering coverage of racial health inequities is crucial, they suggested, for this reason. They wanted to show, in short, that members of racialized populations can experience health problems without becoming social problems and can develop solutions of value to everyone. Oscar Gandy *et al.* (1997) argue in the case of black/white inequalities that audiences are more likely to invoke blame-the-victim perspectives when causal mechanisms are not addressed. Kim *et al.* (2010) similarly suggest that pinning inequities on individual behavior may limit public support for policies that attempt to eliminate racial/ethnic inequities. Taylor-Clark *et al.* note that the majority of the stories they examined focusing on African American healthcare inequalities described no responsible causal agent and that approximately half "did not report actors who are working to ameliorate healthcare inequalities" and failed to "call on any actor to address disparities" (2007:405). These patterns suggest why efforts by these and other mediators to shape health news are both so important and so precarious.

The research, institutions, and programs created by people like López, Jackson, Montoya, and Gallegos are central in much reporting that foregrounds race and ethnicity. Such programs are popular material for journalists, because they infuse stories with a positive spin that, journalists assume, will appeal to audiences: stories "about taking charge and facing . . . risks head on," in the words of NBC anchor Brian Williams.[47] Journalists typically build stories about "social problems" around initiatives to *solve* those problems. These mediators are often pictured as remedying failures of biocommunicability, bridging gaps that purportedly isolate racialized populations from biomedical knowledge. In the NBC story on Latino/a health in Chicago, peer educator Rosa and sociologist Giachello make biocommunicable gaps seem real and causal but surmountable. After Bazell speaks of a "cultural divide," Rosa says on camera, "I'm just like them, they have confidence in me; they trust me." Rosa then teaches residents to read nutritional labels. Being "just like them"—and possessing symbolic capital conferred by their training—enables mediators to bring fellow Latinos/as into the biocommunicability loop. Such figures function as mediators in two senses: mediating between biomedical science and "the community," and between racialized populations and the audience—imagined as predominately white and middle class. They speak about race and cultural differences while reassuring audiences that barriers can be bridged and racial and ethnic others brought within dominant norms of health citizenship and biocommunicability.

Important elements of the racialized biocommunicability explored earlier in this chapter persist. Racialized subjects are typically presented as not being properly integrated into biocommunicable circuits unless they join the programs featured in the stories. The NBC story on Latinos/as in Chicago emphasizes that participants' need to learn nutritional basics, "something that is not always easy, especially for someone who has moved from another country."[48] But portrayals of masses of ignorant brown bodies are generally absent; and participants in these programs often look happy and active. The mediators themselves, of course, are presented as active, authoritative participants in the flow of biomedical knowledge. In some cases the stories are also complicated by a secondary focus on structural factors in health disparities, which professional mediators introduce. Just as the 2009 NBC story on Chicago mentioned jobs with poor access to health insurance and food deserts, a 1 December 2008 NBC story on diabetes and obesity among Latina women showed the director of a program called Mujeres en Acción taking Bazell on a tour of a mainly Latino/a neighborhood; for women who live there, she explained, it may be unsafe to walk.

Professional status gives first-line mediators—researchers and program directors—authoritative voices and influence over the storyline. When laypersons were mediators, however, their role was much more restricted. One story from NBC Affiliate KCRA in Sacramento[49] asserted that 54 million people have pre-diabetes "and many of them don't even know it." It focused on peer educator Gary King, an African American with type 2 diabetes. King is presented positively; he is clearly not understood as one "doesn't even know." The story is an opportunity for him to promote his program, saying (as he holds up chess pieces), "We're hoping to turn pawns into kings." As the story goes on, however, a white American Diabetes

Association spokeswoman plays the authoritative role of transmitting biomedical information, while King describes his family history and efforts to confront diabetes. Race and ethnicity are never mentioned, but the common cultural association between disease and ethnicity is invoked as King says, shifting for the first time into African American Vernacular English, "I miss them ribs; them pork chops." Even as stories featuring mediators generally avoid strongly negative versions of stereotypes, appeals to cultural reasoning are also evident, sometimes reframed as offering positive health advantages.

Michelle Obama's childhood obesity initiatives represent an unusual but prominent example of an intervention by a lay mediator. Her media presence is in general seen as a symbol of "post-racism"—a symbol of a discourse that asserts the passing of rigid racial inequalities. Focusing on the fight against obesity put Obama on a consensual terrain where she was unlikely to be portrayed—as she was in much coverage of Barack Obama's first campaign—as an "angry black woman" raising racial grievances. Stories on her Let's Move! campaign often made no explicit reference to race, portraying happy multiracial images of fitness. Ralina Joseph, however, has argued that Obama's strategic use of post-racial discourse should be seen as a form of resistance to the erasure in public discourse of racialized populations and issues of racial inequality. "Michelle Obama," she argues, "uses the *very tools* of postidentity to argue *against* the tenets of postidentity" (2011:59).

Let's Move! injected African American identity into the discourse of fitness in particularly subtle and important ways, troubling the "unbearable whiteness" usually attached to images of fitness (as in the *SDU-T* Health section). She appears "visibly Black while living healthily"[50]—a rare image in mainstream media reporting. This quotation, like the "unbearable whiteness" phrase, comes from African American blogger Erika Nicole Kendall, editor of BGG2WL: Black Girl's Guide to Weight Loss, which challenges fitness/whiteness connections and critiques patient-consumer discourses about individual choice. While mainstream media rarely reference the "black and green" health culture represented by activists like Kendall, Obama can make challenges to standard connections between race, health, and nutrition newsworthy. In March 2009, Obama enlisted Washington-area school children to cultivate an organic garden on the White House lawn. CNN's report included soundbites from the usual—white—faces of the sustainable food movement, chef Alice Waters, for example, but center stage went to Obama and an "army of fifth graders" who were multiracial but predominately African American. In April of 2011 she partnered with singer Beyoncé on a video that similarly centered on both children of color and African American popular culture. "Let's Move" is set in a school cafeteria. It begins with a chubby, light-skinned child and a thinner Black child moving to the center of the floor where they begin to dance to Beyoncé's hip-hop tune, and are joined by Beyoncé and a chorus overwhelmingly made up of children of color (Figure 6.4). Obama was often seen in news reports dancing to popular music associated with African American culture with similar groups of children.

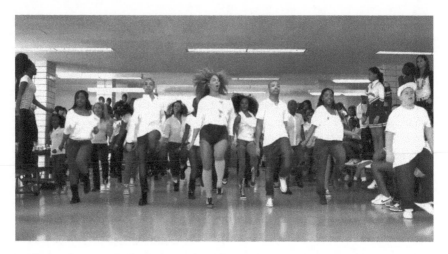

FIGURE 6.4 Beyoncé dances with a chorus mainly made up of children of color in the 2011 "Let's Move!" video. Part of the NABEF's Flash Workout.

Deracializing health

Here's the paradox we're tracing: health news is an important arena for constructing race at the same time that stories in which race is an overt, central focus are relatively uncommon. A search of the Vanderbilt Television New Index and Abstracts, covering the evening news on ABC, CBS, NBC, and CNN, for racial references from 1 January 2000 through 31 December 2013, using all combinations of the term African American, Latino, Hispanic, Asian American, and Native American with Health and Medicine, reveals, after culling irrelevant stories, about 34 health-related stories that mention race and ethnicity directly, some short or only briefly touching on these themes. Health and medicine are central foci of the evening news; if you search "Medicine" during this period, there are over 11,000 stories; those that evoke race and ethnicity form a tiny percentage indeed. In our historical *NYT* and *Chicago Tribune* sample, 4 percent of health stories referred to African Americans or blacks as a group and 2.3 percent to Latinos/as or Hispanics. News coverage largely projects health and medicine as arenas in which race enters only under particular, unusual circumstances. The dominant pattern of racial representation in health news is thus *overt deracialization*, sometimes involving the invisibility of race and ethnicity and sometimes the construction of an ideal, "post-racial" vision of diversity and inclusiveness.

Some stories construct a universalist biological essentialism that imagines individual human bodies admitting of characteristics of age, gender, sexuality, disability, or other categories, but not race. Breast cancer stories thus often construct "women" as a homogeneous, naturally defined category; those on prostate cancer construct "men" in equally post-racial terms. (A male/female gender binary just seems self-evident, universal, and exhaustive.) Diabetes affects "the elderly" or "children" in ways that render differences of race and class irrelevant. An Atlanta

Fox affiliate ran a story entitled "Men's Health Problems" on 12 August 2010.[51] In the anchor's words, "research shows men just don't make it in to see their doctor as often as they should." Seemingly projecting a homogenous affective and biological status to persons occupying the status of "men," neither racial differentials in access to healthcare nor the co-construction of categories of race, gender, and sexuality (Gutiérrez 1991; Stoler 1995) complicate a gender binary.

Race also often disappears through a different universalizing rhetoric: the effects of individual choices. ABC Boston affiliate WCVB produced a story on 2 November 2010 that reported claims by a nutritional "expert" that "fat genes" are "not an excuse to be overweight." Suggesting that what really matters are individuals' nutritional choices, the story echoes the neoliberal logic of, in Emily Martin's (1994) terms, flexible bodies, registers of individual agency and responsibility that lie at the core of contemporary frameworks of biomedicalization. Flourishing in self-help columns, lifestyle and health sections, and health segments of television news broadcasts, such stories advance patient-consumer biocommunicability—readers or viewers are receiving what the WCVB anchor called "the secret ingredients" that teach viewers how to overcome "fat genes." The visuals show the slender, blond, elegantly dressed reporter and nutritionist walking through a supermarket, contrasting their bodies with those of obese and overweight shoppers; all are cut off above the shoulders—a standard technique in television coverage of obesity (Figure 6.5). This camera framing makes the race and ethnicity of "overweight bodies" difficult to determine, though if the viewer looks closely they represent the multiracial mix typical of most health stories. The role of white reporter and nutritionist would seem to reinforce the association of fitness with whiteness.

Other stories project forces acting on vast populations, abstracting racial and ethnic patterns. US "epidemics" of obesity and diabetes are sometimes characterized as the effects of aggressive marketing of unhealthy food and drink. A CBS News segment on 8 August 2002 argues that educating individuals to adopt better nutrition and exercise "just hasn't worked" due to how the food industry "hooks" children on fast foods. The segment focuses on a "victim of McDonalds" who is suing McDonalds and other fast-food outlets. Although the plaintiff appears African American, there is no discussion of race. Stories periodically characterize the effects of lack of health insurance. An NBC story on uninsured Americans[52] interviews a

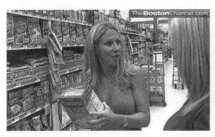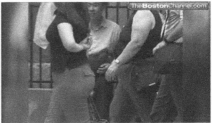

FIGURE 6.5   Two slim blondes give nutritional advice; outside, a multiracial cast of headless fat bodies. WCVB, 2 Nov. 2010.

waitress, Rosa, who reports that her diabetes was inadequately treated due to lack of insurance. Racial differentials in access to health insurance are not mentioned. Much coverage of New York City Mayor Michael Bloomberg's proposal to ban the sale of sugary beverages over 16 fluid ounces by delis, fast-food restaurants, and other facilities similarly focused on obesity as applying to all consumers.

News stories commonly project health and medicine as post-racial through visual images of a multiracial *dramatis personae*. An ABC local news broadcast from Baltimore outlined how women can reduce breast cancer risk. Although most patients were white, an African American physician was the central professional voice, alongside white physicians and X-ray technicians. A local ABC affiliate in New Haven, Connecticut reported on genetic testing that personalizes treatment regimes; it features an Asian American journalist and a medical team with white and Latino/a members led by a Latino immigrant, a highly specialized physician.[53] Stories commonly build series of images of patients or laypersons-in-the-street, constructing a multiracial "anybody" or abstract individual. In our collection of local and national television stories on diabetes and obesity, most stories made no mention of race, and also avoided any clear racial association in the images. This does not happen by chance. Kathy Knight, the network producer profiled in Chapter 2, when asked where they found the people appearing in "character-driven stories," explained that PR offices for research institutions and pharmaceutical companies knew what TV needed and provided articulate patients and researchers. She continued, "They know that diversity is very important to us, and that we really strive to show a real picture of what's happening out there in the country." The findings presented in Table 6.1, showing that the great majority of crucial speaking characters in television health coverage are white, qualify this picture. Nevertheless, the combination in much health news of scripts void of any reference to race or ethnicity, let alone racial health inequities, and racially diverse casts of professionals, patients, and potential patients projects a vision of post-racial biological citizenship (Petryna 2002; Rose and Novas 2005).

"It's stunning to hear that": covering racism in medicine

"We Americans like to think we have the world's best healthcare," said the anchor of the CBS Evening News, introducing a Weekend Journal feature about race and healthcare.[54] "We also like to think that we've created a largely color-blind society. Worthy ideals, but not entirely true." Studies that point to racism in health systems were particularly challenging to the dominant post-racialism ideal that structures most health and medical reporting. We close this chapter by looking at news coverage of biomedical racism. As we mentioned, two studies released in 2002 drew significant attention to racial health inequities: a CDC study of racial differences in health outcomes (Keppel, Pearcy, and Wagener 2002) and the Institute of Medicine's *Unequal Treatment* (Smedley, Stith, and Nelson 2002). The latter was commissioned by Congress, largely at the insistence of the Congressional Black Caucus, and, according to Darryl Jackson, one of our "mediators," thanks to the initiative of the National Medical Association. Jackson helped shape the report's impact by his strong media presence. *Unequal Treatment* was covered widely but not prominently in the press, with short articles appearing on inside pages of newspapers. On television, only one network, CBS, carried the story. Since 2002, mentions of medical racism interrupt overt deracialization only occasionally.

A CBS Weekend Journal story[55] formed the exception that proves the rule. Pegged to a study showing that minorities were less likely to be treated for pain, it featured a Latina who visited a physician for stomach pain, only to have the doctor ask, "How much did you have to drink last night?" The doctor scoffed and left, she says, when she told him she didn't drink. An African American doctor stated, "You wouldn't think healthcare would exhibit that level of racism," before confirming that research showed clear disparities in the treatment given to patients of different races. Even the strongest medical racism stories almost always contain such expressions of surprise, referencing the assumption that medicine is post-racial. In a lengthy CNN story,[56] Dr. Sanjay Gupta interviews three African Americans, asking them to raise their hands if they believe the medical system is racist. All three do, a bit hesitantly, as if saying, "What do you think?" Gupta says, "It's stunning to hear that. I think that maybe you think about people waiting longer in clinics or seeing different doctors each time, but to say it's *racist* is a pretty remarkable thing." His surprise, clearly not shared by his interviewees, identifies him with audiences that assume a post-racial medical system, an assumption that makes it difficult for this sort of message to circulate more broadly.[57]

In November 2007, NBC did a week-long Nightly News series on "African-American Women: Where They Stand." Two of the five reports featured Chief Medical Correspondent Dr. Nancy Snyderman. The first, aired on 27 November, fit within Epstein's (2007) "difference and inclusion" paradigm, mentioning racism only indirectly. Snyderman reported that doctors had been using a model to estimate breast cancer risk developed in 1989 and based on "data gathered solely from white women." Interviewing an African American woman diagnosed with an early-onset, aggressive form of cancer and two researchers working on breast cancer in Africa, Snyderman argued that breast cancer may be a "completely different disease" for African Americans. Snyderman wraps up:

> Early detection really matters, and if you're a black woman and you have a family history of early-onset breast cancer, you really need to consider getting breast cancer screening. . . . Talk to your doctor about your risk. And, Brian, I cannot drive it home enough, clinical trials matter. This is not experimentation. This is how doctors and scientists gather information. We need people of all ages and races in these very important trials.

Here, Snyderman briefly acknowledges a history of racial medical inequality, urging African Americans to make the individual choice to get screened and participate in clinical trials.

Two days later, anchor Brian Williams introduced Snyderman's second story as a "powerful piece of reporting":

> It's about what happens when a black woman and a white woman, similar in every other way, walk into a hospital with the same ailment, in this case heart disease. Black women are more likely to get it, less likely to receive quality treatment for it.

Snyderman gives statistics on heart disease among African American women, then focuses on one patient. "In New York, the message to get healthy is taking a little longer to sink in for Deborah Jackson. So her physician, Dr. Lori Mosca, decided to scare her straight." The patient recounts how her doctor took her to observe an open-heart surgery. Snyderman continues, "Deborah faces an uphill battle, as several studies show a troubling disparity, that black women are less likely than whites to receive quality care." Snyderman continues, "Dr. Mosca says, it's time the medical community does a better job of bridging the gap between race and medicine." The story continues with a soundbite from Mosca, "It may be related to communication issues, and us, really, in the medical establishment, not reaching out to the communities in the way we should and the patients the way that we should."

Snyderman concludes: "So here is the bottom line: you really have to come to your doctor's office with a list of questions written out and bring someone with you," standard active patient-consumer advice.

> And Brian, I hesitate to put it all on the patient, but we have to put that four-letter word, 'race,' on the table, because we're talking about disparity. We can no longer just give it lip service. And now really there has to be recognition and action.

Williams interrupts, "A kind of racism institutionalized, baked into the medical system." "It's so baked in," Snyderman goes on, "that we make assumptions about each other. It's not that doctors want to make the wrong decisions. We make assumptions that we really don't have the right to make. And that's when people fall through the cracks." "It's a crime in this case," Williams concludes. "Powerful piece of reporting, as we said."

Lacking a clear "peg," Snyderman clearly decided to cover this story because she thought it important. Williams' dramatic opening and closing frames suggest that television news is uncomfortable with such stories, however. Snyderman has trouble fitting the story into the conventions of reporting that she normally deploys masterfully. The story starts out essentially reproducing the common "out of the loop" portrayal, attributing racial disparities to biocommunicable failure—describing how physician Mosca sent Jackson to watch open heart surgery to "scare her straight"—before shifting abruptly to medical racism. In her commentary, Snyderman moves back into her familiar role of advising viewers on how to "take charge" of their own health as patient-consumers, only then to apologize for putting the onus on the patient, even as she calls for action on medical racism.

Unequal Treatment and subsequent studies have never been adequately integrated into health coverage. Take the multitude of stories on racialized minorities' purported reluctance to visit doctors or that project them as "people who might be uncomfortable in a medical clinic" (quoting a *SDU-T* story about an outreach program directed to African Americans, carried out in churches).[58] These stories rarely mention racism or invoke *Unequal Treatment*, instead displacing inequities from the medical system to "culture." Many stories on African Americans refer to the Tuskegee syphilis experiment in the 1930s (Jones 1981) as having engendered African American disengagement from biomedical treatment and mainstream biocommunicability. Two months after *Unequal Treatment* appeared, *SDU-T* reporter Cheryl Clark quoted researchers connecting Tuskegee with conspiracy theories that HIV/AIDS is a government plot to kill African Americans, generating "'suspicion about research'" that leads fewer minorities to participate in clinical trials.[59] An *NYT* article on the racial gap in breast cancer survival rates stressed that "many of the women admit to never getting a mammogram and avoiding doctors." It observes, "Years of racial discrimination and distrust of the medical establishment dating back to the Tuskegee, Ala., syphilis experiments on black men in the 1930s continue to influence health decisions made by African-American families in the South."[60] Beyond failing to mention that the "experiment" only ended in 1972, such projections fail to consider that the effects of one example of unconscionable abuses that ended over three decades before might exert less direct influence on efforts to seek care than ongoing experiences of discriminatory treatment by medical professionals, including the acts of infantilization and reprimands delivered in response to what are deemed patients' biocommunicable failures. In projecting health inequities as belonging to the past, such stories buttress white stereotypes of racialized populations.

Conclusion

We have traced a heterogeneous range of ways that race enters into biomediatization. They are, however, far from the only ways the story could be told. One of the most deeply rooted ways that health and has been tied to race in the United States is through race-based social movements. The Black Panthers— still regarded as a key symbol of African American resistance—co-constructed with journalists and officials an image of militancy and violence (Rhodes 2007). Although some of the Panthers' major foci were challenging health inequities through providing healthcare, critiquing medicalization, exploring complementary and alternative treatments, and focusing on maternal and infant nutrition (Nelson 2013), these received little mainstream media attention. Access to healthcare for farm workers and their families was of central importance to the United Farm Workers, and the Chicano Movement pressed for equal access more generally. Chicano anger (see Romano-V 1968) over Madsen's (1964) and

Rubel's (1966) reproduction of cultural logics that depicted Mexican Americans as relying on healers and notions of the evil eye and fright sickness rather than on biomedicine would seem to spring, in part, from how these works erased contemporaneous Chicano/a struggles for access to healthcare and significantly lower access to doctors and hospitals.

Some social movements focus on environmental racism, organizing coalitions of professionals and laypersons for documenting the unequal distribution of toxic hazards and pressing for environmental justice (Bullard 1990; Brown *et al.* 2011). In Chapter 1 we summarized two of the rare stories that focus on such collaborations, both in the *SDU-T*. These were examples of public sphere biocommunicability in which African American and Latino/a San Diego-area residents teamed up with the Health and Environment Action Network to document exposure to metal plating and lead poisoning and demand action.[61] Native American nations, largely invisible in US health news, have in some cases challenged environmental racism and, recently, have used casino and mineral revenues to set up their own healthcare systems.

Highlighting such efforts would impact how people construct both health and racial difference. Nevertheless, the most common pattern is overt deracialization. As many scholars have recently observed, the dominant discourses about race and ethnicity today are discourses of "post-racism" (Ono 2010; Bonilla-Silva 2010) These take many forms; as Joseph (2011:58) noted, "post-identity. . . is presented in the mainstream media somewhere along the spectrum from fact to aspiration," and can be used in the service of a variety of political and cultural projects. In the case of health and medicine, the general ideology of post-racism is reinforced by strong assumptions about the universalism of medicine and science. These vary, again, from assumptions that science simply stands apart from racial difference and understands a biological human body that has no social characteristics, to a normative conviction that medicine should serve all equally across social differences.

The deracialization of health news can be admirable. For example, it is noteworthy that mainstream journalists largely rejected the racialization of the H1N1 pandemic as a Mexican or immigrant threat, despite the persistence of anti-immigrant rhetoric in social media, conservative blogs, and comments sections of newspaper and television websites. But deracializing health news and projecting a post-racial medical ideal have their dangers. Herman Gray (2004) was among the first to point this out, in the context of *The Cosby Show*, an early fictional representation of an African American health professional: portrayals of American society as post-racial, of racialized subjects as happily integrated into the dominant society, can obscure social inequalities and hierarchies, can make those who suffer from those inequalities seem individually to blame and those who contest them ungrateful and out of touch with reality. Post-racial representations, as Tyrone Forman (2004:44) argues, contribute to a climate of racial apathy among whites, a "lack of feeling or indifference toward societal racial and ethnic inequality and lack of engagement with race-related social issues." While "mediators" succeed in getting media coverage, usually quite favorable, for their programs and prompting journalists and officials to address racial health inequities, and while journalists like Gupta or Snyderman may express sincere dismay over the reality of racial disparities in health outcomes and institutional racism in the health system, the truth is that these themes enter the news agenda only on rare occasions, often with obvious discomfort and apology to the audience. Journalistic conventions often make it difficult for strong, coherent stories to be built around these themes.

Given both the degree of racial segregation in the United States and the general association of health issues with notions of privacy and confidentiality (as codified in the Health Insurance Portability and Accountability Act Privacy Rule), people who are not health professionals usually lack direct knowledge of how people who live on the other side of racial, ethnic, class, sexual, or disability borders think about health and disease, of how others acquire and circulate health knowledge and how they pursue wellness and react to illness, and the barriers that they face. The centrality of HIV/AIDS to representations of gay men and Haitians in the 1980s provides a striking example of how important media representations can be for just this reason and of their effects on policies, epidemiology, everyday interactions, and forms of resistance (Epstein 1996; Farmer 1992; Treichler 1999).

It is not only laypersons alone who learn about patient populations through health news. It seems highly likely that negative perceptions by physicians of African American and Latino/a patients' biocommunicable capacities—cited as a factor producing unequal treatment (Smedley *et al.* 2002)—are affected by clinicians' reception of health news. Charles' interview with his physician (Chapter 2) pointed to how biocommunicability, race, and class enter into perceptions of patients. Richards embraced patient-consumer communicability, remarking that he was delighted when his patients brought material they found in media sources—including advertising—into his examining room. But there was a catch: most of his patients "are the last people who will get information over the Internet." Referring to them as "poor or elderly" sidestepped another dimension. Located near Richmond, CA, many of these patients are low-income Latinos/as and particularly African Americans. Richards' wish that more patients brought printouts from websites or inquired about pharmaceutical advertisements suggests that his faith in the patient-consumer model was more aspirational than universal, that it applied only to a minority of his patients, those not included in particular demographics. Despite his commendable commitment as a private practitioner to treat patients who could pay nothing (which ended when he was forced to join an HMO), they did not seem to qualify for this communicably exalted status. That class, age, and race entered into the way he constructed patients in biocommunicable terms does not prove that Richards treated them differently; on this score, we have no data. More broadly, the role of news coverage in shaping physicians' communicable constructions of patients certainly does not emerge apart from the influence of medical training, continuing medical education courses, "cultural competence" training, professional publications, and other factors. Nevertheless, Richards' remarks suggest that biomediatization, race, and class intersect in important ways in diagnosis and treatment; these connections cry out for more research.

Researchers have documented the pervasiveness of an ideological pattern underlying US "racial formations" (Omi and Winant 1986) that turns white racial identities into an unmarked baseline, a racial position that seems to precede and stand outside of discourses of race. Charles Mills argued that this process amounts to a "racial contract" based on an "inverted epistemology," requiring both implicit recognition of how society is structured through racial inequalities (1997:18) and a "structured blindness" (1997:19) emanating from the public dogma that a race-less social contract includes everyone. George Lipsitz (2006, 2011) suggested that whiteness exerts not just ideological but substantial material effects, spatialized through segregation, affording advantages in housing, education, credit, insurance, and other areas, like a credit transferred at birth through racial identity. Given that whiteness confers health benefits—as measured in terms of access to care, quality of care, and health outcomes, turning white subjects into normative neoliberal patient-consumers and parading bodies of various races across the screen but failing to address how race shapes health protects white biomedical privilege. Taylor-Clark et al. (2007) suggest that a growth in news coverage of African American healthcare inequalities and of public awareness of the issue between 1994 and 2004 went hand-in-hand, however, with a decrease in public support for actions taken by the federal government to address them.[62] Examining both halves of the racialization process—the overt deracialization of most coverage and the character of stories that racialize health—helps us understand this connection between greater awareness and diminished support for state intervention. The period in question is, of course, one in which conservative demands to eliminate any forms of affirmative action went, to change the metaphor, fist-in-glove with efforts to undermine state responsibility in favor of market mechanisms.[63]

Several notes of caution are in order. We are clearly not saying that health journalists are responsible for these complex and consequential phenomena: biomediatization is co-produced by medical and media professionals and others, including laypersons. Moreover, our analysis has insisted throughout that there is no singular, simple, stable pattern underlying biomediatization. H1N1 is not diabetes. Class, gender, and sexuality are crucial. Biocommunicable models, which are recurrent and abstracted patterns, do not exist in isolation, and the biocommunicable cartographies that emerge in individual stories often combine and sometimes contradict them in complicated ways. The actors we have referred to as mediators use incredible skill as biomediatizers, often aided by PR/media consulting firms or ex-journalists employed by their institutions, working within these unequal patterns of (non-)representation to draw the attention of policymakers, funders, and members of mass audiences who might have a "pretty negative" (López) view of Latinos/as and African Americans to racial inequities and efforts to confront them. Nevertheless, some—but not all—of the articles that most directly reproduced the biocommunicable underpinnings of racial stereotypes were written by Latino/a journalists and relied primarily on Latino/a professionals.

Analyzing the complex way that racialization unfolds in biomediatization leads us to conclude that *it matters which stories appear in news coverage*. The predominant focus on individual risk factors, lifestyle issues, and patient-consumer biocommunicability goes hand-in-hand with the predominant non-representation of racial and ethnic difference in diverting attention from structural factors. By their very rarity, pieces that highlight race and ethnicity become figures that stand out sharply against this race-shouldn't-matter ground. As George Lipsitz (2011:112) put it with biting parsimony, "people who *have* problems *are* problems" in white imaginaries, and the image of biocommunicable failure plays a large role in effecting this transformation from victim to unsanitary subject to threat.

Notes

1 Immigration coverage is complex and probably has changed considerably depending on the political conjuncture. See Benson (2013).
2 This material was found by looking at stories categorized under health on clipsyndicate. com, on which many local television stations post their stories.
3 "Report Sounds Alarm on Child Accidents," 10 Dec. 2008:A12.
4 Reported by Sabriya Rice on CNN's website, "Hip-Hop for the Heart Sends a Culturally Sensitive Message," http://edition.cnn.com/2009/HEALTH/02/20/minorities.disease/index.html, accessed 13 Jun. 2012.
5 myFOX Health: Eating Disorder Uptick, KMSP FOX 9 Minneapolis, 30 Nov. 2010.
6 "Woman Battles Anorexia After 20 Years," KSTU FOX13 Salt Lake City, 20 May 2010.
7 Sabrina Tabernese, "Women Hit Hard as Toll Rises in Overdoses from Pain Pills," 3 Jul. 2013:A1, 3; see also Deborah Sontag, "Heroin's Small-Town Toll, and a Mother's Pain." *NYT*, 11 Feb. 2014:A1, 13.
8 National HIV, WWLP NBC 22 Springfield MA, 24 Jun. 2010.
9 17 Jun. 2009.
10 Emily Bazar, "Town's High Heart Procedure Rates Raise Questions on Treatment, Costs," *San Francisco Chronicle*, 4 Sept. 2011:A1, 14–15.
11 This figure is for 2010, taken from the United States Census Bureau, State and County QuickFacts, http://quickfacts.census.gov/qfd/states/06/0613945.html, accessed 18 Jul. 2015.
12 CBS, "AIDS: Getting the Message," Inside Sunday, 12 Jun. 1988.
13 Donald G. MacNeil, Jr., 5 Dec. 2013:A1.
14 Carla Rivera, 19 May 2002:B1.
15 A critique of a similar program in New York City in 2013 can be found in DasGupta (2013). These kinds of campaigns, DasGupta argues, typically convey an image of "marginalized bodies out of control, unable to care for themselves or their children."
16 Roni Caryn Rabin, "Heart Failure Strikes Blacks More Often and at Younger Ages, Study Finds," 18 Mar. 2009:A15.
17 "Study: Blacks Suffer Heart Failure at Alarmingly High Rates," 23 Mar. 2009.
18 See for example Krieger (2003) and Williams (1999).
19 Kim Painter, "Study: Black Professionals More Likely to Skimp on Sleep," 10 Sept. 2013.
20 For examples of many discussions in this area, see Duster (1990), Epstein (2007), Lewontin, Rose, and Kam (1984), Montoya (2011), Reardon (2005), and Tallbear (2013).
21 From this vast literature, see Epstein (1996), Treichler (1999), and, for a South African comparison, Fassin (2007).
22 Louise Story, "A Niche Strategy Under Siege," 6 Jun. 2007:D1, 4.
23 Gerard Flynn and Susan Scutti, 21 Aug. 2014.
24 "The Long and Ugly Tradition of Treating Africa as a Dirty, Diseased Place," 25 Aug., 2014, http://www.washingtonpost.com/blogs/monkey-cage/wp/2014/08/25/othering-ebola-and-the-history-and-politics-of-pointing-at-immigrants-as-potential-disease-vectors/.
25 Adam Nossiter, "Fear of Ebola Breeds a Terror of Physicians," A1.

26 Dave Phillips, "Assurances Are Given and a Deputy Goes Home, but Ebola Fears Persist," 10 Oct. 2014:A1.

27 Normitsu Onishi, "Back to the Slums of His Youth, to Defuse the Ebola Time Bomb," 14 Sept. 2014:A1, 17.

28 Patricia Turner is researching rumors connecting Obama with Ebola.

29 http://www.foxnews.com/opinion/2014/10/09/ebola-outbreak-why-obama-is-allowing-ebolaphobia-to-spread.html, accessed 8 Jul. 2015.

30 Reid (2005:111) analyzes the often problematic nature of these kinds of health education campaigns directed at racialized communities.

31 "Man's Death Shows Immigrants' Faith in 'Healers,'" 2 May 2002:A6. The first phase of our research, as noted in the Introduction, focused on the *SDU-T*.

32 Fouhy, "Latinos Developing Diabetes at a Fast Rate."

33 17 Apr. 2002:B3.

34 3 Jul. 2002:A1.

35 Irma Cota, "Improving Health Care for Children of Migrant Workers," *SDU-T*, 22 Mar. 2002: B11.

36 Yilmaz (2014) recounts how another story on Latinos/as by the *SDU-T*'s Leonel Sánchez was restructured in the effort to appeal to white readers. In the case he discusses it involves turning a story with political implications into a de-ethnicized human interest story.

37 Hector Becerra, "Program is Fighting Teenage Pregnancy," 8 Jan. 2004:B3.

38 Denise Nelesen, "Programs Tell Latinos about Diabetes," *SDU-T*, 7 Jun. 2003:E5.

39 Healthcare reform stories are excluded here; most of the people appearing in those stories are male politicians.

40 2 Oct. 2007.

41 The material used for this analysis was not initially collected with the intent of doing quantitative content analysis; we simply saved the Health section of our daily paper, a bit sporadically at first, as we moved in and out of working on this project, then more regularly. The sample could be described as a non-systematic, semi-random sample. All photographs of people were coded, except photos of body parts excluding the face. Race and ethnicity were coded on the basis of both physical appearance and information provided in the caption and article. People in crowd shots with more than ten people were not coded, nor were people in the background of photos.

42 All translations from the Spanish by Charles.

43 See for example Heyman, Núñez, and Talavera (2009), Horton (2014), Horton and Barker (2009), and López (2005).

44 We note the striking difference in the perceptions of the Mexican, largely indigenous, farmworkers studied by Seth Holmes (2013:273), who told him that "'Pesticides only affect white Americans.'"

45 See Krieger (2011) for one influential discussion of these complexities.

46 These are pseudonyms.

47 1 Dec. 2008.

48 Greenhalgh and Carney (2014:268) argue that programmatic interventions and "the ubiquitous media messages" target Latinos and Latinas as triggering the US "obesity epidemic" due to a purported "lack of knowledge about healthy eating and [the] failure of Latinos to 'step up' and question their own behaviors and beliefs." They argue that journalists fail to recognize structural barriers tied to migration and difficulties in obtaining more than low-wage jobs with minimal benefits. The examples we have cited suggest, however, that attention to structural factors and what are portrayed as individual and cultural failings are *both* evident in US health news.

49 21 Sept. 2010.

50 "The Unbearable Whiteness of Eating: How the Food Culture War Affects Black America," BGG2WL, 28 Mar. 2012.

51 Fox. Health Watch: Men's Health Problems. WAGA FOX 5, Atlanta GA 8/12/2010, http://www.clipsyndicate.com/video/playlist/12394/1630411?title=health, accessed 11 Jun. 2012.

52 10 Feb. 2003.

53 3 Nov. 2010.

54 11 May 2002.

55 11 May 2002.

56 20 Jul. 2009.

57 Hoberman (2007) summarizes resistance to critiques of medical racism, including euphemistic ways of addressing the issue often employed by liberal physicians and researchers.

58 Victoria Carlborg, "Body and Soul: Churches to Host Health Conferences," 3 Apr. 2002:NI-7. One of the few actions taken by the Department of Health and Human Services in response to the Institute of Medicine Report (which was generally downplayed by political appointees in the Bush administration) was to organize a Take a Loved-One to the Doctor Day, set for 24 Sept. 2002. ABC radio co-sponsored the campaign, deploying its urban radio stations. An AP story, "Go to the Doctor: Federal Officials Hoping to Reduce Racial Health Gap," 18 Apr. 2002, quoted African American radio host Tom Joyner as saying "Drag them (to the doctor) if you have to. And afterward, hey, have a barbeque—watch the pork, cut down on the fat and cholesterol." This approach to addressing racial disparities obviously took the onus off health professional and institutions, though the AP article went on to summarize other findings of the Institute of Medicine report.

59 "Minorities Less Likely to Join Trials for AIDS Drugs," 2 May 2002:A6.

60 Tara Parker-Pope, "Tackling a Racial Gap in Breast Cancer Survival," 20 Dec. 2013:A1, 22.

61 Chen (2012) explores the complicated ways that lead gets connected with racial representation.

62 Kim *et al.* (2010), who charted newspaper coverage of racial and ethnic disparities in general between 1996 and 2005, suggest that coverage peaked in 1998 and declined from that point through 2005.

63 For a striking example of how contemporary forms of racial difference and the privatization of health services came together in the aftermath of Hurricane Katrina, see Adams (2013b).

CONCLUSION

This book centers on two concepts, biocommunicability and biomediatization. We use these concepts to make a case for the importance of health news as a site not merely for the transmission of health information, but for the formation of fundamental concepts of health and its "publics," not to mention citizenship, the state, the market, and more.

Bicommunicability refers to the cultural models of health knowledge and its circulation that are projected in health news, along with myriad other sites. The image of biocommunicable failure we traced in Chapter 6 is a particularly dramatic illustration of why it is important to think critically about biocommunicability. As a way of representing racial otherness, it is widespread and persistent. Strongly evident in US Ebola coverage starting in 2014, it was partially muted in later Ebola coverage as stories that positioned ex-patients and traditional healers as effective communicators of biomedical messages about the disease began to challenge it. But it reappears regularly, as in mid-2015, when the *NYT* portrayed West Africans' irrational fears and mistrust of doctors as impeding clinical trials of Ebola vaccines and treatments.[1] It is certainly not confined to US health news. We referred to its prominent visibility in a 1992–93 cholera epidemic in Venezuela's Delta Amacuro rainforest. Health officials and journalists collaboratively explained away extremely high morbidity and morality by claiming that "the indigenous Warao culture" placed rainforest residents in a biocommunicable circuit dominated by "shamans," rendering people classified as indigenous incapable of understanding physicians' advice on cholera prevention, including basic hygiene. This biocommunicable cartography became so firmly ingrained that it was readily recycled in 2007–8 when a mysterious disease—probably bat-transmitted rabies—killed scores of children and young adults.[2]

Why would images of biocommunicable failure provide such a powerful way to represent not just racial health inequities but race and health in general?

Biomedical authority models project medical knowledge as embodying hierarchically organized ways of knowing and acting. Individuals and populations have similarly long been evaluated with respect to their perceived rationality and agentivity through what is projected as their communicative capacity. Bauman and Briggs (2003) trace the roots of modern notions of language and communication to John Locke's (1959[1690]) separation of knowledge into the distinct and separate "provinces" of nature and language. Locke's insistence that they required separate epistemologies, now vested in science and linguistics—and that strict boundary-work was required to separate both from politics—formed the basis for the language versus medicine binary that is still going strong. As Bauman and Briggs suggest, this formulation repositioned language and communication as the use of abstract signs selected for their ability to precisely, transparently, and rationally convey thoughts. At the same time that boundary-work overtly separated language from political and social relations, how individuals speak became one of the most important sites for evaluating their rationality, modernity, and ability to participate in civil society.

At the same time that health inequalities figured importantly in the politics of whiteness in the United States, linguistic anthropologists have analyzed predominant identifications of whiteness and Americanness with English, as manifested in Official English policies and attacks on public uses of other languages (Woolard 1989), seemingly humorous deployment of Spanish words by monolingual English speakers (Hill 2008), and xenophobic acts of aggression: "This is the United States—speak English!" (Zentella 2003). Generations of scholars have traced efforts to brand varieties of English tied to African American identities as substandard and deficient, as rendering their speakers irrational and illogical.[3] The image of biocommunicable failure thus combines bio and communication forms of racialization powerfully, merging what are projected as two seemingly separate modes of evaluating rationality, agency, and modernity into one. It is accordingly far from surprising that racialized perceptions of biocommunicable success and failure enter significantly into structuring clinical interactions.

Projections of biocommunicability are complex, as we have seen, both in the representation (or erasure) of racial difference specifically, and in health news more generally. Projections of lay passivity and ignorance compete and sometimes mix with projections of agency and competence. These projections are highly consequential, and the role of health news in producing them deserves far more attention from scholars and practitioners alike than it has received to date.

Biomediatization

As we noted in the Introduction, the rapidly growing literature on mediatization at times parallels accounts of medicalization, projecting a growing colonization of other social spheres by respectively "the media" and "medicine." On the surface, these interpretations appear contradictory. Sorting out what happens where these two processes come together, understanding what we have called "biomediatization," requires going beyond formulations that project a linear process of influence between clearly bounded social fields. Recent works on mediatization have emphasized the importance of moving away from formulations that conceive of media as influencing other social fields from the *outside*, substituting media logics for those of other social fields (e.g. Deacon and Stanyer 2014; Marcinkowski and Steiner 2014.) Couldry (2012) argues that understanding mediatization requires going beyond "mediacentric" forms of analysis that isolate the role of media from wider social processes. We build on that work by looking at mediatization and biomedicalization simultaneously, by placing both media and biomedicine in larger social contexts of capitalism, for example, or racial formations, and by understanding health news as *co-produced* by journalists, biomedical professionals, public relations professionals, social activists, and many other actors.

Biomediatization takes place in a context, as Clarke *et al.* (2003) have argued, in which biomedical institutions are not only expanding their social influence, but also, as part of this process of expansion, becoming entangled with other social fields—not only with media but with business, government, education, and more—and becoming increasingly complex internally. Mediatization is a key part of the process by which this expansion of social influence takes place. If biomedicine is reshaping our conceptions of health, illness, life, death, and the body, transforming capitalism, and catalyzing new forms of citizenship—these effects are produced to a large extent through the media—not only through marketing and advertising, as documented by Dumit (2012) and others, but also through health news. At the same time, mediatization can be seen as a *consequence* of the increasing complexity of biomedicine. As biomedical fields have become increasingly complex internally, increasingly interconnected with other social fields, and as their social impact has grown, raising the stakes for a wide range of actors, the diverse range of actors now involved in biomedicine are more likely to be drawn into mediated public spheres, sometimes by their own choice, to try to expand markets, shape policies, etc., sometimes by other actors, including, in many cases, journalists.[4] Here we have detailed ethnographically how biomedical institutions use or interact with media in attempting to manage their relations with the complex range of actors with which they are involved—government regulators, investors, patient-advocacy organizations, and social movements, resulting in the complex relationships through which bodies, diseases, and treatments are co-produced.

We have also detailed the ways in which journalists interact with and enter into biomedical institutions. We have seen that they are heavily influenced by biomedicine, with a heavy presence of biomedical "experts" as "primary definers"; with specialist health reporters often deeply integrated into biomedical cultures; and physicians serving as "medical editors" on television news. We have also seen that health journalism is highly complex and often highly active. Very often, health news involves not settled, unitary results of either scientific research or market logics, but social conflicts involving wide ranges of actors both inside and outside biomedicine—clinicians may come into conflict with pharma companies over the pricing of medications, for example, or conflicting alliances of scientists, physicians, pharma companies, consumer groups, and patient advocacy organizations may mobilize to influence the outcome of a regulatory decision. These conflicts are shaped by the presence of news media, by the fact that health issues are considered highly newsworthy, and that actors compete for access to the news media in order to get public attention, at the same time that they seek to avoid negative scrutiny. And in these cases, journalists play a highly active role in mediating among competing perspectives.

Biomediatization, then, involves neither the colonization of media by biomedicine, nor the other way around, but the creation of a complex field of boundary-objects and hybrid practices. We could view the centrality of communicative practices in biomedicine as having rendered any claims to professional autonomy, either of journalism or of medicine, as obsolete: perhaps they have now simply *merged*. The problem is that we could not have been in dialogue with health journalists, health officials, clinicians, patients, and others for over a decade—not to mention (in Charles' case) living with a physician and training graduate students in a PhD program divided between a medical school and an anthropology department—without coming face-to-face with a major problem of this claim. Even as medical and media domains are deeply enmeshed, boundary-work is equally central, consisting of daily efforts to make these domains appear separate. CNN's charter health journalist Donald Schultz distances himself from Bristol-Meyer advertising, even as he acknowledges the "conflicts" that emerged. Susan Norris, San Diego's Public Health Officer, declared that her extensive dedication to biomediatization was evidence-based and complained about media sensationalism, even as she acknowledged, sotto voce, that politicians could press her into portraying access to ER facilities in ways that violated her best judgment as a public health professional and acknowledged her dependence on media to accomplish public health objectives. Linda Kelly asserted that the health of her readers was "their doctor's problem, not my problem," even as she stressed her commitment to evidence-based medicine and took pride in health professionals' comments that her articles had sometimes been more effective in inducing patients to follow biomedical guidelines than the urgings of clinicians or public health officials. Such boundary-work was evident not only in our conversations with journalists and health professionals but in nearly every health news story.

We have never suggested that such apparent contradictions turn either journalistic or medical logics into false consciousness, into proof of bad faith or professional malfeasance. We have rather argued that there is something deeper and more interesting going on here. Biomediatization points to how the practices of health journalists, public health officials, clinicians, researchers, patients, and others are imbricated. The extensive boundary-work performed by these actors can never stabilize clear separations between these practices, and we would be seriously misled if we were to accept them uncritically as a basis for analyzing biomediatization. Nevertheless, this boundary-work is a real and central part of the biomediatization process we have traced in this book.

Biomediatization and biocommunicability beyond US borders

As we noted in the Preface, our research took us to various parts of Latin America, particularly Cuba and Venezuela, and involved partnerships with colleagues in Argentina and Mexico. Dan is collaborating with researchers in Italy and Norway. Charles conducted research in Singapore. Nevertheless, we chose to focus on bio-mediatization in the United States here. The reason is simple: there was too much to be documented and too many complexities to be explored to try to launch a global comparison right off the bat. We are well aware that the US case is distinctive in many ways: the US has highly commercialized media and health systems, direct-to-consumer drug advertising, and powerful pharma and biotech industries. US health institutions at all levels generally have embedded PR/media professionals. Moreover, the political process is distinctive in important ways, from the role of lobbyists and corporate campaign contributions to the strength of "national security" institutions. We do think, however, that documenting biomediatization in different political, health, and media systems is quite important. We thus offer a few preliminary generalizations, based on our own fieldwork, collaborations with colleagues in other countries, and the published literature in order to stimulate what we hope will be a broad and deep current of further research.

One initial observation is that health news is everywhere: we have found no country in which news coverage of health is absent. It is flourishing in the shift to digital media. It may not, however, be as central in some parts of the world as in the United States. Francescutti, Martínez Nicolás, and Tucho Fernández (2011), for example, find much more limited health content in television news in Spain than we did in the US. At the same time, "service journalism"—of which health news is often an important component—is growing in many systems (Hanusch 2012). Thus, even as there may be countries where health news is more or less dominant, it may also vary across "platforms," between print, radio, and television forms of "traditional" media, not to mention the mix of glocal (simultaneously local and global) Internet and social media venues.

Second, many of the patterns of biomediatization we have described seem to be present in much of the world at the same time that variation is evident in their extent and the specific networks and practices through which they are enacted. Marchetti's (2010) analysis of the mediatization of medicine in France—the most extensive previous analysis we know of—similarly describes an increasingly important mediating role for journalists and an increasingly complex process of co-production of health information. His analysis does give the impression, though, that in the French case the role of political actors and therefore political journalism is relatively greater than in the United States. "All medical institutions," he writes in his conclusion, "have developed a communication practice (*travail de communication*) to legitimate their work to their interlocutors in politics and the state" (2010:168).

Eduardo Menéndez and Renée Di Pardo (2009), whose exhaustive study of health coverage in Mexico focused on the ten newspapers with the greatest national circulation, stressed that stories largely pictured physicians as the source of knowledge about health. They found a dominant negative quality in health news, which often characterized the public health system as a "catastrophe." Remarkably, not only left and right politicians but public health officials themselves—not to mention scholars—collaborated in producing this impression. We found, in contrast, that US coverage was primarily positive. Other patterns were more similar, like an important effect of organized social interest groups on health news agendas. Menéndez and Di Pardo found, much like US biomedical authority coverage, that laypersons are largely constructed in Mexican print news as bystanders, waiting for specialists with medical knowledge to pass it along to them (via reporters)—rather than as being themselves producers of knowledge about health.

Charles' research in Singapore suggested health is much less biomediatized there than in the United States. As in most of the world, there is no direct-to-consumer pharmaceutical advertising. Very few health institutions have persons trained as journalists on staff, even at the higher levels of the Ministry of Health. The exception is the robust biotech and pharmaceutical sector (Ong in press), whose media efforts are directed at least as much at global as Singaporean audiences. Journalists are not constantly inundated by press releases or contacts from people pitching stories; much more dependent on enterprise reporting, extensive links between professionals in this island nation-state enable journalists to search for story ideas. Singapore is not a single-payer system, but the Ministry attempts to guarantee access to healthcare for all. Despite these differences, however, health news looks rather like US coverage, consisting of a mix of biomedical-authority and patient-consumer stories. The leading national newspaper, the *Straits Times*, has a weekly Mind and Body section that is packed with patient-consumer stories and columns, much like the *SDU-T*.

The biomedical authority/passive patient model is evident everywhere we have looked, regardless of whether the politico-economic system is classified as socialist or capitalist, the health system single-payer or market oriented, media institutions are government owned or for-profit. As we suggested in Chapter 4, this type of biocommunicability predominates during what are characterized as health crises. A comparison of H1N1 coverage in April–July 2009 in Argentina, the United States, and Venezuela pointed to a similar pattern of positioning health professionals as knowledge producers in all three countries, despite differences in political, health, and media institutions.[5] Differences are also apparent, even within this pattern. In those three countries, public health authorities were overwhelmingly portrayed in positive terms, although nearly 32 percent of Argentine stories were negative in tone, versus 17.5 percent for the United States and a surprisingly low 8.2 percent for Venezuela, despite intense criticism of the socialist government by opposition media.

The reporting of the 2009 H1N1 pandemic may well have been studied more extensively across media systems than any other health story; in H1N1 coverage, there seems to be evidence of a common pattern in much of the world of heavy coverage dominated by the messages of global public health authorities. At the same time, that event showed important differences rooted in the nature of the media/ politics/public health nexus in different countries. Cornia *et al.* (2015), in a rare comparative analysis, found that Swedish media presented the pandemic in consensual terms, treating the actions of public health authorities as technical and non-political; Italian media followed partisan lines, praising or condemning the public health response depending on their relation to the party in power; and the British media played a watchdog role, criticizing many aspects of the public health response but not following partisan lines. In parallel to our analysis of H1N1 biomediatization in the United States, Menéndez (2010) suggested that health professionals and journalists collaborated in producing a sense of alarm and in juggling tremendous uncertainty and the perceived imperative to intervene.

Patient-consumer biocommunicability is often much less visible than in the United States; as would be expected, it is virtually absent in Cuba. Nevertheless, biocommunicable models do not correlate one-to-one with either political or healthcare systems. Charles' research in Cuba did not suggest that news coverage in the government press was revolutionary; largely linear and didactic, it projected Cuban citizens primarily as in constant need of injections of health knowledge. He found there a different model, which he called *logros de la revolución* ("achievements of the revolution"), that projected health professionals as producing health knowledge and healthcare through intense revolutionary commitment; laypersons were largely cast as spectators, watching admiringly and gratefully benefitting from care. In interviews, however, many laypersons projected themselves as being just as knowledgeable as their physicians, due to having paid close attention to the plethora of health news in the Cuban press throughout their lives (Briggs 2011a). Given President Hugo Chávez's emphasis on popular participation in shaping revolutionary ideologies and practices, Charles and Clara had suspected that government-owned and -controlled newspapers and television stations in Venezuela would project laypersons as participating in the production and circulation of health knowledge. Despite intense polarization in the political system and large differences between opposition and government media in nearly all other arenas, however, government and opposition media differed very little in how they covered health.

Biomediatization, health, and justice

We make no claim here to be clairvoyant or omniscient, to be able magically to see and analyze what is invisible to others. Indeed, it took us twelve years to reach the point where we had learned enough about biomediatization and had devised what we think are valuable ways of thinking about it to feel comfortable drawing our work to a close and presenting this book. Working in a cross-disciplinary fashion has been crucial, not only combining insights but challenging each other's premises and forms of disciplinary boundary-work. We built our own network of journalists, researchers, health officials, clinicians, and laypersons, and most of the insights contained in this book were inspired by our interlocutors. We have tried to acknowledge these contributions specifically in many cases, but they inevitably go beyond what we can attribute in this way. This book is a collaborative product, even as it is clearly limited by what we did and whom we met as well as the many other things we could have done and possible interlocutors with whom we did not speak.

Our work is analytic, attempting to document areas about which too little is known, reveal their complexities, and explore ways of understanding them. We have tried to avoid the reductionism and moralism that would underlie any over-arching evaluative position. Starting with PR/marketing consultant Jeff Harrison, we have found all of the practices and perspectives we encountered complex and fascinating. Although some coverage, particularly stories stigmatizing immigrant and racialized individuals and populations, made us uncomfortable, we have not set ourselves up as judges of right versus wrong, professional versus unprofessional practices, or naïve versus sophisticated viewpoints or forms of participation, trying to elevate some individuals or classes of actors above any others. Indeed, if bio-mediatization is consequential—and we think it is—then a better goal would be to stimulate all parties to go beyond assumptions of a media versus medical divide and the relegation of news coverage to the status of secondary representations of technoscientific and medical facts. We hope to have inspired readers to think more critically about biomediatization and to engage in debates about its place in shaping health, capitalism, and social relations.

As we prepare to leave these issues in your hands, we think it fair to offer some reflections about what we see as problems that might be fruitfully addressed in sub-sequent research. As we have suggested throughout, stories project a very limited number of biocommunicable subject positions and use them in constructing the characters they introduce and interpellating readers, viewers, and listeners. Being projected as a consumer-patient is very different than being recruited as a passive patient or as a citizen-participant in public sphere debates; they offer very different types of what we can call *biocommunicable citizenship*. And both of these projected subject positions is different than being classified as coming from a population that has purportedly excluded itself from biocommunicable citizenship, whose mem-bers are characterized as needing to recuperate their citizenship through individual remedial action, usually participation in health programs and internalization of the knowledge and biocommunicable models the managers of those programs deem appropriate. Being judged as a biocommunicable failure—and thus possibly classi-fied as an unsanitary subject who is responsible for his or her own health problems and as a potential threat to family members, neighbors, and the body politic—places people in a highly stigmatized position. As our interviews suggested, stigmatized subjects are less commonly interpellated than represented, placed implicitly outside the story's audience, often construed as a homogenous category, as a "they."

Nevertheless, the implications extend to all persons, including those who are not health or media professionals. In the biomedical authority model, the priv-ileged status of knowledge producer is granted to some, denied to most. This strikes us as problematic. A better point of departure would be to view all of us as knowledge producers, as having something worthwhile to contribute to under-standing health, even if the contributions we can offer are distinct. The correlation between poorer health outcomes and diminished access to healthcare on the one hand and biocommunicable stigma on the other seems the most problematic. Our immigrant focus groups were extremely instructive here; participants had extensive knowledge of health problems and of available health services, as well as their shortcomings. By designating them in advance as ignorant subjects in need of injections of knowledge, the biomediatization process produced ignorance—the ignorance of policymakers and practitioners regarding what these individuals could contribute to debates. Insofar as biomedical authority models project laypersons as being required to grasp biomedical information in some two to three minutes or a thousand words of text, assimilate it, and turn it into new ways of acting and relating to others, we are all doomed to failure. Health communication is accordingly like development projects, designed to fail (Ferguson 1990).

Patient-consumer models are more complex in this regard. Laypersons are seldom precisely positioned as knowledge makers; their job is rather to use biomedical knowledge—as provided by their doctors or perhaps a television advertisement—to identify their risk factors and then search out knowledge provided by a wide range of sources, evaluate them all critically, and then make rational decisions about which pills, treatments, and the like to consume. Health thus becomes another arena in which citizenship is demonstrated through consumption (García Canclini 2001). Some stories construct patient-consumers as comparative shoppers, finding out what birth facilities hospitals offer and deciding which most suits their tastes. When patients are trained to ask questions of their doctors, both to understand better but also to make sure that doctors are on the ball, or, like Kathleen Turner, to find out which doctors truly are knowledgeable and help to bring them up to speed about a condition, this role comes to border on participation in knowledge production. Even then, the cost seems to be reducing an active role in ecologies of health knowledge and healthcare to individuals pursuing their own self-interest and a thorough marketization of health. We have commented in various places, particularly Chapter 6, on the naturalization of race and class privilege, inequities of access to healthcare, and unequal treatment in largely reserving the role of patient-consumer to middle-class whites. Moreover, it is, like biomedical authority communicability, a pretty daunting job to grasp the full range of available forms of knowledge about health, including different biomedical specialties, complementary and alternative medicine, food supplements, dietary regimes, exercise programs, and the like, sort out truth from "hype," marketing, and malfeasance, and make complex medical decisions. We have the illusion of freedom, but are doomed again to failure.

Public sphere models of biocommunicability, we have shown, are more common than people imagine. Health news is often treated as "political," though much reporting projects a restricted public sphere in which the active participants are biomedical insiders. There is also a strong tendency to shift attention away from structural causes of health and illness, focusing instead, if not on biology and technology, then on individual behavior and "health education." Menéndez and Di Pardo (2009) similarly pointed out that the majority of Mexican print stories pictured the causes of disease as individual, particularly as the product of behaviors and personal circumstances, thereby detracting attention from structural factors. The model most appealing to us in many ways is less common, but not unknown—this is the kind of public sphere model centered on social movements. Here it is not self-interest that seems to motivate people but participation in collective debates and the fostering of collective welfare, understood in various ways. No population, including physicians, enjoys a completely privileged status. Laypersons, like the woman in San Diego's Barrio Logan (see Figure 1.4, p. 45), are sometimes explicitly represented as knowledge producers, although their participation often gets qualified as being, as the director of HEAN, the environmental activist organization, put it, not "hard scientific information" but a combination of science, "commonsense," and "demand for change." In cancer cluster stories, journalists may elevate laypersons to the status of primary biomediatizers, only to demote them again to the status of scientifically uninformed subjects once state-employed scientists take charge. We should not romanticize these social-movement-oriented stories; they are generally reported when health and media professionals—albeit with activist bents—participate in the same techniques of building relationships with journalists, figuring out news angles that will appeal to journalists, and recruiting laypersons. As the HEAN director suggested, in trying to figure out how to make a story "sexy enough for TV" and to avoid getting covered only in print or on "some obscure web post board or something," she looks for a figure that will appeal to journalists:

> I think a mom who's talking about her child who's been lead poisoned is a hell of a lot more effective than, you know, some corporation that says they don't want to pay for getting the lead out of candy.

This example suggests a strong note of caution. In suggesting that the role of knowledge producer not be restricted to small cadres of health professional elites, we are not issuing a call for individual empowerment. The illusion of individual empowerment is, of course, the ideological "platform" for creating new pharma marketing strategies, for empowering individuals to identify with diseases, quantify their own symptoms, ask the right questions of their doctor, and request the medication featured in the ad. It gets fused with the patina of social movements in the work of patient advocacy groups that are so often sponsored by pharmaceutical corporations (Stokes 2008). As Taussig, Rapp, and Heath (2003) skillfully document, convergences between social movements, scientific research, and clinical intervention through discourses and technologies of genetics can extend both individualism and forms of normalization imposed on bodies classified as abnormal. Medicine is structured in hierarchical terms, and it would be utopian if not foolish to suggest that health news should dress it up as an egalitarian world in which everyone's opinion counts just the same. Similarly, greater openness to debate must be tempered with keeping the precarity as well as the power of biomedical authority in mind. One of the most common responses we got from laypersons when asking about health news was fear and uncertainty. "I'm terrified," one woman noted in thinking about news coverage of shifting recommendations. As we suggested in Chapter 5, high levels of distrust in pharma go together with faith that prescription drugs make lives people's lives better, not to mention massive consumption of medications. Just as we have insisted all along that biomediatization and biocommunicability are complex, suggestions for critical interventions must be equally nuanced and sophisticated.

For us, denials of biocommunicable citizenship and the imposition of biocommunicable stigma are crucial issues, given the way they affect clinical judgments and policy decisions. Few spaces are available in dominant biomediatization processes that allow people the right of reply when they have been denigrated. Here comments sections in on-line news provide important opportunities, along with social media, blogs, and Internet sites. Critical voices that emerge in such contexts are, however, likely to encounter aggressively xenophobic and racist discourses that are often inserted in response to calls made by the moderators of highly partisan on-line forums to stack comments sections with particular messages. We have encountered social movement organizations that monitor news coverage of racial and sexual minorities and the disabled and expose what they see as abuses.

The demands placed upon the ideal active patient-consumer are just as daunting as those of the passive patient. Tracing biocommunicable models has enabled us to pinpoint how they project the bio and communicative dimensions as separate, subordinating the latter, only to bring them together in such a way that being projected as a communicative failure in relation to health knowledge seems to provide direct evidence of failure as a biomedical citizen. We hope to have made a significant contribution here to public debates and policy as well as scholarship by helping to open up biocommunicable models and biomediatization practices to critical scrutiny. Scholars and journalists alike have frequently decried the dangers of allowing PR/media consultants to invisibly orchestrate not just news coverage but medical journal articles and even research and clinical trials. What we have added here is awareness of the crucial role that biocommunicable models play in these debates by constructing biomedical knowledge and non-knowledge, its producers and receivers, sites and temporalities, in particular sorts of ways, as well as by our efforts to document the complex practices used in seeming to bring these models to life. We have similarly suggested that calls for greater transparency or for enhanced fidelity of health stories to clinical and epidemiological "facts" reproduce the very reifications that make it possible to present corporate, state, and other communicative interventions as simply the outpouring of new discoveries, necessary efforts to save publics from ignorance, misinformation, or panic, or the key to freedom and self-fulfillment.

If it takes a network to do biomediatization, it will take coalitions to foster broader debates and open up new collaborative possibilities. Journalists play powerful roles here. We would hope that more space could be created for journalistic self-reflexivity, a space that is greatly restricted by how journalists generally place their own roles in the background and by how health professionals cast journalists as, ideally, just transporters or translators of medical facts. We have argued that singling out journalists for critical scrutiny is mistaken. Forms of stigma tied to biocommunicable models spring out of clinical and public health sites into public discourses and debates through news coverage of health and then reenter as health professionals and patients alike use their experiences as readers and viewers in structuring clinical interactions. Focusing critical attention on complex intersections between biocommunicable models, assumptions about patients' communicative abilities, and clinical practices could form a major contribution to the broad shift from "cultural competency" to "structural competency" in medical education (Metzl and Hansen 2014). As Dutta (2008, 2010) has argued, public health relies on health communication strategies that reproduce both local and global inequalities. If, as the public health officials we interviewed in San Diego County suggested, health news reaches many more people than health education, efforts to overcome health inequities are not likely to succeed if they project the people facing the worst health conditions as being unable to learn or to participate in public debates and contribute to finding new solutions.

In short, we offer no magic bullet, no one-size-fits-all prescription for better health and communication. In the end, however, we would like to encourage efforts to question the power of biocommunicable models and biomediatization practices that are based on commonsense notions about where medicine ends and media begin. All of us are part of biomediatization networks, and we all fall under the spell of biocommunicable models. That's not the problem. The issue is that we need to sit down together, all of us, and talk about how about they shape our fundamental assumptions about what is knowledge and what is non-knowledge, about who knows, who needs to listen, and who is just plain tuned out.

For journalists, biocommunicable models can foster standardized storylines and lists of characters at the same time that they make it more difficult to conceive of new types of sources. Challenging dominant biocommunicable models can thus lead to more innovative health journalism. For clinicians, there are keys here for better diagnosis and treatment by curtailing stereotypical judgments about patients' communicative capacities and enhancing clinician–patient exchanges. If patients are constructed as valuable partners in the construction of knowledge about health—both by clinicians and in health news—they will be much more likely to be capable partners in constructing and carrying out treatment plans. For public health professionals, constructing "the public" as either in constant need of injections of biomedical knowledge or as self-interested maximizers of information and services might thwart the possibility of stimulating a deeper sense among laypersons of being able to contribute actively to facing both individual and collective health problems; it similarly might open up the possibility of creating healthier health policies. For laypersons, we hope that a look inside biocommunicability and biomediatization could help fuel not demands for drugs but demands to be taken seriously as fellow participants in the production of health knowledge and help generate tactics for responding creatively and effectively when faced with denigrating biocommunicable projections, whether in examining rooms, news stories, or heath communication programs. Finally, we hope that scholars have found new research foci, new analytic possibilities, and a broader range of ways to contribute to public debates, public policies, and clinical practices.

We accordingly hope that readers will pull these arguments out of the pages of this book and bring them into their living rooms, news rooms, examining rooms, conference tables, and classrooms. Doing so, to repurpose the title of our book, will make health public in a refreshing new way.

Notes

1 Norimitsu Onishi and Sheri Fink, "Vaccines Face Same Mistrust that Fed Ebola," 13 Mar. 2015.
2 The literature on colonialism and medicine suggests that projections of hygiene, medical knowledge, reliance on physicians *versus* other practitioners, and health-related practices have been central means of producing and rationalizing racial and ethnic hierarchies for centuries (Anderson 2006; Arnold 1993; Hunt 1999).
3 For examples, see Labov (1972), Morgan (2002), and Perry and Delpit (1998).
4 At the same time, we do not share many of the assumptions of the structural-functionalism within which their discussion is framed; our argument is parallel in some ways to that of Marcinkowski and Steiner (2014), who write

> The higher the internal complexity of a social system and the greater the diversity of the resulting demands, the greater is the need for attention and acceptance, and the more important its ability to observe and effectively stimulate the issue-structure of mass-mediated communication.

5 The Argentine analysis was conducted by Anahi Sy and Hugo Spinelli. Health professionals were dominant sources in each country, accounting for 54.5 percent of Argentine, 51.3 percent of US, and 61.2 percent of Venezuelan citations.

REFERENCES

Aalberg, Toril, Jesper Strömbäck, and Claes de Vreese. 2012. The Framing of Politics as Strategy and Game: A Review of Concepts, Operationalizations, and Key Findings. *Journalism* 13(2):162–178.

Abu-Lughod, Lila. 2005. *Dramas of Nationhood: The Politics of Television in Egypt*. Chicago: University of Chicago Press.

Adams, Vincanne. 2013a. Evidence-Based Global Public Health: Subjects, Profits, Erasures. In *When People Come First: Critical Studies in Global Health*, João Biehl and Adriana Petryna, eds., 54–90. Princeton, NJ: Princeton University Press.

———. 2013b. *Markets of Sorrows, Labors of Faith: New Orleans in the Wake of Katrina*. Durham, NC: Duke University Press.

Allison, Tom. 2009. Paranoia Pandemic: Conservative Media Baselessly Blame Swine Flu Outbreak on Immigrants, www.mediamatters.org, accessed April 27.

Altheide, David L., and Robert P. Snow. 1979. *Media Logic*. Beverly Hills, CA: Sage.

Anderson, Warwick. 2006. *Colonial Pathologies: American Tropical Medicine, Race, and Hygiene in the Philippines*. Durham, NC: Duke University Press.

Angeli, Elizabeth L. 2012. Metaphors in the Rhetoric of Pandemic Flu: Electronic Media Coverage of H1N1 and Swine Flu. *Journal of Technical Writing and Communication* 42(3):203–222.

Appadurai, Arjun. 1988. Putting Hierarchy in Its Place. *Cultural Anthropology* 3(1):36–49.

Arnold, David. 1993. *Colonizing the Body: State Medicine and Epidemic Disease in Nineteenth-Century India*. Berkeley: University of California Press.

Arrow, Kenneth J. 1963. Uncertainty and the Welfare Economics of Health Care. *The American Economic Review* 53(5):941–973.

Askew, Kelly, and Richard R. Wilk, eds. 2002. *The Anthropology of Media: A Reader*. Malden, MA: Blackwell.

Atlani-Duault, L., A. Mercier, C. Rousseau, P. Guyot, and J.P. Moatti. 2015. Blood Libel Rebooted: Traditional Scapegoats, Online Media, and the H1N1 Epidemic. *Culture, Medicine and Psychiatry* 39:43–61.

Austin, J.L. 1962. *How to Do Things with Words*. Cambridge, MA: Harvard University Press.

Baker, Lee D. 1998. *From Savage to Negro: Anthropology and the Construction of Race, 1896–1954*. Berkeley: University of California Press.

Barker, Kezia. 2012. Influenza Preparedness and the Bureaucratic Reflex: Anticipating and Generating the 2009 H1N1 Event. *Health and Place* 18:701–709.

Bauer, Martin. 1998. The Medicalization of Science News: From the 'Rocket-Scalpel' to the 'Gene-Meteorite' Complex. *Social Science Information* 37(4):731–751.

Bauman, Richard, and Charles L. Briggs. 2003. *Voices of Modernity: Language Ideologies and the Politics of Inequality*. Cambridge: Cambridge University Press.

Bell, Susan E., and Anne E. Figert. 2012. Medicalization and Phamaceuticalization at the Margins: Looking Backward, Sideways and Forward. *Social Science and Medicine* 75:775–783.

Bennett, W. Lance. 1990. Toward a Theory of Press-State Relations in the United States. *Journal of Communication* 40(2):103–127.

Benson, Rodney. 2013. *Shaping Immigration News: A French-American Comparison*. New York: Cambridge University Press.

Benson, Rodney, and Neveu, Erik, eds. 2005. *Bourdieu and the Journalistic Field*. Cambridge: Polity.

Biehl, João. 2005. *Vita: Life in a Zone of Abandonment*. Berkeley: University of California Press.

Bird, S. Elizabeth, ed. 2010. *The Anthropology of News and Journalism: Global Perspectives*. Bloomington: Indiana University Press.

Blakely, Debra. 2006. *Mass Mediated Disease: A Case Study Analysis of Three Flu Pandemics and Public Health Policy*. Lanham: Lexington Books.

Block, Alex Ben. 2012. 'Dr. Oz' and 'Ellen' See Ratings Growth; 'Kelly and Michael' Topping 2011 in Demo. *The Hollywood Reporter* Nov. 7 2012.

Boas, Franz. 1965[1911]. *The Mind of Primitive Man*. New York: Free Press.

Bonilla-Silva, Eduardo. 2010. *Racism without Racists: Color-Blind Racism and Racial Inequality in Contemporary America* (3rd Ed.). Lanham, MD: Rowman and Littlefield.

Boston Women's Health Collective. 1971. *Our Bodies, Ourselves: A Course by and for Women*. Boston: New England Free Press.

Bourdieu, Pierre. 1993. *The Field of Cultural Production*. New York: Columbia.

——. 1996. *On Television*. New York: The New Press.

Bowker, Geoffrey C., and Susan Leigh Star. 1999. *Sorting Things Out: Classification and Its Consequences*. Cambridge, MA: MIT Press.

Boyer, Dominic. 2005. *Spirit and System: Media, Intellectuals and the Dialectic in Modern German Culture*. Chicago: University of Chicago Press.

——. 2013. *The Life Informatic: Newsmaking in the Digital Era*. Ithaca, NY: Cornell University Press.

Brainard, Curtis. 2013. Sticking with the Truth: How 'Balanced' Coverage Helped Sustain the Bogus Claim that Childhood Vaccines Can Cause Autism. *Columbia Journalism Review*, May/June, 19–21.

Brechman Jean M., Chul-joo Lee, and Joseph N. Cappella. 2011. Distorting Genetic Research about Cancer: From Bench Science to Press Release to Published News. *Journal of Communication* 61:496–513.

Breilh, Jaime. 2003. *Epidemiología Crítica: Ciencia Emancipadora e interculturalidad*. Buenos Aires: Lugar Editorial.

——. 2008. Latin American Critical ('Social') Epidemiology: New Settings for an Old Dream. *International Journal of Epidemiology* 37:745–750.

Briggs, Charles L. 2005. Genealogies of Race and Culture and the Failure of Vernacular Cosmopolitanisms: Rereading Franz Boas and W.E.B. Du Bois. *Public Culture* 17(1):75–100.

——. 2010. Pressing Plagues: On the Mediated Communicability of Virtual Epidemics. In *Plagues and Epidemics: Infected Spaces Past and Present*, D. Ann Herring and Alan C. Swedlund, eds., 39–59. Oxford: Berg.

——. 2011a. All Cubans are Doctors! News Coverage of Health and Bioexceptionalism in Cuba. *Social Science and Medicine* 73:1037–1044.

——. 2011b. Communicating Biosecurity. *Medical Anthropology* 30(1):6–29.

——. 2012. What We Should Have Learned from Américo Paredes: The Politics of Communicability and the Making of Folkloristics. *Journal of American Folklore* 125(495):91–110.

Briggs, Charles L., and Clara Mantini-Briggs. 2003. *Stories in the Time of Cholera: Racial Profiling during a Medical Nightmare*. Berkeley: University of California Press.

Briggs, Charles L., and Daniel C. Hallin. 2007. Biocommunicability: The Neoliberal Subject and its Contradictions in News Coverage of Health Issues. *Social Text* 25(4):43–66.

——. 2010. Health Reporting as Political Reporting: Biocommunicability and the Public Sphere. *Journalism* 11:149–165.

Briggs, Charles L., and Mark Nichter. 2009. Biocommunicability and the Biopolitics of Pandemic Threats. *Medical Anthropology* 28(3):189–198.

Brown, Phil, Rachel Morello-Frosch, and Stephen Zavestoski. 2011. *Contested Illnesses: Citizens, Science, and Health Social Movements*. Berkeley: University of California Press.

Bullard, Robert D. 1990. *Dumping in Dixie: Race, Class, and Environmental Quality*. Boulder: Westview Press.

Caduff, Carlo. 2012. The Semiotics of Security: On the Biopolitics of Informational Bodies in the United States. *Cultural Anthropology* 27(2):333–357.

——. 2015. *The Pandemic Perhaps: Dramatic Events in a Public Culture of Danger*. Oakland: University of California Press.

CDHS (California Department of Health Services). 2004. *2004 West Nile Activity in California*. http://www.westnile.ca.gov/news.php?id=54, accessed 31 March 2007.

Carey, James W. 1989. *Communication as Culture: Essays on Media and Society*. Winchester, MA: Unwin Hyman.

Cartwright, Lisa. 2013. How to Have Social Media in an Invisible Pandemic. In *The International Encyclopedia of Media Studies*, Angharad N. Valdivia, ed., Vol. V. Malden, MA: Blackwell.

CDC (Centers for Disease Control and Prevention). 2002. *Crisis and Emergency and Risk Communication*. Atlanta: CDC.

——. 2007[2006]. *Crisis and Emergency and Risk Communication: Pandemic Influenza*. Atlanta: CDC.

Chadwick, Andrew. 2013. *The Hybrid Media System: Politics and Power*. New York: Oxford University Press.

Chakrabarty, Dipesh. 2000. *Provincializing Europe*. Princeton, NJ: Princeton University Press.

Chávez, Leo R. 2001. *Covering Immigration: Popular Images and the Politics of the Nation*. Berkeley: University of California Press.

——. 2006. Imagining the Nation, Imagining Donor Recipients: Jesica Santillan and the Public Discourse of Belonging. In *A Death Retold: Jessica Santillan, the Bungled Transplant, and Paradoxes of Medical Citizenship*, Keith Wailoo, Julie Livingston, and Peter Guarnaccia, eds., 276–296. Chapel Hill: University of North Carolina Press.

——. 2013. *The Latino Threat: Constructing Immigrants, Citizens and the Nation*. Palo Alto, CA: Stanford University Press.

Chen, Mel Y. 2012. *Animacies: Biopolitics, Racial Mattering, and Queer Affect*. Durham, NC: Duke University Press.

Chew, Cynthia, and Gunther Eysenbach. 2010. Pandemics in the Age of Twitter: Content Analysis of Tweets during the 2009 H1N1 Outbreak. *PLoS ONE* 5(11):e14118.

Clarke, Adele E., Janet K. Shim, Laura Mamo, Jennifer Ruth Fosket, and Jennifer R. Fishman. 2003. Biomedicalization: Technoscientific transformations of health, illness, and U.S. biomedicine. *American Sociological Review* 68:161–194.

Clarke, Christopher. 2008. A Question of Balance: The Autism-Vaccine Controversy in the British and American Elite Press. *Science Communication* 30(1):77–107.

Clarke, Juanne N., and Michelle M. Everest. 2006. Cancer in the Mass Print Media: Fear, Uncertainty and the Medical Model. *Social Science and Medicine* 62:2591–2600.

Cohen, Deborah, and Phillip Carter. 2010. WHO and the Pandemic Flu 'Conspiracies.' *BMJ* 340:c2912.

Cohen, Lawrence. 2002 [2001]. The Other Kidney: Biopolitics beyond Recognition. In *Commodifying Bodies*, Nancy Scheper-Hughes and Loic Wacquant, eds., 9–29. London: Sage.

———. 2011. Migrant Supplementarity: Remaking Biological Relatedness in Chinese Military and Indian Five-Star Hospitals. *Body and Society* 17(2–3):31–54.

Cohen, Lizabeth. 2008. *A Consumer's Republic: The Politics of Mass Consumption in Postwar America.* New York: Knopf.

Cole, Jonathan R. 1988. Dietary Cholesterol and Heart Disease: The Construction of a Medical 'Fact.' In *Surveying Social Life: Essays in Honor of Herbert H. Hyman,* Hubert J. Gorman, ed. Middletown, CT: Wesleyan University Press.

Collier, Stephen J., and Andrew Lakoff. 2015. Vital Systems Security: Reflexive Biopolitics and the Government of Emergency. *Theory, Culture and Society* 32(2):19–51.

Collier, Stephen J., Andrew Lakoff, and Paul Rabinow. 2004. Biosecurity: Towards an Anthropology of the Contemporary. *Anthropology Today* 20(5):3–7.

Conrad, Peter. 1992. Medicalization and Social Control. *Annual Review of Sociology* 18:209–232.

———. 2007. *The Medicalization of Society: On the Transformation of Human Conditions into Treatable Disorders.* Baltimore: Johns Hopkins University Press.

Cornia, Alessio, Marina Ghersetti, Paolo Mancini, and Thomas Odén. 2015. The Partisans, the Technocrats, and the Watchdogs: Domestication in Media Coverage of the Swine Flu Pandemic in 2009. *Journalism Studies* in press.

Couldry, Nick. 2012. *Media, Society and World: Social Theory and Digital Media Practice.* Cambridge: Polity Press.

Couldry, Nick, and Andreas Hepp. 2013. Conceptualizing Mediatization: Contexts, Traditions, Argument. *Communication Theory* 23(3):191–202.

County of San Diego Board of Supervisors. 2004. *San Diego County Child and Family Health and Well-Being: Report Card 2004.* San Diego, CA: County of San Diego Health and Human Services Agency.

Da Silva Madeiros, Flavia Natércia, and Luisa Massarani. 2010. Pandemic on the Air: A Case Study on the Coverage of New Influenza A-H1N1 by Brazilian Prime Time TV News. *Journal of Science Communication* 9(3).

Dahwood, Fatima S. et al. 2012. Estimated Global Mortality Associated with the First 12 Months of 2009 Pandemic H1N1 Virus Circulation: A Modeling Study. *Lancet Infectious Disease* 12:687–695.

Danz, Shari M. 2000. A Nonpublic Forum or a Brutal Bureaucracy? Advocates' Claims of Access to Welfare Center Waiting Rooms. *New York University Law Review* 75(4):1004–1044.

Das, Veena. 2015. *Affliction: Health, Disease, Poverty.* New York: Fordham University and Oxford University Press.

DasGupta, Sayatani. 2013. Controlling Portions, Controlling Pregnancies: Race and Class Panic in New York City Public Health Campaigns. 3 April 2013. http://storiesaregoodmedicine. blogspot.com/2013/04/controlling-portions-controlling.html, accessed 15 July 2015.

Dávila, Arlene. 2001. *Latinos, Inc.: The Marketing and Making of a People.* Berkeley: University of California Press.

Davis, Kathy. 2007. *The Making of Our Bodies, Ourselves: How Feminism Travels Across Borders.* Durham, NC: Duke University Press.

Davis, Mike. 2005. *The Monster at Our Door: The Global Threat of Avian Flu.* New York: Henry Holt.

Deacon, David, and James Stanyer. 2014. Mediatization: Key Concept or Conceptual Bandwagon? *Media, Culture and Society* 36(7):1032–1044.

DeBruin, Debra, Joan Liaschenko, and Mary Faith Marshall. 2012. Social Justice in Pandemic Preparedness. *American Journal of Public Health.* 102(4):586–591.

De Genova, Nicholas. 2005. *Working the Boundaries: Race, Space, and "Illegality" in Mexican Chicago.* Durham, NC: Duke University Press.

Du Bois, W.E.B. 1990[1903]. *The Souls of Black Folk.* Chicago: A.C. McClurg.

Dumit, Joseph. 2003. *Picturing Personhood: Brain Scans and Biomedical Identity.* Princeton, NJ: Princeton University Press.

———. 2012. *Drugs for Life: How Pharmaceutical Companies Define Our Health.* Durham, NC: Duke University Press.

Duster, Troy. 1990. *Backdoor to Eugenics.* New York: Routledge.

Dutta, Mohan J. 2008. *Communicating Health: A Culture-Centered Approach.* Cambridge, UK: Polity.

———. 2010. The Critical Cultural Turn in Health Communication: Reflexivity, Solidarity and Praxis. *Health Communication,* 25:534–539.

Dutta, Mohan J., and Ambar Basu. 2011. Culture, Communication, and Health: A Guiding Framework. In *The Routledge Handbook of Health Communication,* Teresa L. Thompson, Roxanne Parrott, and Jon F. Nussbaum, eds., 320–334. New York: Routledge.

Ecks, Stefan. 2013. *Eating Drugs: Psychopharmaceutical Pluralism in India.* New York: NYU Press.

Enanoria, Wayne T.A., Adam W. Crawley, Winston Tseng, Jasmine Furnish, Jeannie Balido, and Tomás Aragón. 2013. The Epidemiology and Surveillance Response to Pandemic Influenza A (H1N1) among Local Health Departments in the San Francisco Bay Area. *BMC Public Health* 13:276.

Entman, Robert M. 1993. Framing: Toward Clarification of a Fractured Paradigm. *Journal of Communication* 43(4):51–58.

Entman, Robert M., and Rojecki, Andrew. 2000. *The Black Image in the White Mind.* Chicago: University of Chicago Press.

Epstein, Steven. 1996. *Impure Science: AIDS, Activism, and the Politics of Knowledge.* Berkeley: University of California Press.

———. 2007. *Inclusion: The Politics of Difference in Medical Research.* Chicago: University of Chicago Press.

Esser, Frank, and D'Anglo P. 2006. Framing the Press and Publicity Process in U.S., British and German General Election Campaigns: A Comparative Study of Metacoverage. *International Journal of Press/Politics* 11(3):44–66.

Ettema, James S., and Theodore L. Glasser 1998. *Custodians of Conscience: Investigative Journalism and Public Virtue.* New York: Columbia University Press.

Fadiman, Anne. 1997. *The Spirit Catches You and You Fall Down: A Hmong Child, Her American Doctors, and the Collision of Two Cultures.* New York: Noonday Press.

Farmer, Paul. 1992. *AIDS and Accusation: Haiti and the Geography of Blame*. Berkeley: University of California Press.

——. 1999. *Infections and Inequalities: The Modern Plagues*. Berkeley: University of California Press.

Fassin, Didier. 2007. *When Bodies Remember: Experiences and Politics of AIDS in South Africa*. Berkeley: University of California Press.

——. 2012. *Humanitarian Reason: A Moral History of the Present*. Rachel Gomme, transl. Berkeley: University of California Press.

Ferguson, James. 1990. *The Anti-Politics Machine: "Development," Depoliticization, and Bureaucratic Power in Lesotho*. Cambridge: Cambridge University Press.

Field, Hyman, and Patricia Powell. 2001. Public Understanding of Science versus Public Understanding of Research. *Public Understanding of Science* 10:421–426.

Fineberg, Harvey V. 2008. Preparing for Avian Influenza: Lessons from the "Swine Flu Affair." *Journal of Infectious Diseases* 197:S14-18.

Fogarty, Andrea S., Kate Holland, Michelle Imison, R. Warwick Blood, Simon Chapman, and Simon Holding. 2011. Communicating Uncertainty: How Australian Television Reported H1N1 Risk in 2009: A Content Analysis. *BMC Public Health* 11:181.

Forman, Tyrone A. 2004. Color-Blind Racism and Racial Indifference: The Role of Racial Apathy in Facilitating Enduring Inequalities. In *The Changing Terrain of Race and Ethnicity*, Marisa Krysan and Amanda Lewis, eds., 43–66. New York: Russell Sage Foundation.

Foucault, Michel. 1997. The Birth of Biopolitics. In *Ethics: Subjectivity and Truth*, Paul Rabinow, ed., pp.73–80. New York: New Press.

Francescutti, Luis Pablo, Manuel Martínez Nicolás, and Fernando Tucho Fernández. 2011. La información sanitaria en los telediarios. *Cuadernos de Investigación* No. 1. Madrid: Universidad Rey Juan Carlos.

Fraser, Christophe et al. 2009. Pandemic Potential of a Strain of Influenza A(H1N1): Early Findings. *Science* 324:1557–1561.

Fraser, Nancy. 1990. Rethinking the Public Sphere: A Contribution to the Critique of Actually Existing Democracy. *Social Text 25/26*, 56–80.

Friedman, Lester D., ed. 2004. *Cultural Sutures: Medicine and Media*. Durham: Duke University Press.

Fullwiley, Duana. 2011. *The Enculturated Gene: Sickle Cell Health Politics and Biological Difference in West Africa*. Princeton, NJ: Princeton University Press.

Gabe, Jonathan, Simon Williams, Paul Martin, and Catherine Coveney. 2015. Pharmaceuticals and Society: Power, Promises and Prospects. *Social Science and Medicine* 131:193–198.

Gagnon, Marc-André, and Joel Lexchin. 2008. The Cost of Pushing Pills: A New Estimate of Pharmaceutical Promotion Expenditures in the United States. *PLoS Medicine* 5(1):29–33.

Gandy, Oscar H. 1980. Information in Health: Subsidized News. *Media, Culture and Society* 2(2):103–115.

Gandy, Oscar H., Jr., Katharina Kopp, Tanya Hands, Karen Frazer, and David Philips. 1997. Race and Risk: Factors Affecting the Framing of Stories about Inequality, Discrimination, and Just Plain Bad Luck. *Public Opinion Quarterly* 61(1):158–182.

Gans, Herbert J. 1979. *Deciding What's News: A Study of CBS Evening News, NBC Nightly News, Newsweek, and Time*. New York: Vintage.

García Canclini, Néstor. 2001. *Consumers and Citizens: Globalization and Multicultural Conflicts*. Minneapolis: University of Minnesota Press.

Geertz, Clifford. 1972. Religion as a Cultural System. In Reader in Comparative Religion: An Anthropological Approach, William A. Lessa, Evon Z. Vogt, eds., third edition, 167–178. Harper and Row, New York.

Gieryn, Thomas F. 1983. Boundary-Work and the Demarcation of Science from Non-Science: Strains and Interests in Professional Ideologies of Scientists. *American Sociological Review* 48(6):781–795.

Gilliam, Franklin D., Shanto Iyengar, Adam Simon, and Oliver Wright. 1996. Crime in Black and White: The Violent, Scary World of Local News. *Harvard International Journal of Press/Politics* 1(3):6–23.

Ginsburg, Faye D., Lila Abu-Lughod, and Brian Larkin, eds. 2002. *Media Worlds: Anthropology on New Terrain.* Berkeley: University of California Press.

Gitlin, Todd. 1980. *The Whole World is Watching: Mass Media in the Making and Unmaking of the New Left.* Berkeley: University of California Press.

González, Daniel, and Yvonne Wingett. 2009. Swine-Flu Outbreak Fuels More Debate About Securing Border. *The Arizona Republic,* April 29 2009.

Gordon, Avery F. 1997. *Ghostly Matters: Haunting and the Sociological Imagination.* Minneapolis: University of Minnesota Press.

Gray, Herman. 2004. *Watching Race: Television and the Struggle for Blackness* (Second ed.). Minneapolis: University of Minnesota Press.

Greenhalgh, Susan, and Megan A. Carney. 2014. Bad Biocitizens? Latinos and the US "Obesity Epidemic." *Human Organization* 73(3):267–276.

Gusterson, Hugh. 1996. *Nuclear Rites: A Weapons Laboratory at the End of the Cold War.* Berkeley: University of California Press.

Gutiérrez, Félix, and Wilson, Clint C. 1980. The Demographic Dilemma. *Columbia Journalism Review,* 17, Jan./Feb.:1979.

Gutiérrez, Ramón. 1991. *When Jesus Came, the Corn Mothers Went Away: Marriage, Sexuality, and Power in New Mexico.* Stanford: Stanford University Press.

Habermas, Jürgen. 1996. Civil Society and the Political Public Sphere. In Jürgen Habermas, *Between Facts and Norms: Contributions to a Discourse Theory of Law and Democracy.* Cambridge, MA: MIT Press.

Hacking, Ian. 2007. Kinds of People: Moving Targets. *Proceedings of the British Academy* 151:285–318.

Hall, Stuart, Chas Critcher, Tony Jefferson, John Clarke, and Brian Roberts. 1978. *Policing the Crisis: Mugging, the State, and Law and Order.* London: Macmillan.

Hallin, Daniel C. 1986. *The 'Uncensored War': The Media and Vietnam.* New York: Oxford University Press.

——. 1992. Sound Bite News: Television Coverage of Elections, 1968–1988. *Journal of Communication* 42(2):5–25.

——. 1994. *We Keep America on Top of the World: Television Journalism and the Public Sphere.* London: Routledge.

——. 2000. Commercialism and Professionalism in the American News Media. In *Mass Media and Society,* James Curran and Michael Gurevitch, eds. (third edition), 218–237. London: Arnold.

Hallin, Daniel C., and Charles L. Briggs. 2015. Transcending the Medical/Media Opposition in Research on News Coverage of Health and Medicine. *Media, Culture and Society* 37(1):85–100.

Hallin, Daniel C., Robert Karl Manoff, and Judy K. Weddle. 1994. Sourcing Patterns of National Security Reporters. *Journalism Quarterly* 70(4):753–766.

Hallin, Daniel C., Marisa Brandt, and Charles L. Briggs. 2013. Biomedicalization and the Public Sphere: Newspaper Coverage of Health and Medicine, 1960s–2000s. *Social Science and Medicine* 96:121–128.

Hamilton, James T. 2004. *All the News That's Fit to Sell: How the Market Transforms Information into News.* Princeton: Princeton University Press.

Hannerz, Ulf. 2004. *Foreign News: Exploring the World of Foreign Correspondents.* Chicago: University of Chicago Press.

Hanusch, Folker. 2012. Broadening the Focus: The Case for Service Journalism as a Field of Scholarly Inquiry. *Journalism Practice* 6(1):2–11.

Harvard Opinion Research Program. 2009. Influenza A(H1N1)/Swine Flu Survey I. Cambridge, MA: Harvard School of Public Health, www.hsph.harvard.edu/news/press-releases/files/Swine_Flu.TOPLINE.pdf, accessed 15 Aug. 2009.

Haughney, Christine. 2012. Today's Key to Selling Magazines: A TV Doctor. *The New York Times*, 6 July 2012, B1.

Hayden, Cori. 2010. The Proper Copy: The Insides and Outsides of Domains Made Public. *Journal of Cultural Economy* 3(1):85–102.

Healy, David M. 2004. *Let Them Eat Prozac: The Unhealthy Relationship between the Pharmaceutical Industry and Depression.* New York University Press.

——. 2006. The New Medical Oikumene. In *Global Pharmaceuticals: Ethics, Markets, Practices*, Petryna, Adriana, Andrew Lakoff, and Arthur Kleinman, eds., 61–84. Durham, NC: Duke University Press.

Heath, Deborah, Rayna Rapp, and Karen-Sue Taussig. 2004. Genetic Citizenship. In *A Companion to the Anthropology of Politics*, David Nugent and Joan Vincent, eds., 152–167. Malden, MA: Blackwell.

Henrich, Natalie, and Bev Holmes. 2011. What the Public Was Saying about the H1N1 Vaccine: Perceptions and Issues Discussed in On-Line Comments during the 2009 H1N1 Pandemic. *PLoS ONE* 6(4):3 18479.

Hepp, Andreas. 2012. *Cultures of Mediatization.* Cambridge: Polity.

——. 2013. The Communicative Figurations of Mediatized Worlds: Mediatization Research in Times of the 'Mediatization of Everything'. *European Journal of Communication* 28:615–629.

Heyman, Josiah McC., Guillermina Gina Núñez, and Victor Talavera. 2009. Healthcare Access and Barriers for Unathorized Immigrants in El Paso County, Texas. *Family and Community Health* 32(1):4–21.

Hill, Jane H. 2008. *The Everyday Language of White Racism.* Chichester, UK: Wiley-Blackwell.

Hilton, Shona, and Kate Hunt. 2010. UK Newspapers' Representations of the 2009–10 Outbreak of Swine Flu: One Health Scare Not Over-Hyped by the Media? *Journal of Epidemiological Community Health* 65:941–946.

Hinnant, Amanda, María E. Len-Ríos and Rachel Young. 2012. Journalistic Use of Exemplars to Humanize Health News. *Journalism Studies* 14(4):539–554.

Hjavard, Sigurd. 2013. *The Mediatization of Culture and Society.* London: Routledge.

Hoberman, John M. 2007. Medical Racism and the Rhetoric of Exculpation: How Do Physicians Think About Treatment? *New Literary History* 38:3:505–525.

Hodgetts, Darrin, Kerry Chamberlain, Margaret Scammel, Rolinda Karapu, and Linda Waimarie Nikora. 2008. Constructing Health News: Possibilities for a Civic-Oriented Journalism. *Health* 12(1):43–66.

Hoffman, Beatrix, Rachel Grob, and Mark Schlesinger, eds. 2011. *Patients as Policy Actors.* New Brunswick: Rutgers University Press.

Holland, Kate, and R. Warwick Blood. 2013. Public Responses and Reflexivity during the Swine Flu Pandemic in Australia. *Journalism Studies* 14(4):523–538.

Holland, Kate, R. Warwick Blood, Michelle Imison, Simon Chapman, and Andrea Fogarty. 2012. Risk, Expert Uncertainty, and Australian News Media: Public and Private Faces of Expert Opinion during the 2009 Swine Flu Pandemic. *Journal of Risk Research* 15(6):657–671.

Holmes, Seth M. 2013. *Fresh Fruit, Broken Bodies: Migrant Farmworkers in the United States.* Berkeley: University of California Press.

Horton, Sarah. 2014. Debating "Medical Citizenship": Policies Shaping Undocumented Immigrants' Learned Avoidance of the U.S. Health Care System. In *Hidden Lives and Human Rights in the United States,* Lois Ann Lorentzen, ed., Vol. 2, 297–319. Santa Barbara: Praeger.

Horton, Sarah, and Judith C. Barker. 2009. "Stains" on Their Self-Discipline: Public Health, Hygiene, and the Disciplining of Undocumented Immigrant Parents in the Nation's Internal Borderlands. *American Ethnologist* 36(4):784–798.

Hunt, Nancy Rose. 1999. *A Colonial Lexicon of Birth Ritual, Medicalization, and Mobility in the Congo.* Durham, NC: Duke University Press.

Hutchins, Sonja S., Kevin Fiscella, Robert S. Levine, Danielle C. Ompad, and Marian McDonald. 2009. Protection of Racial/Ethnic Minority Populations during an Influenza Pandemic. *American Journal of Public Health* 99(suppl 2):S261-270.

Iyengar, Shanto. 1994. *Is Anyone Responsible?: How Television Frames Political Issues.* Chicago: University of Chicago Press.

Jacobs, Geert. 1999. *Preformulating the News: An Analysis of the Metapragmatics of Press Releases.* Philadelphia: John Benjamins.

Jasanoff, Sheila, ed. 2004. *States of Knowledge: The Co-production of Science and the Social Order.* London: Routledge,

Jasanoff, Shiela, Gerald E. Markle, James C. Petersen, and Trevor Pinch, eds. 1995. *Handbook of Science and Technology Studies.* Thousand Oaks, CA: Sage.

Jensen, Jakob D., Cortney M. Moriarty, Ryan J. Hurley, and Jo Ellen Stryker. 2010. Making Sense of Cancer News Coverage Trends: A Comparison of Three Comprehensive Content Analyses. *Journal of Health Communication* 15:136–151.

Joffe, Héléne. 2011. Public Apprehension of Emerging Infectious Diseases: Are Changes Afoot? *Public Understanding of Science* 20:446.

Joffe, Helene, and Georgina Haarhoff. 2002. Representations of Far-Flung Illnesses: The Case of Ebola in Britain. *Social Science and Medicine* 54:955–969.

Jones, James H. 1981. *Bad Blood: The Tuskeegee Syphilis Experiment.* New York : Free Press.

Joseph, Ralina L. 2011. "Hope is Finally Making a Comeback": First Lady Reframed. *Communication, Culture and Critique* 4(1):56–77.

Jung, Moon-Kie. 2015. *Beneath the Surface of White Supremacy: Denaturalizing U.S. Racisms Past and Present.* Stanford, CA: Stanford University Press.

Kahn, Jonathan. 2005. From Disparity to Difference: How Race-Specific Medicines May Undermine Polices to Address Inequalities in Health Care. *Southern California Interdisciplinary Law Journal* 15(105):105–130.

Kaiser Family Foundation/Pew Research Center. 2009. Health News Coverage in the U.S. Media, January-June 2009. http://www.journalism.org/2009/07/29/health-news-coverage-us-media-early-2009/, accessed 22 Aug. 2014.

Karpf, Anne. 1988. *Doctoring the Media.* London: Routledge.

Kelly, Bridget et al. 2010. Cancer Information Scanning and Seeking in the General Population. *Journal of Health Communication* 15:734–753.

Keppel, Kenneth G., Jeffrey N. Pearcy, and Diane K. Wagener. 2002. *Trends in Racial and Ethnic-Specific Rates for the Health Status Indicators: United States, 1990–98.* Department of Health and Human Services, Centers for Disease Control and Prevention.

Kim, Annice E., Shiriki Kumanyika, Daniel Shive, Vzy Igweatu, and Son-Ho Kim. 2010. Coverage and Framing of Racial and Ethnic Health Disparities in US Newspapers, 1996–2005, *American Journal of Public Health,* Vol. 100, No. S1:S224-S231.

Klinenberg Eric. 2002. *Heat Wave: A Social Autopsy of Disaster in Chicago*. Chicago: University of Chicago Press.

Krieger, Nancy. 2003. Does Racism Harm Health? Did Child Abuse Exist before 1962? On Explicit Questions, Critical Science, and Current Controversies: An Eco-Social Perspective. *American Journal of Public Health* 93:194–199.

———. 2011. *Epidemiology and the People's Health: Theory and Context*. Oxford: Oxford University Press.

Labov, William. 1972. *Language in the Inner City*. Philadelphia: University of Pennsylvania Press.

Lakoff, Andrew. 2008. The Generic Biothreat, or, How We Became Unprepared. *Cultural Anthropology* 23(3):399–428.

Lakoff, Andrew, and Stephen J. Collier, eds. 2008. *Biosecurity Interventions: Global Health and Security in Question*. New York: Columbia University Press.

Landerer, Nino. 2013. Rethinking the Logics: A Conceptual Framework for the Mediatization of Politics. *Communication Theory* 23(3):239–258.

Larkin, Brian. 2008. *Signal and Noise: Media, Infrastructure, and Urban Culture in Nigeria*. Durham, NC: Duke University Press.

Latour, Bruno. 1987. *Science in Action*. Cambridge, MA: Harvard University Press.

Latour, Bruno. 1988. *The Pasteurization of France*. Alan Sheridan and John Law, transl. Cambridge, MA: Harvard University Press.

———. [1993]1991. *We Have Never Been Modern*. Trans. Catherine Porter. Cambridge, MA: Harvard University Press.

Latour, Bruno, and Steve Woolgar. 1979. *Laboratory Life: The Construction of Scientific Facts*. Beverly Hills, CA: Sage.

Lau, Kimberly J. 2000. *New Age Capitalism: Making Money East of Eden*. Philadelphia: University of Pennsylvania Press.

Laurell, Asa Cristina. 1989. Social Analysis of Collective Health in Latin America. *Social Sciences and Medicine* 28:1183–191.

Lawrence, Regina G. 2000. Game-Framing the Issues: Tracking the Strategy Frame in Public Policy News. *Journal of Communication* 17(2):93–114.

———. 2004. Framing Obesity: The Evolution of News Discourse on a Public Health Issue. *Harvard International Journal of Press/Politics* 9(3):56–75.

Lawrence, Regina G., and Matthew L. Schafer (2012). Debunking Sarah Palin: Mainstream News Coverage of 'Death Panels'. *Journalism* 13(6):766–782.

Lederer, Susan E. 2006. Tucker's Heart: Racial Politics and Heart Transplantation in America. In *A Death Retold: Jessica Santillan, the Bungled Transplant, and Paradoxes of Medical Citizenship*, Keith Wailoo, Julie Livingston, and Peter Guarnaccia, eds, 142–157. Chapel Hill: University of North Carolina Press.

Lee, Nancy. 2007. *Curing Consumers: How the Patient Became a Consumer in Modern American Medicine*. Ph.D. dissertation, University of California, San Diego.

Lee, Seow Ting, and Iccha Basnyat. 2013. From Press Release to News: Mapping the Framing of the 2009 H1N1 A Influenza Pandemic. *Health Communication* 28:119–132.

Lengauer, Günther, Frank Esser, and Rosa Berganza. 2012. Negativity in Political News: A Review of Concepts, Operationalizations and Key Findings. *Journalism* 13:179–202.

Lewontin, R.C., Steven Rose, and Leon J. Kam. 1984. *Not in Our Genes: Biology, Ideology, and Human Nature*. New York: Pantheon.

Lippmann, Walter, and Charles Merz. 1920. A Test of the News. *The New Republic* 23(296):1–42.

Lipsitz, George. 2006. *The Possessive Investment in Whiteness: How White People Profit from Identity Politics*. Philadelphia: Temple University Press.

——. 2011. *How Racism Takes Place*. Philadelphia: Temple University Press.

Liu, Brooke Fisher, and Sora Kim. 2011. How Organizations Framed the 2009 H1N1 Pandemic via Social and Traditional Media: Implications for U.S. Health Communicators. *Public Relations Review* 37:233–244.

Lock, Margaret. 2002. *Twice Dead: Organ Transplants and the Reinvention of Death*. Berkeley: Univ. Calif. Press.

Locke, John. 1959[1690]. *An Essay Concerning Human Understanding*. 2 vols. New York: Dover.

Lopes, Felisbela, Teresa Ruão, Sandra Marinho, and Rita Araújo. 2012. A Media Pandemic: Influenza A in Protuguese Newspapers. *International Journal of Healthcare Management* 5(1):19–27.

López, Leslie. 2005. De Facto Disentitlement in an Information Economy: Enrollment Issues in Medicaid Managed Care. *Medical Anthropology Quarterly* 19(1):26–46.

Lowe, Celia. 2010. Viral Clouds: Becoming H5N1 in Indonesia. *Cultural Anthropology* 25(4):625–649.

Lundby, Kurt. 2009. *Mediatization: Concept, Changes, Consequences*. New York: Peter Lang.

Lupton, Deborah. 1995. *The Imperative of Health: Public Health and the Regulated Body*. London: Sage.

——. 1997. *Moral Threats and Dangerous Desires: AIDS in the News Media*. London: Falmer Press.

——. 2012. *Medicine as Culture: Illness, Disease and the Body*, Third Edition. London: Sage.

MacPhail, Theresa. 2014. *The Viral Network: A Pathography of the H1N1 Influenza Pandemic*. Ithaca: Cornell University Press.

Madsen, William. 1964. *Mexican-Americans of South Texas*. New York: Holt, Rinehart and Winston.

Mankekar, Purnima. 1999. *Screening Culture, Viewing Politics: An Ethnography of Television, Womanhood, and Nation in Postcolonial India*. Durham, NC: Duke University Press.

Manoff, Robert Karl. 1989. Modes of War and Modes of Social Address: The Text of SDI. *Journal of Communication* 39(1):59–84.

Marchetti, Dominique. 2010. *Quand la Santé Devient Médiatique: Les Logiques de Production de L'information dans la Presse*. Grenoble: Presses Universitaires de Grenoble.

Marcinkowski, Frank, and Adrian Steiner. 2014. Mediatization and Political Autonomy: A Systems Approach. In *Mediatization of Politics*, Frank Esser and Jesper Strömbäck, eds., 74–89. New York: Palgrave Macmillan.

Martin, Emily. 1994. *Flexible Bodies: Tracking Immunity in American Culture from the Days of Polio to the Age of AIDS*. Boston: Beacon Press.

Martín Barbero, Jesús. 1987. *De los Medios a las Mediaciones: Comunicación, Cultura y Hegemonía*. México: Ediciones G. Gili.

Masco, Joseph. 2006. *The Nuclear Borderlands: The Manhattan Project in Post-Cold War New Mexico*. Princeton: Princeton University Press.

Mazzoleni, Gianpietro. 1995. Towards a 'Videocracy'? Italian Political Communication at a Turning Point. *European Journal of Communication* 10(3):291–319.

Mazzoleni, Gianpietro, and Winfried Schultz. 1999. Mediatization of Politics: A Challenge for Democracy? *Political Communication* 16:247–261.

McCauley, Michael, Sara Minsky, and Kasisomayajula Viswanath. 2013. The H1N1 Pandemic: Media Frames, Stigmatization and Coping. *BMC Public Health* 13:1116.

Menéndez, Eduardo L. 1981. *Poder, Estratificación y Salud: Análisis de las Condiciones Sociales y Económicas de la Enfermedad en Yucatán*. Mexico: La Casa Chata.

———. 2010. Las influenzas por todos tan temidas o de los difíciles usos de conocimiento. *Desacatos* 32:17–34.

Menéndez, Eduardo L., and Renée B. Di Pardo 1996. *De Algunos Alcoholismos y Algunos Saberes: Atención Primaria y Proceso de Alcoholización*. México: CIESAS.

———. 2009. *Miedos, Riesgos e Inseguridades: Los Medios, Los Profesionales y Los Intelectuales en la Construcción Social de la Salúd Como Catástrofe*. Mexico: CIESAS.

Mesch, Gustavo S., Kent P. Schwirian, and Tayna Kolobov. 2013. Attention to the Media and Worry over Becoming Infected: The Case of Swine Flu (H1N1) Epidemic of 2009. *Sociology of Health and Illness* 35(2):325–331.

Metzl, Jonathan M., and Helena Hansen. 2014. Structural Competency: Theorizing a New Medical Engagement with Stigma and Inequality. *Social Science and Medicine* 103:126–133.

Mignolo, Walter. 2011. *The Darker Side of Western Modernity: Global Futures, Decolonial Options*. Durham, NC: Duke University Press.

Mills, Charles W. 1997. *The Racial Contract*. Ithaca, NY: Cornell University Press.

Mol, Annemarie. 2008. *The Logic of Care: Health and the Problem of Patient Choice*. London: Routledge.

Montoya, Michael. 2011. *Making the Mexican Diabetic: Race, Science, and the Genetics of Inequality*. Berkeley: University of California Press.

Morgan, Marcyliena H. 2002. *Language, Discourse and Power in African American Culture*. Cambridge: Cambridge University Press.

Morgan, Susan, Tyler R. Harrison, Lisa Volk Chewning, and Jacklyn B. Habib. 2006. America's Angel or Thieving Immigrant? Media Coverage, the Santillan Story, and Publicized Ambivalence toward Donation and Transplantation. In Keith Wailoo, Julie Livingston, and Peter Guarnaccia, eds. *A Death Retold: Jessica Santillan, the Bungled Transplant, and Paradoxes of Medical Citizenship*, 19–45. Chapel Hill: University of North Carolina Press.

Muhlmann, Géraldine. 2004. *Journalism for Democracy*. Cambridge: Polity.

Nader, Laura. 1972. Up the Anthropologist—Perspectives Gained from Studying Up. In *Reinventing Anthropology*, Dell H. Hymes, ed., 284–311. New York: Pantheon.

National Women's Law Center. 2010. Making the Grade on Women's Health: A State by State Report Card. http://hrc.nwlc.org/.

Navarro, Vicente. 1993. *Dangerous to Your Health: Capitalism in Health Care*. New York: Monthly Review Press.

Nelkin, Dorothy. 1995. *Selling Science: How the Press Covers Science and Technology*. New York: W.H. Freeman.

Nelson, Alondra. 2013. *Body and Soul: The Black Panther Party and the Fight against Medical Discrimination*. Minneapolis: University of Minnesota Press.

Nerlich, Brigitte, and Nelya Koteyko. 2012. Crying Wolf? Biosecurity and Metacommunication in the Context of the 2009 Swine Flu Pandemic. *Health and Place* 18:710–717.

Neustadt, Richard, and Harvey V. Fineberg. 1978. *The Swine Flu Affair*. Washington, DC: U.S. Department of Health, Education and Welfare.

Nguyen, Vinh-Kim. 2010. *The Republic of Therapy: Triage and Sovereignty in West Africa's Time of AIDS*. Durham, NC: Duke University Press.

Nichter, Mark. 1996 [1989]. Pharmaceuticals, the Commodification of Health, and the Health Care-Medicine Use Transition. In Mark Nichter and Mimi Nichter, *Anthropology and International Health: Asian Case Studies*, 265–326. Amsterdam: Gordon and Breach Publishers.

Niederdeppe, Jeff, Erika Franklin Fowler, Kenneth Goldstein, and James Pribble. 2010. Does Local Television News Coverage Cultivate Fatalistic Beliefs About Cancer Prevention? *Journal of Communication* 60:230–253.

Niederdeppe, Jeff, Cabral A. Bigman, Amy L. Gonzales, and Sarah E. Gollust. 2013. Communication About Health Disparities in the Mass Media. *Journal of Communication* 63:8–30.

Nucci, Mary L., Cara L. Cuite, and William K. Hallman. 2009. When Good Food Goes Bad: Television Network News and the Spinach Recall of 2006. *Science Communication* 31(2):238–265.

Omi, Michael, and Howard Winant. 1986. *Racial Formation in the United States: From the 1960's to the 1980's*. New York: Routledge and Kegan Paul.

Ong, Aihwa. In press. *Fungible Life: Uncertainty in the Asian City of Life*. Durham, NC: Duke University Press.

Ono, Kent. 2010. Postracism: A Theory of the 'Post'- as Political Strategy. *Journal of Communication Inquiry* 34(3):227–233.

Paredes, Américo. 1977. On Ethnographic Work among Minority Groups: A Folklorist's Perspective. *New Scholar* 7:1–32.

Parry, Bronwyn. 2012. Domesticating Biosurveillance: 'Containment' and the Politics of Bioinformation. *Health and Place* 18:718–725.

Parsons, Talcott. 1951. *The Social System*. Glencoe: Free Press.

———. 1964. The Professions and Social Structure. In *Essays in Sociological Theory: Pure and Applied*, 34–49. New York: Free Press.

Pedelty, Mark. 1995. *War Stories: The Culture of Foreign Correspondents*. New York: Routledge.

Pellechia, Marianne G. 1997. Trends in Science Coverage of Three US Newspapers. *Public Understanding of Science* 6:49–68.

Perry, Theresa, and Lisa Delpit, eds. 1998. *The Real Ebonics Debate: Power, Language, and the Education of African-American Children*. Boston: Beacon.

Petryna, Adriana. 2002. *Life Exposed: Biological Citizens after Chernobyl*. Princeton: Princeton University Press.

———. 2009. *When Experiments Travel: Clinical Trials and the Global Search for Human Subjects*. Princeton: Princeton University Press.

Petryna, Adriana, Andrew Lakoff, and Arthur Kleinman, eds. 2006. *Global Pharmaceuticals: Ethics, Markets, Practices*. Durham, NC: Duke University Press.

President's Cancer Panel. 2010. Reducing Environmental Cancer Risk: What We Can Do Now. National Institutes of Health. http://deainfo.nci.nih.gov/advisory/pcp/annual-Reports/pcp08-09rpt/PCP_Report_08-09_508.pdf.

Preston, Richard. 1994. *The Hot Zone: The Terrifying True Story of the Origins of the Ebola Virus*. New York: Random House.

Quinn, Sandra Crouse, Supriya Kumar, Vicki S. Freimuth, Donald Musa, Nestor Castaneda-Angarita, and Kelley Kidwell. 2011. Racial Disparities in Exposure, Susceptibility, and Access to Health Care in the US H1N1 Influenza Pandemic. *American Journal of Public Health* 101(2):285–293.

Rabinow, Paul. 1992. Artificiality and Enlightenment: From Sociobiology to Biosociality. In *Incorporations*, Jonathan Crary and Sanford Kwinter, eds., 234–252. New York: Zone.

———. 1996. *Making PCR: A Story of Biotechnology*. Chicago: University of Chicago Press.

———. 1999. *French DNA: Trouble in Purgatory*. Chicago: University of Chicago Press.

Rapp, Rayna. 1999. *Testing Women, Testing the Fetus: The Social Impact of Amniocentesis in America*. New York: Routledge.

Rapp, Rayna, and Faye Ginsburg. 2001. Enabling Disability: Rewriting Kinship, Reimagining Citizenship. *Public Culture* 13(3):533–556.

Rapp, Rayna, Deborah Heath, and Karen-Sue Taussig. 2002. Genealogical Dis-ease: Where Hereditary Abnormality, Biomedical Explanation, and Family Responsibility Meet. In

Relative Values: Reconfiguring Kinship Studies, Sarah Franklin and Susan McKinnon, eds., 384–409. Durham, NC: Duke University Press.

Reardon, Jenny. 2005. *Race to the Finish: Identity and Governance in an Age of Genetics*. Princeton, NJ: Princeton University Press.

Redfield, Peter. 2013. *Life in Crisis: The Ethical Journal of Doctors without Borders*. Berkeley: University of California Press.

Reid, Roddey. 2005. *Globalizing Tobacco Control: Anti-smoking Campaigns in California, France, and Japan*. Bloomington: Indiana University Press.

Reisen, William, Hugh Lothrop, and Robert Chiles, et al. 2004. West Nile Virus in California. *Emerging Infectious Diseases* 10(8):1369–1378.

Rhodes, Jane. 2007. *Framing the Black Panthers: The Spectacular Rise of a Black Power Icon*. New York: Free Press.

Rock, Paul. 1973. News as Eternal Recurrence. In *The Manufacture of News*, Stanley Cohen and Jock Young, eds., 226–243. London: Sage.

Romano-V., Octavio. 1968. The Anthropology and Sociology of the Mexican-Americans: The Distortion of Mexican-American History. *El Grito* 2(1):13–26.

Rose, Nikolas. 2007. *The Politics of Life Itself: Biomedicine, Power, and Subjectivity in the Twenty-First Century*. Princeton: Princeton University Press.

Rose, Nikolas, and Carlos Novas. 2005. Biological Citizenship. In *Global Assemblages: Technology, Politics, and Ethics as Anthropological Problems*, Aihwa Ong and Stephen J. Collier, eds., 439–463. Malden, MA: Blackwell.

Rubel, Arthur J. 1966. *Across the tracks: Mexican-Americans in a Texas City*. Austin: University of Texas Press.

Santa Ana, Otto. 2002. *Brown Tide Rising: Metaphors of Latinos in Contemporary American Public Discourse*. Austin: University of Texas Press.

Saussure, Ferdinand de. 1959. *Course in General Linguistics*, C. Bally, ed. and A. Sechehaye, trans. Chicago: Open Court, pp. 1–23.

Scheper-Hughes, Nancy. 2000. The Global Traffic in Human Organs. *Current Anthropology* 41(2):191–224.

Schudson, Michael. 1993. *Watergate in American Memory: How We Remember, Forget, and Reconstruct the Past*. New York: Basic Books.

———. 2003. *The Sociology of News*. New York: W.W. Norton.

Schulz, Winfried. 2004. Reconstructing Mediatization as an Analytical Concept. *European Journal of Communication* 19(1):87–101.

Schwitzer, Gary. 2009. *The State of Health Journalism In the U.S.* Menlo Park, CA: Henry J. Kaiser Family Foundation.

Seale, Clive. 2002. *Media and Health*. London: Sage.

Shrestha, Sundar S. et al. 2011. Estimating the Burden of 2009 Pandemic Influenza A(H1N1) in the United States (April 2009–April 2010). *Clinical Infectious Diseases* 52(S1):S75-S82.

Signorielli, Nancy. 1993. *Mass Media and Impact on Health: A Sourcebook*. Westport, CN: Greenwood Press.

Skocpol, Theda. 1996. *Boomerang: Health Care Reform and the Turn Against Government*. New York: W.W. Norton.

Slater, Michael D., Marilee Long, Erwin P. Betinghaus, and Janson B. Reineke. 2008. News Coverage of Cancer in the United States: A National Sample of Newspapers, Television, and Magazines. *Journal of Health Communication* 13:523–537.

Smedley, Brian D., Adrienne Y. Stith, and Alan R. Nelson, eds. 2002. *Unequal Treatment: Confronting Racial and Ethnic Disparities in Health Care*. Washington, DC: National Academy Press.

Snow, Catherine, and Charles Ferguson. 1977. *Talking to Children: Language Input and Acquisition.* Cambridge: Cambridge University Press.

Sontag, Susan. 1990. *Illness as Metaphor and AIDS and its Metaphors.* New York: Doubleday.

Specter, Michael. 2013. The Operator: Is the Most Trusted Doctor in America Doing more Harm than Good. *The New Yorker,* Feb. 4.

Staniland, Karen, and Greg Smith. 2013. Flu Frames. *Sociology of Health and Illness* 35(2):309–324.

Star, Susan Leigh. 2010. This is Not a Boundary Object: Reflections on the Origin of a Concept. *Science, Technology and Human Values* 35(5):601–617.

Star, Susan Leigh, and James Griesemer 1989. Institutional Ecology, 'Translations', and Boundary Objects: Amateurs and Professionals in Berkeley's Museum of Vertebrate Zoology, 1907–39. *Social Studies of Science* 19(3):387–420.

Starr, Paul. 1982. *The Social Transformation of American Medicine.* New York: Basic Books.

Stengers, Isabelle. 2005. The Cosmopolitical Proposal. In *Making Things Public: Atmospheres of Democracy,* Bruno Latour and Peter Weibel, eds., 994–1004. Cambridge, MA: MIT Press.

Stephenson, Niamh, Mark Davis, Paul Flowers, Casimir MacGregor, and Emily Waller. 2014. Mobilising "Vulnerability" in the Public Health Response to Pandemic Influenza. *Social Science and Medicine* 102:10–17.

Stocking, George W., Jr. 1968. *Race, Culture, and Evolution: Essays in the History of Anthropology.* New York: Free Press.

Stokes, Ashli Quesinberry. 2008. The Paradox of Pharmaceutical Empowerment: Healthology and On-line Public Relations. In *Emerging Perspectives in Health Communication: Meaning, Culture and Power,* Heather M. Zoller and Mohan J. Dutta, eds., 335–356. New York: Routledge.

Stoler, Ann Laura. 1995. *Race and the Education of Desire: Foucault's History of Sexuality and the Colonial Order of Things.* Durham, NC: Duke University Press.

Strömbäck, Jesper. 2008. Four Phases of Mediatization: An Analysis of the Mediatization of Politics. *International Journal of Press/Politics* 13(3):228–246.

Stryker, Jo E., Karen M. Emmons, and Kasisomayajula Viswanath. 2007. Uncovering Differences Across the Cancer Control Continuum: A Comparison of Ethnic and Mainstream Cancer Newspaper Stories. *Preventive Medicine* 44:20–25.

Subervi, Federico, Lucila Vargas, and L. Brody. 1998. *What's is the Diagnosis? Latinos, Media and Health: A Study of Health Coverage in Latino Newspapers, Television and Radio News, 1997–1998.* Menlo Park, CA: Kaiser Family Foundation.

Sunder Rajan, Kaushik. 2006. *Biocapital: The Constitution of Postgenomic Life.* Durham, NC: Duke University Press.

Szasz, Andrew, and Michael Meuser. 1997. Environmental Inequalities: Literature Review and Proposals for New Directions in Research and Theory. *Current Sociology* 45:99–120.

Tallbear, Kimberly. 2013. *Native American DNA: Tribal Belonging and the False Promise of Genetic Science.* Minneapolis: University of Minnesota Press.

Tan, Emily. 2007. Looking for Health Info Online? WebMD Isn't the Only Option. *Advertising Age,* July 30.

Tapia, Ruby C. 2011. *American Pietàs: Visions of Race, Death, and the Maternal.* Minneapolis: University of Minnesota Press.

Taussig, Karen-Sue, Rayna Rapp, and Deborah Heath. 2003. Flexible Eugenics: Technologies of the Self in the Age of Genetics. In *Genetic Nature/Culture: Anthropology and Science beyond the Two Culture Divide,* Alan Goodman, Deborah Heath, and Susan Lindee, eds., 58–76. Berkeley: University of California Press.

Taussig, Michael. 1993. *Mimesis and Alterity: A Particular History of the Senses.* NY: Routledge.

Taylor, Janelle S. 2003. The Story Catches You and You Fall Down: Tragedy, Ethnography, and Cultural Competence. *Medical Anthropology Quarterly* 17(2):159–181.

Taylor-Clark, Kalahn Alexandra, Felicia E. Mebane, Gillian K. SteelFisher, and Robert J. Blendon. 2007. News of Disparity: Content Analysis of News Coverage of African American Healthcare Inequalities in the USA, 1994–2004. *Social Science and Medicine* 65:405–417.

Treichler, Paula A. 1999. *How to Have Theory in an Epidemic: Cultural Chronicles of AIDS.* Durham, NC: Duke University Press.

Turow, Joseph. 2010. *Playing Doctor: Television, Storytelling and Medical Power. Second Edition.* Ann Arbor: University of Michigan Press.

Tyndall Report. n.d.a. http://tyndallreport.com/decadeinreview/, accessed 20 Aug. 2014)

Tyndall Report. n.d.b. http://tyndallreport.com/yearinreview2013/health/, accessed 22 Aug. 2014)

Underwood, Doug. 1993. *When MBAs Rule the News Room: How the Marketers and Managers are Reshaping Today's Media.* New York: Columbia University Press.

Ungar, Sheldon. 1998. Hot Crisis and Media Reassurance: A Comparison of Emerging Diseases and Ebola Zaire. *British Journal of Sociology* 49(1):36–56.

——. 2008. Global Bird Flu Communication: Hot Crisis and Media Reassurance. *Science Communication* 29(4):472–497.

Urban, Greg. 2001. *Metaculture: How Culture Moves through the World.* Minneapolis: University of Minnesota Press.

Vargas, Lucila. 2000. Genderizing Latino News: An Analysis of a Local Newspaper's Coverage of Latino Current Affairs. *Critical Studies in Media Communication* 17(3):261–293.

Vargas, Lucila, and Bruce dePyssler. 1999. U.S. Latino Newspapers as Health Communication Resources. *Howard Journal of Communication* 10(3):189–205.

Vasterman, Peter L.M., and Nel Ruigrok. 2013. Pandemic Alarm in the Dutch Media: Media Coverage of the 2009 Influenza A(H1N1) Pandemic and the Role of Expert Sources. *European Journal of Communication* 28(4):436–453.

Verhoeven, Piet. 2008. Where has the Doctor Gone? The Mediatization of Medicine on Dutch Television, 1961–2000. *Public Understanding of Science* 17:461–472.

Wagner-Egger, Pascal, Adrian Bangerter, Ingrid Gilles, Eva Green, David Rigaud, Franciska Krings, Christian Staerklé, and Alain Clémence. 2011. Lay Perceptions of Collectives at the Outbreak of the H1N1 Epidemic: Heroes, Villains and Victims. *Public Understanding of Science* 20(4):461–476.

Wailoo, Keith, Julie Livingston, and Peter Guarnaccia, eds. 2006. *A Death Retold: Jessica Santillan, the Bungled Transplant, and Paradoxes of Medical Citizenship.* Chapel Hill: University of North Carolina Press.

Waitzkin, Howard. 2000. *The Second Sickness: Contradictions of Capitalism Health Care.* Lanham, MD: Rowman and Littlefield.

——. 2011. *Medicine and Public Health at the End of Empire.* Boulder, CO: Paradigm.

Wald, Priscilla. 2008. *Contagious: Cultures, Carriers, and the Outbreak Narrative.* Durham, NC: Duke University Press.

Walsh-Childers, Kim, Heather Edwards, and Stephen Grobmeyer. 2011. Covering Women's Greatest Health Fear: Breast Cancer Information in Consumer Magazines. *Health Communication* 26:209–220.

West, Emily. 2006. Mediating Citizenship through the Lens of Consumerism: Frames in the American Medicare Reform Debates of 2003–2004. *Social Semiotics* 16(2):243–261.

Williams, David R. 1999. Race, Socioeconomic Status, and Health: The Added Effects of Racism and Discrimination. *Annals of the New York Academy of Sciences* 896:173–188.

Williams, Raymond. 1980. Base and Superstructure in Marxist Cultural Theory. In Raymond Williams, *Problems in Materialism and Culture*. London: Verso.

Williams, Simon J., Paul Martin, and Jonathan Gabe. 2011. The Pharmaceuticalization of Society? A Framework for Analysis. *Sociology of Health and Illness* 33(5):710–725.

Winett, Liana Blas, and Regina Lawrence. 2005. The Rest of the Story: Public Health, the News, and the 2001 Anthrax Attacks. *International Journal of Press/Politics* 10(3):3–25.

Wood, Susan F., and Kristin L. Perosino. 2008. Increasing Transparency at the FDA: The Impact of the FDA Amendments Act of 2007. *Public Health Reports* 123:527–530.

Woolard, Kathryn A. 1989. Sentences in the Language Prison: The Rhetorical Structuring of an American Language Policy Debate. *American Ethnologist* 16(2):268–278.

Yilmaz, Ferruh. 2014. Ideology at Work in (the Production of) the News on Ethnic Minorities. *Studies in Media and Communication* 2(1), http://dx.doi.org/10.11114/smc.v2i1.325, accessed 12 July 2015.

Zaller, John, and Dennis Chiu. 1996. Government's Little Helper: U.S. Press Coverage of Foreign Policy Crises, 1945–1991. *Political Communication* 13:385–405.

Zentella, Ana Celia. 2003. José Can You See: Latin@ Responses to Racist Discourse. In *Bilingual Games: Some Literary Investigations*, Doris Sommer, ed., 51–66. New York: Palgrave Macmillan.

Zola, Irving Kenneth. 1972. Medicine as an Institution of Social Control. *Sociological Review* 20:487–504.

INDEX

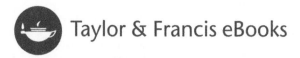